Atlas of
INFECTIOUS
DISEASES

Volume X

CARDIOVASCULAR INFECTIONS

Atlas of
INFECTIOUS DISEASES

Volume X

CARDIOVASCULAR INFECTIONS

Editor-in-Chief

Gerald L. Mandell, MD

Professor of Medicine
Owen R. Cheatham Professor of the Sciences
Chief, Division of Infectious Diseases
University of Virginia Health Sciences Center
Charlottesville, Virginia

Editor

Oksana M. Korzeniowski, MD

Professor of Medicine
Division of Infectious Diseases
Allegheny University of the Health Sciences
Hospital Epidemiologist
Allegheny University Hospitals–MCP
Philadelphia, Pennsylvania

With 17 contributors

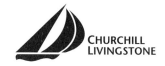

DEVELOPED BY CURRENT MEDICINE, INC.
PHILADELPHIA

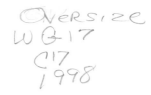
CURRENT MEDICINE
400 MARKET STREET, SUITE 700
PHILADELPHIA, PA 19106

Library of Congress Cataloging-in-Publication Data

Cardiovascular infections / editor-in-chief, Gerald L. Mandell;
editor Oksana M. Korzeniowski; with 26 contributors.
    p. cm.—(Atlas of infectious diseases; v. 10)
  Includes bibliographical references and index.
  ISBN 0-443-07750-9
  1. Cardiovascular system—Infections—Atlases. I. Mandell, Gerald L.
II. Korzeniowski, Oksana M., 1945– . III. Series.
  [DNLM: 1. Cardiovascular Diseases—pathology—atlases.
2. Cardiovascular Diseases—etiology—atlases. 3. Communicable Diseases—
complications—atlases. WG 17 C267 1998]
RC678.C37 1998
616.1'07—dc21
DNLM/DLC
for Library of Congress
                                                             97-15076
                                                               CIP

Development Editor: ....Lee Tevebaugh

Editorial Assistant: ....Scott Thomas Hurd

Art Director: ....Paul Fennessy

Design and Layout: ....Patrick Ward, Christine M. Keller,
                                                      Jerilyn Bockorick, and Robert LeBrun

Illustration Director: ....Ann Saydlowski

Illustrator: ....Beth Starkey

Production Manager: ....Lori Holland

Typesetting: ....John Tomcavage

Managing Editor: ....Lori J. Bainbridge

Indexer: ....Ann Cassar

Printed in Hong Kong by Paramount Printing Group Limited.

10 9 8 7 6 5 4 3 2 1

PREFACE

The diagnosis and management of patients with infectious diseases are based in large part on visual clues. Skin and mucous membrane lesions, eye findings, imaging studies, Gram stains, culture plates, insect vectors, preparations of blood, urine, pus, cerebrospinal fluid, and biopsy specimens are studied to establish the proper diagnosis and to choose the most effective therapy. The *Atlas of Infectious Diseases* is a modern, complete collection of these images. Current Medicine, with its capability of superb color reproduction and its state-of-the-art computer imaging facilities, is the ideal publisher for the atlas. Infectious diseases physicians, scientists, microbiologists, and pathologists frequently teach other health-care professionals, and this comprehensive atlas with available slides is an effective teaching tool.

Oksana Korzeniowski is an expert in internal medicine and infectious diseases with special emphasis on cardiovascular infections. She has assembled an international panel of authors who have contributed striking and informative images to aid in our understanding and management of these complex infections.

Gerald L. Mandell, MD
Charlottesville, Virginia

CONTRIBUTORS

Harry Acquatella, MD
Professor of Medicine
Universidad Central de Venezuela
Centro Medico
Caracas, Venezuela

Henry F. Chambers, MD
Professor of Medicine
University of California, San Francisco
Attending Physician
San Francisco General Hospital
San Francisco, California

C. Glenn Cobbs, MD
Professor Emeritus
Department of Medicine
University of Alabama at Birmingham
Chief, Medical Service
Veterans Administration Medical Center
Birmingham, Alabama

Adnan S. Dajani, MD
Professor
Department of Pediatrics
Wayne State University
Director, Division of Infectious Diseases
Children's Hospital of Michigan
Detroit, Michigan

Adolf W. Karchmer, MD
Professor of Medicine
Harvard Medical School
Chief, Division of Infectious Diseases
Beth Israel Deaconess Medical Center
Boston, Massachusetts

Oksana M. Korzeniowski, MD
Professor of Medicine
Division of Infectious Diseases
Allegheny University of the Health Sciences
Hospital Epidemiologist
Allegheny University Hospitals–MCP
Philadelphia, Pennsylvania

Matthew E. Levison, MD
Professor of Medicine
Allegheny University of the Health Sciences
Chief, Division of Infectious Diseases
Allegheny University Hospitals–MCP
Philadelphia, Pennsylvania

William J. Lewis, MD
Clinical Assistant Professor
Division of Infectious Diseases
University of Oklahoma
Staff Physician
Tulsa Infectious Diseases Clinic
Tulsa, Oklahoma

Frederick Masoudi, MD
Fellow
Department of Medicine
Division of Cardiology
University of Colorado
Denver, Colorado

José M. Miró, MD, PhD
Associate Professor of Medicine
University of Barcelona
Senior Specialist
Infectious Diseases Unit
Hospital Clínic i Provincial
Barcelona, Spain

Judith A. O'Donnell, MD
Assistant Professor of Medicine
Division of Infectious Diseases
Allegheny University of the Health Sciences
Philadelphia, Pennsylvania

Cathal O'Sullivan, MB, MRCP
Fellow
Division of Infectious Diseases
University of Alabama at Birmingham
Birmingham, Alabama

Robert J. Sherertz, MD
Professor
Division of Infectious Diseases
Bowman Gray School of Medicine
Hospital Epidemiologist
North Carolina Baptist Hospital
Winston-Salem, North Carolina

Alexis B. Sokil, MD
Associate Professor of Medicine
Allegheny University of the Health Sciences
Director, Noninvasive Cardiac Imaging
Allegheny University Hospitals–MCP
Philadelphia, Pennsylvania

Kathryn A. Taubert, PhD
Associate Professor
Department of Physiology
University of Texas Southwestern
Senior Scientist
American Heart Association
Dallas, Texas

William A. VanDecker, MD
Assistant Professor of Medicine
Division of Cardiology
Allegheny University of the Health Sciences
Associate Director, Noninvasive Cardiac Imaging
Allegheny University Hospitals–MCP
Philadelphia, Pennsylvania

Walter R. Wilson, MD
Professor of Internal Medicine
Mayo Medical School
Chair, Division of Infectious Diseases
Mayo Clinic
Rochester, Minnesota

CONTENTS

CHAPTER 1

Infective Endocarditis and Other Vascular Infections in Intravenous Drug Abusers

José M. Miró
Walter R. Wilson

PARENTERAL DRUG ADDICTION, especially intravenous (IV) heroin abuse, represents an important challenge to health programs in most developed countries [1,2]. Infective endocarditis (IE) is one of the most severe complications of IV drug addiction [2–8], and IV drug addiction is one of the most important causes of IE in urban medical centers in developed countries. IE in IV drug abusers (IVDAs) is responsible for 5% to 20% of hospital admissions and for 5% to 10% of the total death rate in this group [5–8]. The incidence of IE in IVDAs in the AIDS era is decreasing, probably due to precautions taken to avoid HIV acquisition [7].

Staphylococcus aureus is the etiologic agent in most cases (60% to 70%) [2–8]. In order of frequency, other isolated organisms are: streptococcus (viridans streptococci, group A streptococcus) and enterococcus (15% to 20%), *Pseudomonas aeruginosa*, *Serratia marcescens* and other gram-negative rods (<10%), and *Candida* species (<2%) [2–9]. The source of these bacteria or fungi is the inoculation of the microorganism from the drug user's own skin or from the contamination of the drugs, the diluents, and/or the injection equipment [4–7]. The tricuspid valve is most frequently affected (>50%), followed by the left valves (mitral and aortic) (20% to 30%). Pulmonic valve infection is rare (<1%) [2–8]. Left and right valves are simultaneously affected (mixed IE) in 5% to 10% of cases. Only 10% to 30% of IVDAs have underlying cardiac pathology, mainly involving the mitral and aortic valves [3–7].

Clinical manifestations of IE are variable depending on the side of the heart involved [2–7]. IVDAs with right-sided IE have predominantly pulmonary symptoms, whereas the clinical features of patients with left-sided IE are similar to those described in endocarditis on the native valve in the non–drug-addicted population. Diagnosis of IE in IVDAs is made according to the clinical, microbiologic, and echocardiographic criteria recently described by Durack and coworkers [10].

In most recent studies, the mortality for IE in IVDAs ranges between 5% and 30% [2,4–7]. Prognosis depends on the site of cardiac involvement [2–8]. The prognosis in right-sided IE is usually good (mortality, <5%; surgery, <2%). Patients with tricuspid valve vegetations >2 cm [11] and with adult respiratory distress syndrome [12] have higher mortality. Left-sided IE, particularly when the aortic valve is involved, worsens the prognosis considerably (mortality, 20%–30%; surgery, 15%–25%) [2–8]. IE caused by gram-negative bacilli or fungi has the worst prognosis. Heart failure and systemic embolisms (mainly in the central nervous system) are the main causes of death [2–8]. Compared with the general population with IE, IVDAs have a higher incidence of recurrent IE most likely due to continued use of IV drugs [2–7]. For this reason, surgical indications and the type of surgery should be critically assessed in order to avoid the development of prosthetic IE in IVDAs. In case of tricuspid surgery, most surgeons choose total or partial valve resection without valve replacement as the procedure of choice [7,13]. Recently, a new approach has been successfully performed to avoid the use of any synthetic material by transplanting cryopreserved mitral homografts into the tricuspid position [14].

The prevalence of HIV-1 infection among IVDAs with IE is high, ranging between 40% and 75% [15,16]. HIV infection does not worsen the prognosis of surgery in HIV-infected IVDAs with IE [17,18]. HIV-infected IVDAs who are severely immunosuppressed (<200 CD4 cells/µL) or who have AIDS are more likely to die from endocarditis than those whose HIV infection is asymptomatic and who have >200 CD4 cells/µL [16]. Finally, opportunistic infections related to AIDS also should be considered in HIV-1–infected IVDAs with endocarditis who are severely immunosuppressed.

INFECTIOUS COMPLICATIONS OF INTRAVENOUS DRUG ABUSE

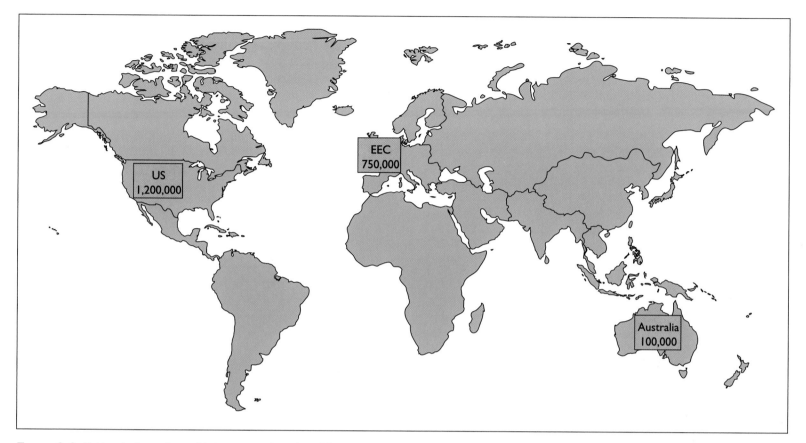

FIGURE 1-1 Estimated number of intravenous heroin addicts in developed countries. Parenteral drug addiction represents an important challenge to health programs in most developed countries. It involves approximately 1.2 million people in the United States (US), 750,000 in the European Economic Community (EEC) countries, and 100,000 in Australia [1,2]. Most parenteral drug abusers are young adults (20 to 35 years of age), and the male-to-female case ratio is 3:1 [2–8]. In general, parenteral drug abusers choose the intravenous route of injection of heroin ("main liners") and, with less frequency, the subcutaneous route ("skin poppers") [2,4,5]. Other drugs (morphine, pentazocine, cocaine, amphetamines, and benzodiazepines) are used less frequently, although the use of cocaine combined with heroin in intravenous injection ("speed ball") has been increasing in recent years [2,4,5]. In some geographic areas (*eg*, Detroit and Chicago), the consumption of a particular kind of drug, such as pentazocine and tripelennamine, can predominate.

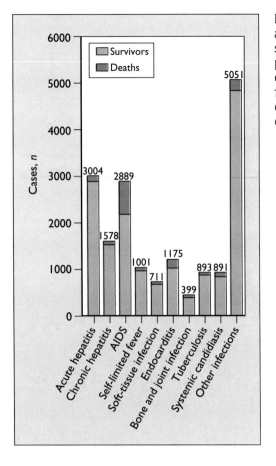

FIGURE 1-2 Type of infectious complications and mortality in Spanish intravenous drug abusers (IVDAs) reported between 1977 and 1991. Infectious complications are responsible for 60% to 80% of hospital admissions and for 20% to 30% of deaths in parenteral drug abusers [19]. Heroin or cocaine overdoses, AIDS, and infective endocarditis are the main causes of mortality [20]. Of more than 17,000 infections in IVDAs from 72 participating hospitals, hepatitis, AIDS, soft-tissue infections, infective endocarditis, tuberculosis, and systemic candidiasis were the most frequent. Infective endocarditis occurred in 7% of IVDAs [8].

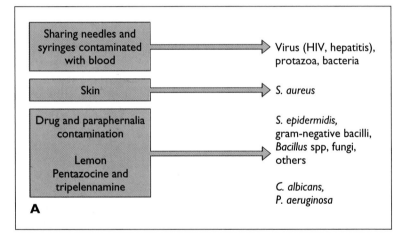

FIGURE 1-3 Sources of infections in intravenous drug abusers (IVDAs). **A,** Source of the microorganisms. The intravenous injection of heroin and cocaine is a risk factor for *Staphylococcus aureus* bacteremia. It has been suggested that this organism probably originates from the drug user's own skin [7,21–24]. In contrast, other bacteria and fungi may be derived from the drugs, adulterants, injection equipment, or the diluents (tap water, lemon juice, saliva) [24–26]. *Pseudomonas aeruginosa* infections have been directly associated with parenteral usage of pentazocine and tripelennamine [27,28]. This association explains the greater incidence of *P. aeruginosa* infections in the geographic areas where this drug is popular. Lemon juice needed to dissolve "brown heroin" is contaminated by *Candida albicans* from the drug abuser's oropharynx and is the source of infection in the case of systemic candidiasis [29,30]. IVDAs can acquire any microorganism circulating in the blood (including malaria) and any viral disease (hepatitis B, C, and D viruses and HIV) as a result of sharing injection equipment. **B,** Scarified forearm with pigmented veins in a heroin abuser with *S. aureus* endocarditis. (*continued*)

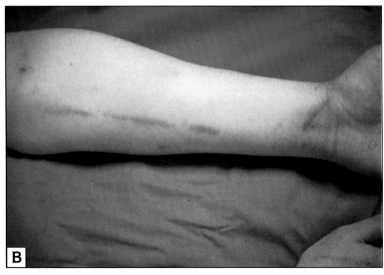

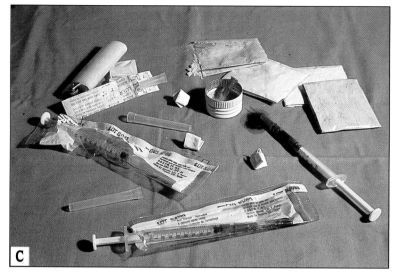
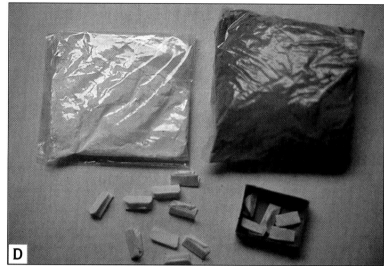

FIGURE 1-3 (*continued*) **C**, Syringes and other paraphernalia used by parenteral drug abusers. **D**, Confiscated packages of white and brown heroin and "street" heroin samples (in small packets).

INCIDENCE, ETIOLOGY, AND PATHOGENESIS

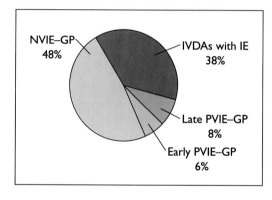

FIGURE 1-4 Types of infective endocarditis in 779 consecutive episodes diagnosed in two tertiary teaching hospitals in Barcelona between 1975 and 1992. The first cases of infective endocarditis (IE) complicating intravenous drug addiction were reported in the United States in the 1930s [5]. Currently, intravenous drug addiction is one of the most important causes of IE in urban medical centers in developed countries [7,31]. The incidence in the United States ranges between 2% and 5% per year [2,3,7], with cocaine abusers having the highest risk [32]. IE in intravenous drug abusers (IVDAs) is responsible for 5% to 20% of hospital admissions and for 5% to 10% of the total death rate in this group [2,5,7,8]. IVDAs often have recurrent endocarditis [2,5,7]. The incidence of IE in IVDAs in the AIDS era is decreasing, probably due to changes in the routes of drug administration, increased use of sterile needles and syringes, and reduced sharing of injection equipment [7]. GP—general population; NVIE—native valve infective endocarditis; PVIE—prosthetic valve endocarditis. (*Adapted from* Tornos and Miró [31].)

Etiology of IE in Spanish intravenous drug abusers	
	Episodes, *n* (%)*
Staphylococcus aureus[†]	1138 (74%)
Coagulase-negative staphylococci	44 (3%)
Viridans streptococci	94 (6%)
Enterococci	21 (1.5%)
Other streptococci	37 (2%)
Pseudomonas aeruginosa	12 (<1%)
Other gram-negative aerobes	11 (<1%)
Other organisms	4
Candida spp	18 (1%)
Polymicrobial IE	44 (3%)
Culture-negative IE	106 (7%)

*Total number of episodes = 1529.

[†]Methicillin-susceptible *Staphylococcus aureus* >95%.

IE—infective endocarditis.

FIGURE 1-5 Etiology of infective endocarditis (IE) in 1529 episodes involving Spanish intravenous drug abusers (IVDAs) between 1977 and 1993. *Staphylococcus aureus* was the etiologic agent in almost 75% of cases, with 95% being methicillin-susceptible *S. aureus* (MSSA). Streptococci were isolated in about 10% of cases; the viridans group and the enterococci are the most common species. Pseudomonas and gram-negative bacilli were unusual in Spain, whereas *Candida* IE represented 1% of cases. IE was polymicrobial and culture negative in 3% and 7% of cases, respectively. These data are in accordance with the data reported in the literature [2–7,33]. In order of frequency, *S. aureus* is the etiologic agent in 60% to 70% of cases (usually MSSA); streptococci (viridans streptococci, group A streptococcus) and enterococcus in 15% to 20%; *Pseudomonas aeruginosa*, *Serratia marcescens*, and other gram-negative rods in <10%; and *Candida* species in <2% [2–7,33]. Endocarditis with polymicrobial infection is reported in about 5% of cases. Endocarditis with negative blood cultures is reported in 5% to 10% of cases [2–7,33]. (*Adapted from* Miró *et al.* [33].)

Types of valves involved in infective endocarditis in Spanish intravenous drug abusers	
Valve involved	**Episodes, *n* (%)***
Right side	1199 (79%)
Tricuspid valve	1045 (68%)
Pulmonic valve	14 (1%)
Tricuspid valve + pulmonary valve	8
Unknown	132
Left side	254 (16%)
Aortic valve	103 (7%)
Mitral valve	98 (6%)
Mitral valve + aortic valve	27
Mural/coarctation of aorta	3
Unknown	24
Mixed infective endocarditis	76 (5%)

*Total number of episodes = 1529.

FIGURE 1-6 Types of valves involved in 1529 episodes of infective endocarditis (IE) in Spanish intravenous drug abusers between 1977 and 1993. IE was right-sided or mixed in 84% of the episodes. The tricuspid valve was affected in almost all cases of right-sided IE. The pulmonic valve was involved in 2% of cases. On the left side of the heart, the aortic and mitral valves were equally affected. These data are consistent with the data reported in the literature in which the tricuspid valve is the most frequently affected (>50% of cases), followed by the mitral and aortic valves (20% to 30%), whereas pulmonic valve infection is rare (<1%) [2–7,33]. Left and right valves are simultaneously affected (mixed IE) in 5% to 10% of cases. Only 10% to 30% of intravenous drug abusers have underlying cardiac pathology, mainly involving the mitral and aortic valves [2–7,33]. (*Adapted from* Miró *et al.* [33].)

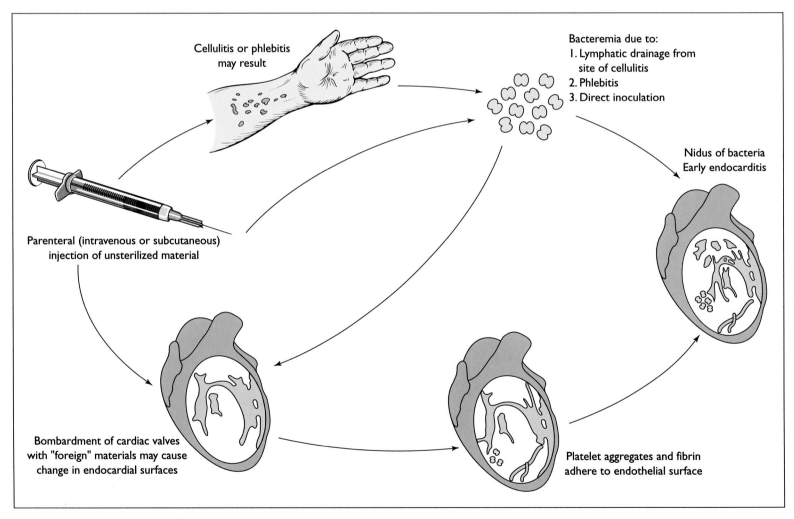

FIGURE 1-7 Postulated pathogenesis of infective endocarditis in intravenous drug abusers (IVDAs). The reason for tricuspid valve predominance in IVDAs with infective endocarditis is unknown, although it is most likely due to the endothelial damage caused by the continuous bombardment of the tricuspid valve by impurities contained in the injected drugs or adulterants [9]. However, pathologic studies of tricuspid valves from IVDAs who died of causes unrelated to infective endocarditis showed normal valves [7]. Attempts to reproduce tricuspid valve endocarditis in the rabbit model by injecting "street" heroin over several weeks followed by a high inoculum of *Staphylococcus aureus* have been unsuccessful [7,34].

CLINICAL MANIFESTATIONS

Clinical manifestations of IE in intravenous drug abusers			
	Right-sided IE, % (*n*=100)	Mixed IE, % (*n*=12)	Left-sided IE, % (*n*=31)
Fever	98	100	90
Cardiac murmurs	51	75	87
Heart failure	1	25	13
Pulmonary symptoms	70	50	—
Central nervous system compromise	6	17	26
Renal insufficiency	7	8	7
Musculoskeletal pain	32	17	23
Peripheral vascular phenomena	3	25	52

IE—infective endocarditis.

FIGURE 1-8 Clinical manifestations of 143 episodes of infective endocarditis (IE) in intravenous drug abusers (IVDAs) diagnosed at the Hospital Clinic of Barcelona (Spain) between 1979 and 1991. IVDAs with right-sided IE presented with pulmonary symptoms in 70% of cases [2–7]. The murmur of tricuspid insufficiency only appeared in about half of the patients. IVDAs with left-sided IE resemble the non–drug- addicted population with left-sided IE [2–7]. Murmurs, underlying heart disease, left heart failure, systemic emboli, and peripheral valvular phenomena were frequently present. (*Adapted from* Miró *et al.* [33].)

Injection-Related Injury

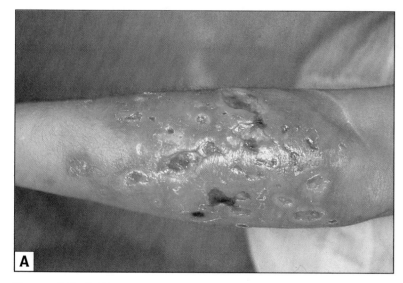

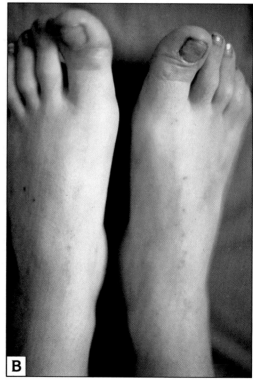

FIGURE 1-9 A, Forearm cellulitis and skin ulcers manifested in a parenteral cocaine abuser aged 32 years who developed septic thrombophlebitis. Cocaine has a potent vasoconstriction effect and used subcutaneously can produce deep ulcers, such as in this patient. **B,** Feet veins with injection tracks on a heroin addict with *Staphylococcus aureus* endocarditis. Cellulitis and superficial and profound abscesses are the most frequent skin and soft-tissue infections in intravenous drug abusers [6,8]. With less frequency, necrotizing fasciitis (cocaine is the most important risk factor) and pyomyositis are described. Soft-tissue infections are located at the injection sites, usually in the upper limbs (*panel 9A*), although they can also be located in the lower limbs (*panel 9B*), the neck, and groin [6].

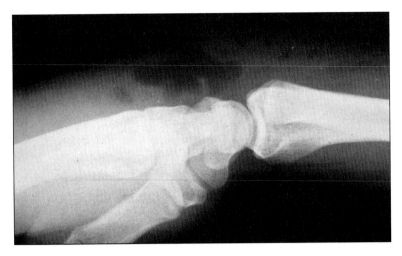

FIGURE 1-10 Wrist radiograph showing gas due to a polymicrobial infection in a heroin abuser who developed *Staphylococcus aureus* septic thrombophlebitis and bilateral pulmonary embolisms. In all intravenous drug abusers, injection-related complications such as bone and joint involvement, septic thrombophlebitis, and false arterial aneurysms should be excluded. *S. aureus* is the most frequently isolated organism. Skin and soft-tissue infections also are caused by streptococcus (group A streptococcus, peptostreptococcus), enterococcus, gram-negative rods, or mixed oral flora with aerobes and anaerobes when intravenous drug abusers use saliva to dissolve drugs [6].

Infective Endocarditis–Associated Phenomena

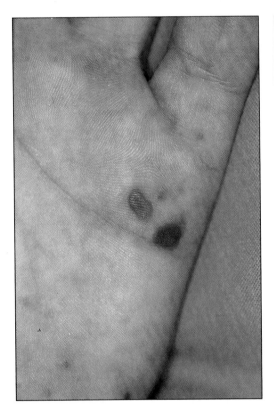

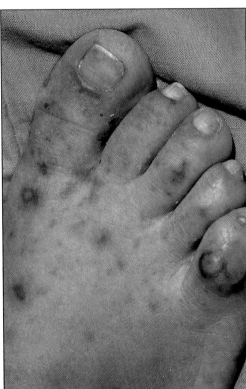

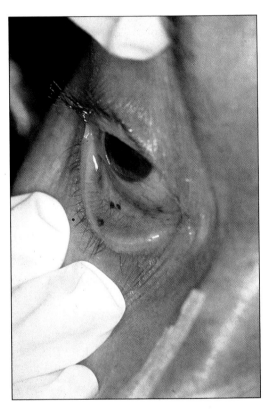

FIGURE 1-11 Hemorrhagic macular skin (Janeway) lesions on the hand of a heroin addict with *Staphylococcus aureus* left-sided endocarditis. Peripheral valvular phenomena are not often found in intravenous drug abusers (IVDAs) with right-sided infective endocarditis [2–7]. Cutaneous or mucosal petechiae, Osler nodes, and Janeway lesions are present in 25% to 45% of IVDAs with left-sided infective endocarditis.

FIGURE 1-12 Hemorrhagic macular and purulent skin lesions on the foot of heroin addict with *Staphylococcus aureus* left-sided endocarditis as the result of septic systemic embolisms.

FIGURE 1-13 Non–drug-addicted man aged 54 years with mitral valve endocarditis caused by *Staphylococcus aureus*. At admission the physical examination showed several cutaneous or mucosal vascular phenomena characteristic of left-sided endocarditis. Petechiae are present in the right conjunctivae.

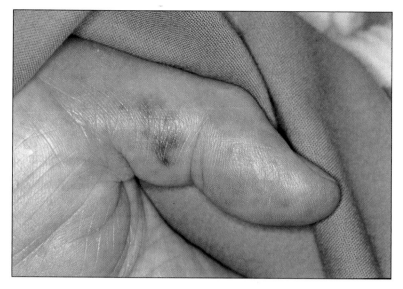

FIGURE 1-14 Tender and purplish nodules in the thumb finger pulp (Osler nodes) and hemorrhagic and erythematous macules (Janeway lesions) in the same finger of the right hand of the patient shown in Fig. 1-13.

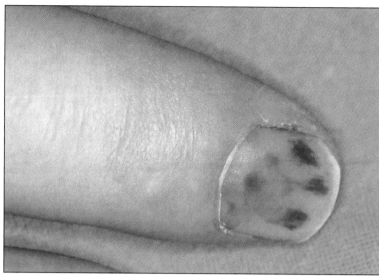

FIGURE 1-15 Splinter hemorrhages in a fingernail. Splinter hemorrhages may be due to simple trauma, but when multiple nails are involved in a patient with infective endocarditis (such as this patient from Fig. 1-13), they represent a vasculitic component of the infection.

VASCULAR INFECTIONS

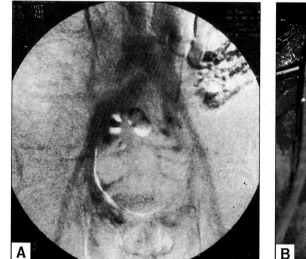

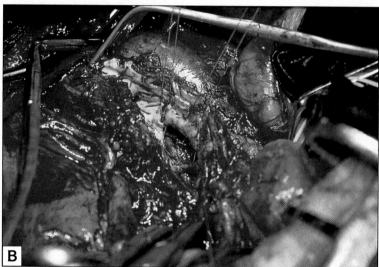

FIGURE 1-16 Peripheral and central vessels used for injection by intravenous drug abusers (IVDAs) frequently become injured or infected. Peripheral septic thrombophlebitis and false arterial aneurysms are the most common vascular infections in IVDAs [2,4–6,35]. Primary mycotic aneurysms are rare and usually related to infective endocarditis [6]. Peripheral septic thrombophlebitis [2–4,6] is generally located on the upper limbs (*see* Fig. 1-9A). Patients usually have fever, chills, and inflammatory signs along the affected vein, which (when compression is applied) suppurates through its proximate opening. Septic pulmonary embolization sometimes occurs and mimics right-sided endocarditis. Infection can extend through the intrathoracic veins. *Staphylococcus aureus* is usually the etiologic agent. Treatment includes antibiotic therapy and resection of the affected vein. False arterial aneurysms [6,35] are mainly located on femoral, subclavian, or jugular arteries. They are the consequence of the lesion originated on the arterial wall when the IVDA tries to inject the drug through the femoral, subclavian, or jugular veins. These aneurysms have to be suspected when a pulsating mass appears on the groin or lower neck areas. The majority of them are infected with *S. aureus* or with polymicrobial flora. Treatment includes prolonged antibiotic therapy and surgical resection of the false aneurysm. **A,** Physical examination of a male heroin addict aged 39 years revealed a continuous murmur on the right abdominal flank, suggesting an arteriovenous communication. The venous digital subtraction angiography showed a wide communication (fistula) between the terminal aorta and the inferior cava vein. **B,** Surgical view of the patient shown in *panel 16A.* A mycotic aneurysm in the aorta fistulized to the inferior cava vein. (*Courtesy of* C. Mestres, MD.)

Chest radiographic manifestations in right-sided infective endocarditis in intravenous drug abusers	
Normal	8%
Pulmonary infiltrates*	75%
Cavitated infiltrates	48%
Pleural effusion†	40%
Cardiomegaly	8%

*Single or multiple peripheral, streaky, or nodular densities.

†Intravenous drug abusers can have empyema and/or pneumothorax.

FIGURE 1-17 Chest radiographic manifestations in 100 episodes of right-sided infective endocarditis (IE) in intravenous drug abusers diagnosed at the Hospital Clinic of Barcelona (Spain) between 1979 and 1991. The diagnosis of right-sided IE is often based on the presence of characteristic radiologic pulmonary infiltrates [4,7]. Although the murmur of tricuspid insufficiency is usually absent in patients with tricuspid IE, chest radiographs reveal single or multiple rounded or segmented pulmonary infiltrates, which may cavitate and become associated with pleural effusion or empyema in more than 75% of cases of right-sided IE [2–7,34]. Pneumothorax is unusual [36]. Peripheral septic thrombophlebitis [2–7,34,37] clinically mimics right-sided IE. (*Adapted from* Miró [34].)

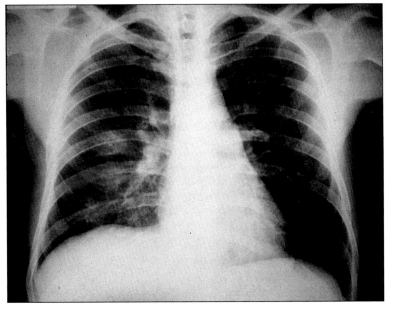

FIGURE 1-18 Chest radiograph of a male intravenous heroin addict aged 25 years with right-sided endocarditis showing three infiltrates in the right lung secondary to septic pulmonary embolizations.

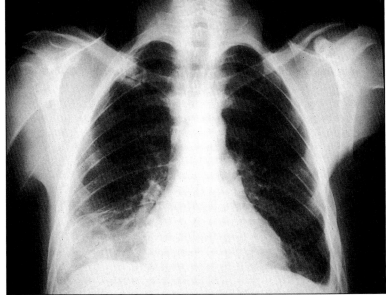

FIGURE 1-19 Chest radiograph of a male intravenous heroin addict aged 30 years with right-sided endocarditis showing bilateral pleural effusions and two cavitated infiltrates in the right lung as the result of lung infarctions.

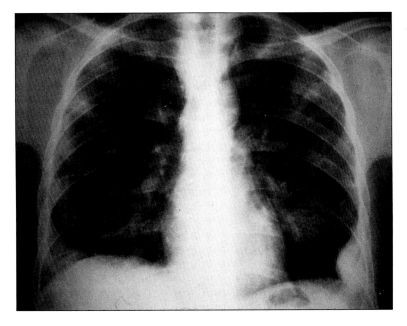

FIGURE 1-20 Chest radiograph showing bilateral cavitary infiltrates and pleural effusion in a male intravenous heroin addict aged 23 years with right-sided endocarditis.

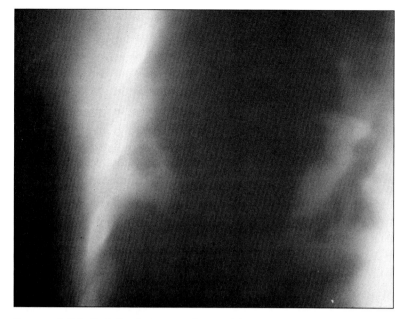

FIGURE 1-21 Detail of chest radiographic tomography of a male intravenous heroin addict aged 29 years with *Staphylococcus aureus* right-sided endocarditis showing a small cavitated infiltrate located in the periphery of the right lung.

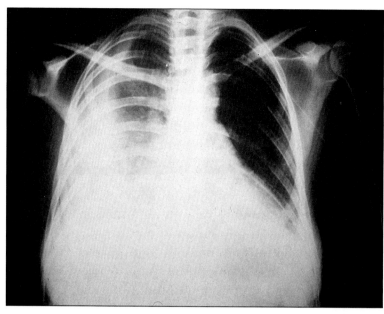

FIGURE 1-22 Chest radiograph of a male intravenous heroin addict aged 27 years with right-sided endocarditis showing a large right pleural effusion (empyema) due to *Staphylococcus aureus*.

COMPLICATIONS

Complications of IE in intravenous drug abusers			
	Right-sided IE, % (*n*=100)	**Mixed IE, %** (*n*=12)	**Left-sided IE, %** (*n*=31)
Left heart failure	—	25	29
Right heart failure	7	8	—
Systemic emboli	—	25	25
Central nervous system involvement*	8	25	32
Renal failure	26	16	29
Septic metastasis	38	50	32
Acute respiratory failure (pulmonary thromboembolisms)	27	25	—
Surgery	4	16	39
Mortality	4	25	19

*Meningitis, stroke.

FIGURE 1-23 Complications in 143 episodes of infective endocarditis (IE) in intravenous drug abusers (IVDAs) diagnosed at the Hospital Clinic of Barcelona (Spain) between 1979 and 1991. Complications of IE reflect the side of the heart involved [3,4,7]. IVDAs with right-sided IE developed acute respiratory failure, septic metastases, and right heart failure. Four percent of the patients studied needed surgery, and 4% died. IVDAs with left sided IE had left heart failure, systemic emboli, central nervous system involvement, and septic metastases. Thirty-nine percent of the patients needed surgery, and 19% died. (*Adapted from* Miró [34].)

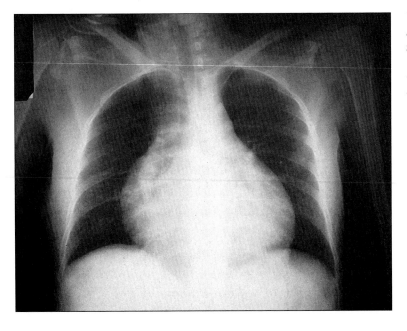

FIGURE 1-24 Chest radiograph of a female intravenous heroin addict aged 28 years with *Staphylococcus aureus* pericarditis showing cardiomegaly due to a purulent pericardial effusion. Purulent pericarditis is an unusual complication of intravenous drug addiction. It needs an early diagnosis and combined medical and surgical therapies for cure.

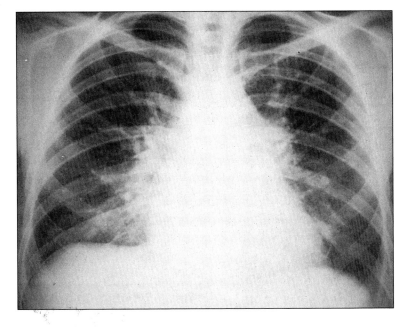

FIGURE 1-25 Chest radiograph of a male intravenous heroin addict aged 32 years with *Staphylococcus aureus* aortic endocarditis showing cardiomegaly, enlarged hilar shadows, and a bilateral interstitial pattern (pulmonary edema) due to left heart failure. Left heart failure is one of the most common complications of aortic valve endocarditis and mandates immediate aortic valve replacement. It is important not to misdiagnose this radiographic picture for *Pneumocystis carinii* pneumonia in intravenous drug abusers with AIDS or for noncardiogenic pulmonary edema related to drug overdoses. One must keep in mind that in *S. aureus* endocarditis the first clinical extracardiac manifestations of infective endocarditis may be due to septic systemic metastases such as brain abscesses (*see* Fig. 1-26), arthritis, or osteomyelitis (*see* Figs. 1-27 and 1-28) [2–7,34].

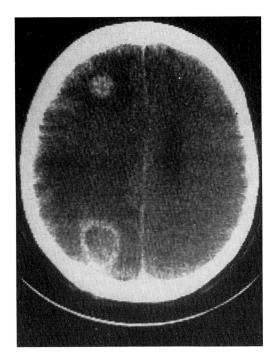

FIGURE 1-26 Cranial computed tomography of a heroin addict with *Staphylococcus aureus* endocarditis showing two brain abscesses located in the left frontal and occipital areas. Both nodular and ring-enhancing lesions are surrounded by edema. It is important not to misdiagnose pyogenic brain abscesses for opportunistic infections (*eg*, toxoplasmosis) or tumors (lymphoma) in intravenous drug abusers with AIDS.

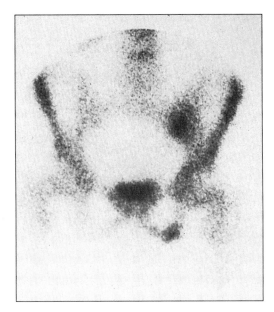

FIGURE 1-27 Bone scintigram with 99mTc-methylene diphosphonate in a heroin addict with *Staphylococcus aureus* tricuspid endocarditis showing left sacroiliac joint and ischium uptake due to septic metastasis.

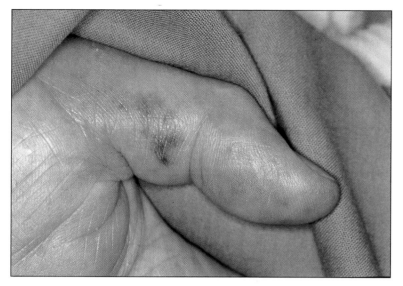

FIGURE 1-14 Tender and purplish nodules in the thumb finger pulp (Osler nodes) and hemorrhagic and erythematous macules (Janeway lesions) in the same finger of the right hand of the patient shown in Fig. 1-13.

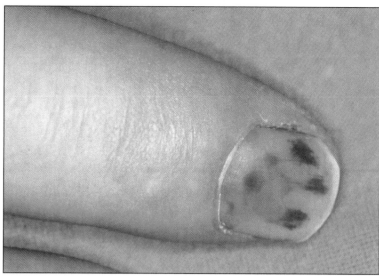

FIGURE 1-15 Splinter hemorrhages in a fingernail. Splinter hemorrhages may be due to simple trauma, but when multiple nails are involved in a patient with infective endocarditis (such as this patient from Fig. 1-13), they represent a vasculitic component of the infection.

VASCULAR INFECTIONS

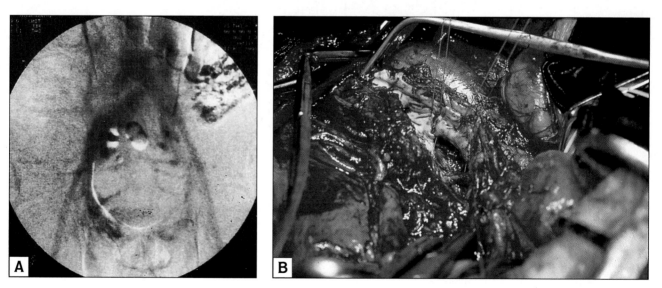

FIGURE 1-16 Peripheral and central vessels used for injection by intravenous drug abusers (IVDAs) frequently become injured or infected. Peripheral septic thrombophlebitis and false arterial aneurysms are the most common vascular infections in IVDAs [2,4–6,35]. Primary mycotic aneurysms are rare and usually related to infective endocarditis [6]. Peripheral septic thrombophlebitis [2–4,6] is generally located on the upper limbs (*see* Fig. 1-9A). Patients usually have fever, chills, and inflammatory signs along the affected vein, which (when compression is applied) suppurates through its proximate opening. Septic pulmonary embolization sometimes occurs and mimics right-sided endocarditis. Infection can extend through the intrathoracic veins. *Staphylococcus aureus* is usually the etiologic agent. Treatment includes antibiotic therapy and resection of the affected vein. False arterial aneurysms [6,35] are mainly located on femoral, subclavian, or jugular arteries. They are the consequence of the lesion originated on the arterial wall when the IVDA tries to inject the drug through the femoral, subclavian, or jugular veins. These aneurysms have to be suspected when a pulsating mass appears on the groin or lower neck areas. The majority of them are infected with *S. aureus* or with polymicrobial flora. Treatment includes prolonged antibiotic therapy and surgical resection of the false aneurysm. **A**, Physical examination of a male heroin addict aged 39 years revealed a continuous murmur on the right abdominal flank, suggesting an arteriovenous communication. The venous digital subtraction angiography showed a wide communication (fistula) between the terminal aorta and the inferior cava vein. **B**, Surgical view of the patient shown in *panel 16A*. A mycotic aneurysm in the aorta fistulized to the inferior cava vein. (*Courtesy of* C. Mestres, MD.)

Chest radiographic manifestations in right-sided infective endocarditis in intravenous drug abusers	
Normal	8%
Pulmonary infiltrates*	75%
Cavitated infiltrates	48%
Pleural effusion†	40%
Cardiomegaly	8%

*Single or multiple peripheral, streaky, or nodular densities.

†Intravenous drug abusers can have empyema and/or pneumothorax.

FIGURE 1-17 Chest radiographic manifestations in 100 episodes of right-sided infective endocarditis (IE) in intravenous drug abusers diagnosed at the Hospital Clinic of Barcelona (Spain) between 1979 and 1991. The diagnosis of right-sided IE is often based on the presence of characteristic radiologic pulmonary infiltrates [4,7]. Although the murmur of tricuspid insufficiency is usually absent in patients with tricuspid IE, chest radiographs reveal single or multiple rounded or segmented pulmonary infiltrates, which may cavitate and become associated with pleural effusion or empyema in more than 75% of cases of right-sided IE [2–7,34]. Pneumothorax is unusual [36]. Peripheral septic thrombophlebitis [2–7,34,37] clinically mimics right-sided IE. (*Adapted from* Miró [34].)

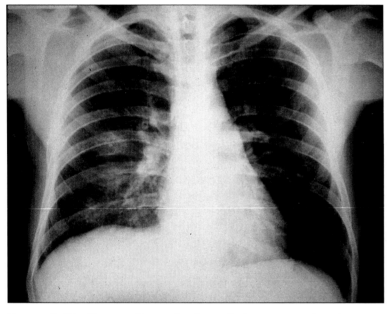

FIGURE 1-18 Chest radiograph of a male intravenous heroin addict aged 25 years with right-sided endocarditis showing three infiltrates in the right lung secondary to septic pulmonary embolizations.

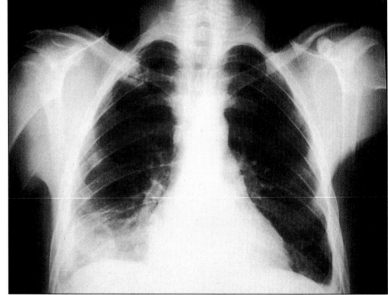

FIGURE 1-19 Chest radiograph of a male intravenous heroin addict aged 30 years with right-sided endocarditis showing bilateral pleural effusions and two cavitated infiltrates in the right lung as the result of lung infarctions.

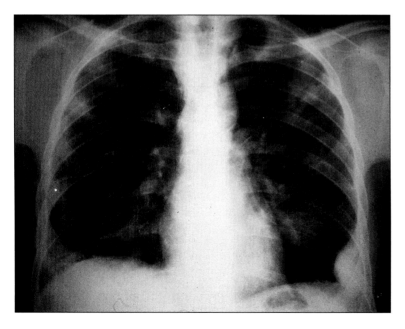

FIGURE 1-20 Chest radiograph showing bilateral cavitary infiltrates and pleural effusion in a male intravenous heroin addict aged 23 years with right-sided endocarditis.

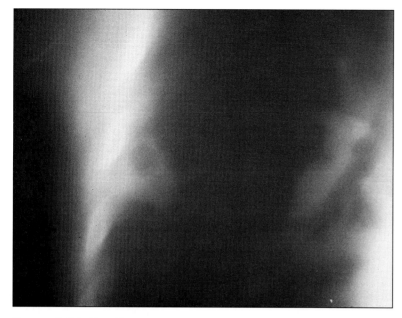

FIGURE 1-21 Detail of chest radiographic tomography of a male intravenous heroin addict aged 29 years with *Staphylococcus aureus* right-sided endocarditis showing a small cavitated infiltrate located in the periphery of the right lung.

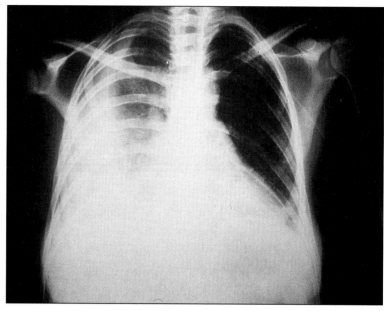

FIGURE 1-22 Chest radiograph of a male intravenous heroin addict aged 27 years with right-sided endocarditis showing a large right pleural effusion (empyema) due to *Staphylococcus aureus.*

COMPLICATIONS

Complications of IE in intravenous drug abusers

	Right-sided IE, % (*n*=100)	Mixed IE, % (*n*=12)	Left-sided IE, % (*n*=31)
Left heart failure	—	25	29
Right heart failure	7	8	—
Systemic emboli	—	25	25
Central nervous system involvement*	8	25	32
Renal failure	26	16	29
Septic metastasis	38	50	32
Acute respiratory failure (pulmonary thromboembolisms)	27	25	—
Surgery	4	16	39
Mortality	4	25	19

*Meningitis, stroke.

FIGURE 1-23 Complications in 143 episodes of infective endocarditis (IE) in intravenous drug abusers (IVDAs) diagnosed at the Hospital Clinic of Barcelona (Spain) between 1979 and 1991. Complications of IE reflect the side of the heart involved [3,4,7]. IVDAs with right-sided IE developed acute respiratory failure, septic metastases, and right heart failure. Four percent of the patients studied needed surgery, and 4% died. IVDAs with left sided IE had left heart failure, systemic emboli, central nervous system involvement, and septic metastases. Thirty-nine percent of the patients needed surgery, and 19% died. (*Adapted from* Miró [34].)

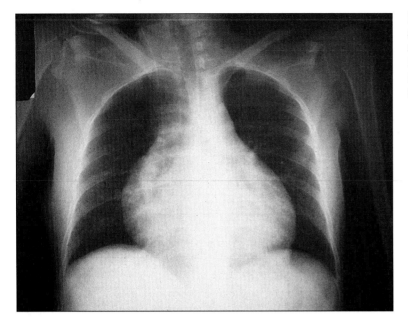

FIGURE 1-24 Chest radiograph of a female intravenous heroin addict aged 28 years with *Staphylococcus aureus* pericarditis showing cardiomegaly due to a purulent pericardial effusion. Purulent pericarditis is an unusual complication of intravenous drug addiction. It needs an early diagnosis and combined medical and surgical therapies for cure.

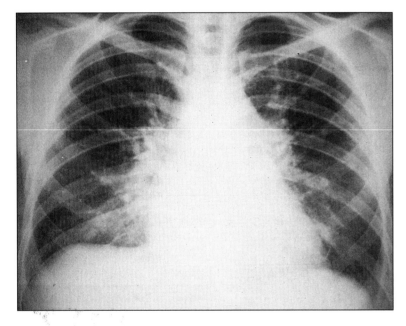

FIGURE 1-25 Chest radiograph of a male intravenous heroin addict aged 32 years with *Staphylococcus aureus* aortic endocarditis showing cardiomegaly, enlarged hilar shadows, and a bilateral interstitial pattern (pulmonary edema) due to left heart failure. Left heart failure is one of the most common complications of aortic valve endocarditis and mandates immediate aortic valve replacement. It is important not to misdiagnose this radiographic picture for *Pneumocystis carinii* pneumonia in intravenous drug abusers with AIDS or for noncardiogenic pulmonary edema related to drug overdoses. One must keep in mind that in *S. aureus* endocarditis the first clinical extracardiac manifestations of infective endocarditis may be due to septic systemic metastases such as brain abscesses (*see* Fig. 1-26), arthritis, or osteomyelitis (*see* Figs. 1-27 and 1-28) [2–7,34].

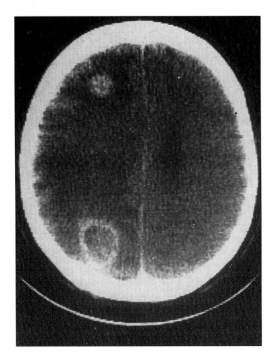

FIGURE 1-26 Cranial computed tomography of a heroin addict with *Staphylococcus aureus* endocarditis showing two brain abscesses located in the left frontal and occipital areas. Both nodular and ring-enhancing lesions are surrounded by edema. It is important not to misdiagnose pyogenic brain abscesses for opportunistic infections (*eg*, toxoplasmosis) or tumors (lymphoma) in intravenous drug abusers with AIDS.

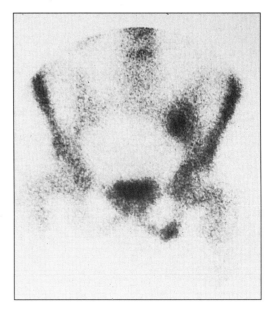

FIGURE 1-27 Bone scintigram with ^{99m}Tc-methylene diphosphonate in a heroin addict with *Staphylococcus aureus* tricuspid endocarditis showing left sacroiliac joint and ischium uptake due to septic metastasis.

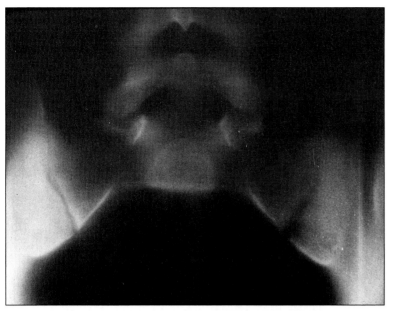

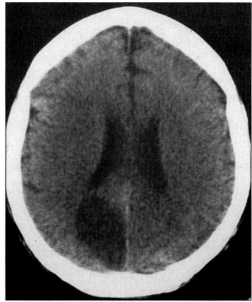

FIGURE 1-28 Radiographic tomography of the sacroiliac joints in a heroin addict with *Staphylococcus aureus* tricuspid endocarditis showing a septic metastasis in the left sacroiliac joint. Note the large bone erosion in both articular faces of the left sacroiliac joint in the same patient shown in Fig. 1-27.

FIGURE 1-29 Cranial computed tomography of a heroin addict with *Staphylococcus aureus* mitral endocarditis showing a brain infarction in the distribution of the left posterior cerebral artery. The left occipital hypodense area represents an ischemic infarction due to a septic embolism. Central nervous system involvement (*eg*, meningitis, stroke) is the main causes of mortality [2–7,33].

FUNGAL INFECTIVE ENDOCARDITIS

Systemic candidiasis in intravenous drug abusers

Country	Episodes, *n*	Cutaneous lesions, *n*	Ocular lesions, *n*	Osteoarticular lesions, *n*	*Candida* endocarditis, *n*
France	137	95	64	28	0
Spain	192	150	106	64	3
Other European Economic Community countries	56	9	53	4	0
Australia	25	18	21	5	0
United States	2	0	1	2	0
Total	395	272 (69%)	245 (62%)	103 (26%)	3 (1%)

FIGURE 1-30 Characteristics of systemic candidiasis in intravenous drug abusers (IVDAs). Intravenous drug addiction is one of the most important predisposing factors for developing fungal endocarditis. Most cases of fungal endocarditis in IVDAs are due to *Candida* species, most frequently *Candida albicans* and *Candida parapsilosis*. Until 1980, only three different clinical syndromes of *Candida* infections in IVDAs were recognized in the United States: endocarditis, bone and joint infections (both usually caused by non-*albicans* species of *Candida*) and endophthalmitis [29]. In 1980, in several western European countries and Australia, there was an outbreak of a new syndrome caused by *C. albicans*, which was related to the use of brown heroin dissolved with lemon juice [29,30]. Clinically, the syndrome is characterized by a variable febrile phase that allows the isolation of *C. albicans* from the blood followed by a characteristic triad of skin pustules and subcutaneous nodes on hairy areas, ocular lesions (chorioretinitis or endophthalmitis), and osteoarticular lesions (chondrocostal), which may appear isolated or concurrently [13]. *Candida* endocarditis occurred in about 1% of cases [29,38]. Microbiologic diagnosis is obtained in 40% to 100% of the cases with the isolation of *C. albicans* from skin or chondrocostal lesions. The main sequelum is the loss of visual acuity. Death is rare and is always related to endocarditis [29]. Amphotericin B with or without 5-flucytosine is the recommended therapy, although patients with isolated skin or chondrocostal lesions may be successfully treated with fluconazole [29]. Surgery is needed if patients have ocular, bone, or endocardial lesions [29]. (*Adapted from* Bisbe *et al.* [29].)

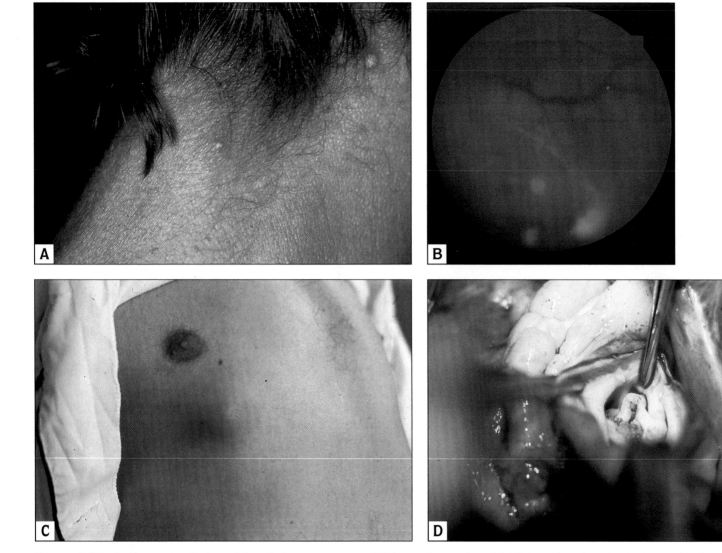

FIGURE 1-31 A, Cutaneous lesions (pustules) on a man aged 35 years addicted to brown heroin who had disseminated candidiasis due to *Candida albicans* and later developed *C. albicans* aortic endocarditis [38]. The patient was treated with intravenous amphotericin B. **B,** *C. albicans* chorioretinitis found at admission on patient shown in *panel 31A*. **C,** Chondrocostal tumor (costochondritis) found at the physical examination of the same patient. **D,** Aortic vegetations found at surgery. Vegetation culture was positive for *C. albicans*. Replacement of aortic valve by an aortic bioprosthesis was performed. (Panels 31A–31C *from* Bisbe *et al.* [29]; with permission.)

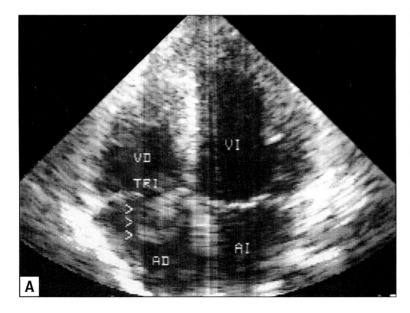

FIGURE 1-32 Combined medical and surgical treatment mandatory for fungal infective endocarditis. Because many of these patients continue using intravenous drugs and return to the hospital with prosthetic valve endocarditis [6], most physicians select total or partial valve resection without valve replacement as the surgical treatment for tricuspid infective endocarditis [7,13]. A new approach to avoid the use of any synthetic material is implantation of a cryopreserved mitral homograph into the tricuspid position [14]. **A,** Transthoracic echocardiography four-chamber view showing a large tricuspid valve vegetation (*arrowheads*). (*continued*)

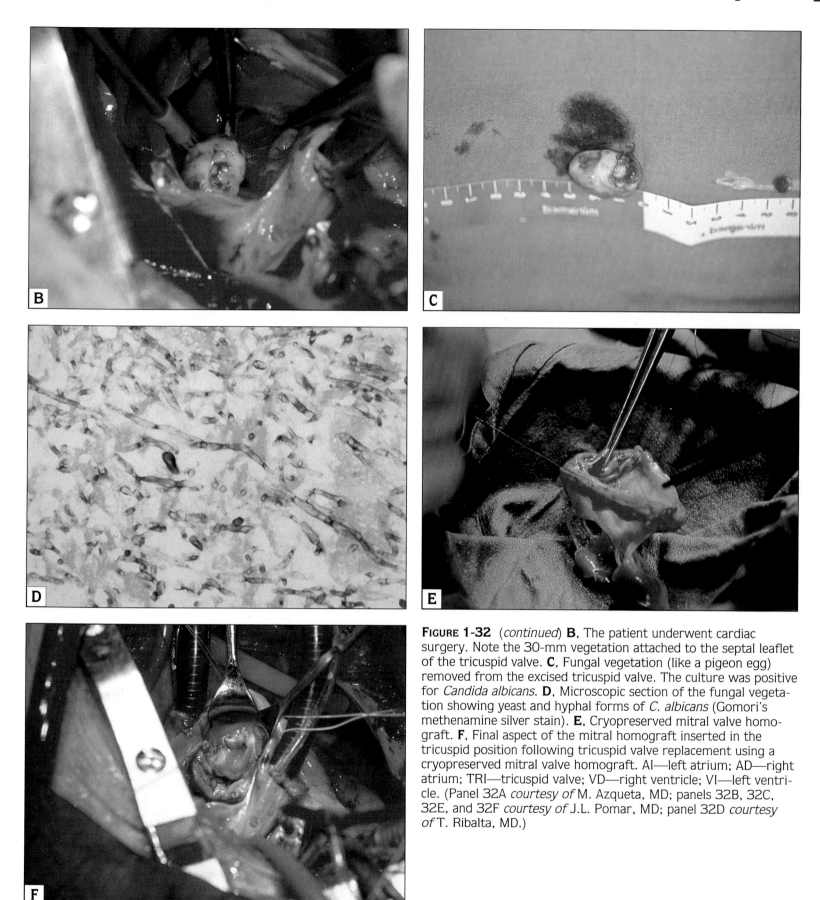

FIGURE 1-32 (*continued*) **B,** The patient underwent cardiac surgery. Note the 30-mm vegetation attached to the septal leaflet of the tricuspid valve. **C,** Fungal vegetation (like a pigeon egg) removed from the excised tricuspid valve. The culture was positive for *Candida albicans*. **D,** Microscopic section of the fungal vegetation showing yeast and hyphal forms of *C. albicans* (Gomori's methenamine silver stain). **E,** Cryopreserved mitral valve homograft. **F,** Final aspect of the mitral homograft inserted in the tricuspid position following tricuspid valve replacement using a cryopreserved mitral valve homograft. AI—left atrium; AD—right atrium; TRI—tricuspid valve; VD—right ventricle; VI—left ventricle. (Panel 32A *courtesy of* M. Azqueta, MD; panels 32B, 32C, 32E, and 32F *courtesy of* J.L. Pomar, MD; panel 32D *courtesy of* T. Ribalta, MD.)

DIAGNOSIS

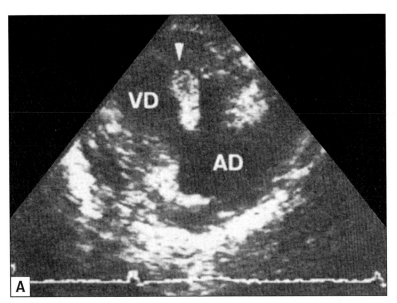

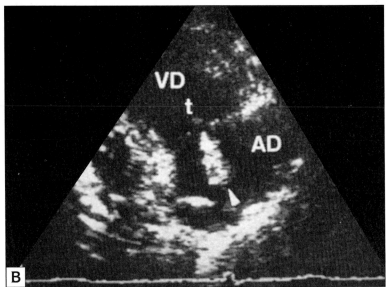

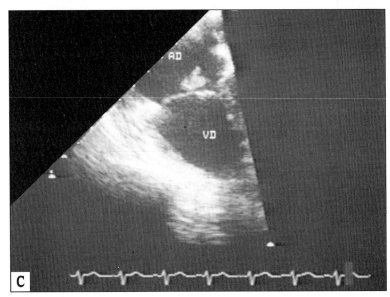

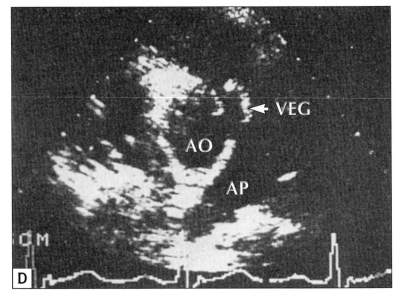

FIGURE 1-33 A and **B**, Transthoracic echocardiograms of a male intravenous (IV) heroin addict aged 25 years with *Staphylococcus aureus* right-sided endocarditis showing a large tricuspid valve vegetation (*arrowheads*). The echocardiogram in *panel 33A* was taken during the diastolic period and the one in *panel 33B* during the systolic period. **C**, Transesophageal echocardiogram of a male heroin addict aged 32 years with *S. aureus* right-sided endocarditis showing a large tricuspid valve vegetation. **D**, Transthoracic echocardiogram of a male IV heroin addict aged 26 years with *S. aureus* right-sided endocarditis showing a pulmonic valve vegetation. Diagnosis of right-sided infective endocarditis in intravenous drug abusers is made on clinical grounds with microbiologic confirmation of bacteria and echocardiographic detection of tricuspid vegetations [10]. Pulmonic endocarditis is unusual and is reported in less than 1% of cases. In right-sided endocarditis, the clinical hallmark is the presence of radiologic pulmonary infiltrates (*see* Figs. 1-18 to 1-22) [2–7,34,37]. Bidimensional echocardiography [39,40] and blood cultures [2–7,33] will confirm the diagnosis in most cases. In right-sided endocarditis, transthoracic echocardiography and transesophageal echocardiography show equal sensitivity (as high as 80%) [11,34,37,41–43]. Blood cultures are positive in 80% to 100% of cases [2–7,33]. AD—right atrium; AO—aortic valve; AP—pulmonary artery; t—tricuspid valve; VD—right ventricle; VEG—vegetation. (*Courtesy of* M. Azqueta, MD.)

OUTCOME

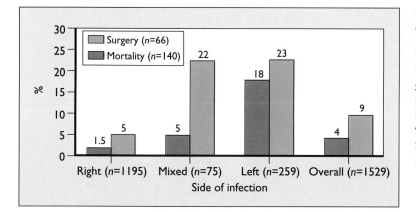

FIGURE 1-34 Incidence of surgery and mortality in 1529 episodes of infective endocarditis in Spanish intravenous drug abusers (IVDAs) according to side of the heart involved. The prognosis of infective endocarditis in IVDAs is dependent on the site of cardiac involvement [2–8]. Overall, 9% of IVDAs died and 4% needed surgery [34]. The prognosis in right-sided infective endocarditis is usually good (mortality, <5%; surgery, <2%) as compared with left-sided endocarditis (mortality, 18%; surgery, 23%). Patients with tricuspid valve vegetations >2 cm [11] and with adult respiratory distress syndrome [12] have a significantly higher mortality (P<0.05). (*Adapted from* Miró *et al.* [33].)

Indications and type of surgery in right-sided infective endocarditis in intravenous drug abusers

Indications
Fungal endocarditis
Persistent or recurrent bacteremia despite optimal antimicrobial therapy
Tricuspid valve vegetations ≥2 cm, recurrent pulmonary emboli, and/or right heart failure (?)
Type of surgery
Partial or total tricuspid valve excision without valve replacement
Vegetectomy
Tricuspid valve replacement
Cryopreserved mitral valve transplantation on tricuspid position

FIGURE 1-35 Indications and type of surgery in right-sided infective endocarditis in intravenous drug abusers. When infective endocarditis involves the tricuspid valve and surgery is required, most surgeons elect total or partial valve resection without valve replacement as the procedure of choice [7,13]. However, long-term follow-up has shown that right-sided heart failure can appear as a consequence of chronic massive tricuspid regurgitation, and in some patients late implantation of a valve prosthesis may be required.

Incidence of recurrent infective endocarditis and delayed surgery in Spanish IVDAs

	Cases, *n*	Ratio per 100 patient-years	*P* value
Recurrent infective endocarditis			
IVDAs (*n*=130)	24	5.3	<0.01
NVIE–GP (*n*=103)	5	1.2	—
PVIE–GP (*n*=21)	1	1.2	—
Delayed surgery			
IVDAs (*n*=130)	3	0.6	<0.01
NVIE–GP (*n*=103)	17	4.4	—
PVIE–GP (*n*=21)	3	4.5	—

GP—general population; IVDAs—intravenous drug abusers; NVIE—native valve infective endocarditis; PVIE—prosthetic valve infective endocarditis.

FIGURE 1-36 Incidence of recurrent infective endocarditis and delayed surgery in Spanish intravenous drug abusers (IVDAs). Compared with the general population diagnosed with an episode of infective endocarditis at the Hospital Clinic of Barcelona between 1979 and 1991 [34], IVDAs had a statistically significant higher incidence of recurrent infective endocarditis (P<0.01), which was most likely due to continued use of intravenous drugs. However, this group also had the lowest incidence of delayed surgery (P<0.01), presumably because of the lower morbidity in patients with predominantly tricuspid valve involvement. (*Adapted from* Miró [34].)

HIV INFECTION AND ENDOCARDITIS

Infective endocarditis in IVDAs with HIV-1

The prevalence of HIV-1 infection ranges between 40% and 75% in urban areas from developed countries.

The incidence of IE in IVDAs in the AIDS era is decreasing, probably due to change in drug administration habits to avoid HIV transmission.

IE in IVDAs has a different clinical picture and outcome depending on HIV status and degree of immunosuppression. HIV-positive IVDAs with IE have a higher ratio of right-sided IE to *Staphylococcus aureus* IE than non–HIV-infected IVDAs. Surgery in HIV-infected IVDAs with IE does not worsen the prognosis.

Overall mortality between HIV-infected or non–HIV-infected IVDAs with IE is similar. However, among HIV-infected IVDAs, mortality is significantly higher in IVDAs severely immunosuppressed (<200 CD4 cells/μL) or with AIDS.

IE—infective endocarditis; IVDAs—intravenous drug abusers.

FIGURE 1-37 Infective endocarditis (IE) in intravenous drug abusers (IVDAs) with HIV-1 infection. Current studies show that the prevalence of HIV in patients with endocarditis is high [15,16]. The full consequences of HIV infection in IE in IVDAs are not yet fully known [6], and few studies have been published on this subject [15–18]. Studies have shown that HIV-infected IVDAs appear to have a higher ratio of right-sided IE to *Staphylococcus aureus* endocarditis than non–HIV-infected IVDAs [16]. Response to antibiotic therapy is similar among HIV-infected or non–HIV-infected IVDAs. Surgery in HIV-infected IVDAs with IE does not worsen the prognosis [17,18]. Overall mortality between HIV-infected or non–HIV-infected IVDAs with IE is similar [15,16]. However, mortality is significantly higher in HIV-infected IVDAs with CD4 cell counts of <200/μL [16]. AIDS patients who also are IVDAs can have multiple simultaneous infections related to either drug abuse or AIDS [2,5,8].

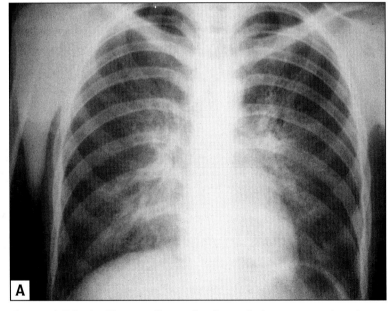
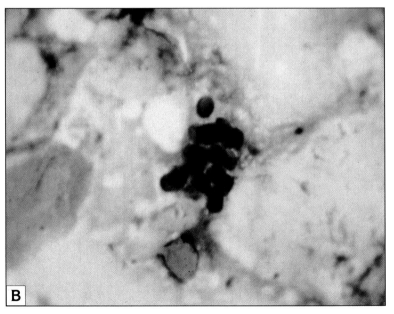

FIGURE 1-38 A, Chest radiograph of a male intravenous heroin addict aged 27 years who was admitted to the hospital due to nonproductive cough, shortness of breath, and fever of 10 days' duration. The physical examination in the emergency room showed oral thrush and needle tracks in the upper extremities. The chest radiograph showed a bilateral interstitial pattern without hilar lymph nodes, cavitation, pleural effusion, or cardiomegaly, suggesting *Pneumocystis carinii* pneumonia (PCP). A sputum induction confirmed the diagnosis showing *P. carinii* cysts. However, the two blood cultures drawn at admission became positive for *Staphylococcus aureus* and a transthoracic echocardiographic examination revealed a tricuspid valve vegetation. HIV serology was positive, and the CD4 cell count was 98/μL. The patient was diagnosed with HIV infection stage C3 (Centers for Disease Control and Prevention criteria, 1993), PCP, and *S. aureus* tricuspid valve endocarditis. Specific therapy was administered for both PCP and endocarditis, and the patient was discharged from the hospital 3 weeks later. **B,** Microscopic view of the sputum induction sample from the patient in *panel 38A* showing a cluster of cysts of *P. carinii* (Gomori's methenamine silver stain). (*Courtesy of* M.E. Valls, MD.)

ACKNOWLEDGMENTS

We are indebted to the staff members of the Infectious Diseases (J.M. Gatell, MD), Pathology (T. Ribalta, MD), Cardiovascular Surgery (J.L. Pomar, MD, and C. Mestres, MD), Echocardiography (C. Pare, MD, and M. Azqueta, MD) and Microbiology (F. Marco, MD, M. Pujol, MD, and M.E. Valls, MD) Units for their help in collecting the slides.

REFERENCES

1. Coutinho RA: Epidemiology and control of AIDS among drug users (plenary conference). Presented at the Fifth International Conference on AIDS. Montreal, 1989.

2. Haverkos HW, Lange WR: Serious infections other than human immunodeficiency virus among intravenous drug abusers. *J Infect Dis* 1990, 156:894–902.

3. Reisberg B: Infective endocarditis in the narcotic addict. *Prog Cardiovasc Dis* 1979, 22:193–204.

4. Sheagren JN: Endocarditis complicating parenteral drug abuse. In *Current Clinical Topics in Infectious Diseases.* Edited by Remington JS, Swartz MN. New York: McGraw-Hill; 1981:211–233.

5. Cherubin CE, Sapira JD: The medical complications of drug addiction and the medical assessment of the intravenous drug user: 25 years later. *Ann Intern Med* 1993, 119:1017–1028.

6. Levine DP, Sobel JD: Infections in intravenous drug abusers. In *Principles and Practice of Infectious Diseases,* 4th ed. Edited by Mandell GL, Bennett JE, Dolin R. New York: Churchill Livingstone; 1995:2696–2709.

7. Sande MA, Lee BL, Millills J, Chambers HF: Endocarditis in intravenous drug users. In *Infective Endocarditis,* 2nd ed. Edited by Kaye D. New York: Raven Press; 1992:345–359.

8. Grupo de Trabajo para el Estudio de las Infecciones en Drogadictos: Estudio multicéntrico de las complicaciones infecciosas en adictos a drogas por vía parenteral en España: Análisis final de 17,592 casos (1977–1991). *Enferm Infecc Microbiol Clin* 1995, 13:532–539.

9. Cannon NJ, Cobbs CG: Infective endocarditis in drug addicts. In *Infective Endocarditis.* Edited by Kaye D. Baltimore: University Park Press; 1976: 111–127.

10. Durak DT, Lukes AS, Bright DK, Duke Endocarditis Service: New criteria for diagnosis of infective endocarditis: Utilization of specific echocardiographic findings. *Am J Med* 1994, 96:200–209.

11. Hecht SR, Berger M: Right-sided endocarditis in intravenous drug users: Prognostic features in 102 episodes. *Ann Intern Med* 1992, 117:560–566.

12. Torres-Tortosa M, González M, Pérez E, *et al.:* Endocarditis infecciosa en heroinónamos en la provincia de Cádiz: Un estudio multicéntrico sobre 150 episodios. *Med Clin (Barc)* 1992, 98:521–526.

13. Arbulu A, Holmes RJ, Asfaw I: Surgical treatment of intractable right-sided endocarditis in drug addicts: 25 years' experience. *J Heart Valve Dis* 1993, 2:129–137.

14. Pomar JL, Mestres C, Paré JC, Miró JM: Management of persistent tricuspid endocarditis with transplantation of cryopreserved mitral homografts. *J Thorac Cardiovasc Surg* 1994, 107:1460–1463.

15. Nahass RB, Weinstein MP, Bartels J, Bocke DJ: Infective endocarditis in intravenous drug users: A comparison of human immunodeficiency virus type 1-negative and -positive patients. *J Infect Dis* 1990, 162:967–970.

16. Pulvirenti JJ, Kerns E, Benson C, *et al.:* Infective endocarditis in injection drug users: Importance of human immunodeficiency virus serostatus and degree of immunosuppression. *Clin Infect Dis* 1996, 22:40–45.

17. Lemma M, Vanelli P, Beretta L, *et al.:* Cardiac surgery in HIV-positive intravenous drug addicts: Influence of cardiovascular bypass on the progression to AIDS. *Thorac Cardiovasc Surg* 1992, 40:279–282.

18. Aris A, Pomar JL, Saura E: Cardiopulmonary bypass in HIV-positive patients. *Ann Thorac Surg* 1993, 55:1104–1108.

19. Scheidegger C, Zimmerli W: Infectious complications in drug addicts: Seven-year review of 269 hospitalized narcotic abusers in Switzerland. *Rev Infect Dis* 1989, 11:486–493.

20. Stoneburner RL, Des Jarlais DC, Benezra D, *et al.:* A larger spectrum of severe HIV-1 related disease in intravenous drug users in New York City. *Science* 1988, 242:916–919.

21. Tuazon CU, Sheagren JN: Staphylococcal endocarditis in parenteral drug abusers: Source of the organism. *Ann Intern Med* 1975, 82:788–790.

22. Tuazon CU, Sheagren JN: Increased rate of carriage of *Staphylococcus aureus* among narcotic addicts. *J Infect Dis* 1974, 129:725–727.

23. Vlahov D, Sullivan M, Astemborski J, Nelson K: Bacterial infections and skin cleaning prior to injection among intravenous drug users. *Public Health Rep* 1992, 107:595–598.

24. Miró JM, Puig de la Bellacasa J, Gatell JM, *et al.:* Estudio de la tasa de portadores cutaneomucosos de estafilococos en heroinómanos del área de Barcelona y de las características microbiológicas de la heroína y material de inyección. *Med Clin (Barc)* 1984, 83:620–623.

25. Tuazon CU, Hill R, Sheagren JN: Microbiological study of street heroin and injection paraphernalia. *J Infect Dis* 1974, 129:327–329.

26. Tuazon CU, Miller H, Shamsuddin D: Antimicrobial activity of street heroin [letter]. *J Infect Dis* 1980, 142:944.

27. Shekar R, Rice TW, Zierdt CH, Kallick CA: Outbreak of endocarditis caused by *Pseudomonas aeruginosa* serotype O11 amount pentazocine and tripelennamine abusers in Chicago. *J Infect Dis* 1985, 151:203–208.

28. Botsford KB, Weinstein RA, Nathan CR, Kabis SA: Selective survival in pentazocine and tripelennamine of *Pseudomonas aeruginosa* serotype O11 from drug addicts. *J Infect Dis* 1985, 151:209–216.

29. Bisbe J, Miró JM, Latorre X, *et al.:* Disseminated candidiasis in addicts who use brown heroin: Report of 83 cases and review. *Clin Infect Dis* 1992, 15:910–923.

30. Miró JM, Puig de la Bellacasa J, Odds FC, *et al.:* Source of the infection in an outbreak of systemic candidiasis in Spanish heroin addicts. *J Infect Dis* 1987, 156:857–858.

31. Tornos MP, Miró JM: Endocarditis infecciosa. In *Tratado de Medicina Interna Farreras-Rozman,* decimotercera edición. Edited by Rozman C. Ediciones Doyma: Barcelona; 1995:605–614.

32. Chambers HF, Morris DL, Täuber MG, Modin G: Cocaine use and the risk of endocarditis in intravenous drug abusers. *Ann Intern Med* 1987, 106:833–836.

33. Miró JM, Cruceta A, Gatell JM: Infective endocarditis (IE) in Spanish IV drug addicts (IVDA): Analysis of 1,529 episodes (1978–1993) [abstr 109]. Presented at the 3rd International Symposium on Modern Concepts in Endocarditis. Boston, MA, 1995.

34. Miró JM: Endocarditis infecciosa en drogadictos: Estudio epidemiológico, clínico y experimental. Tesis doctoral. Universidad de Barcelona, Spain, 1994.

35. McIlroy MA, Reddy D, Markowitz N, Saravolatz LD: Infected false aneurysms of the femoral artery in intravenous drug addicts. *Rev Infect Dis* 1989, 11:578–585.

36. Aguado JM, Arjona R, Ugarte P: Septic pulmonary emboli: A rare cause of bilateral pneumothorax in drug abusers. *Chest* 1990, 98:1320–1324.

37. Weisse AB, Heller DR, Schimenti RJ, Montgomery RL: The febrile parenteral drug user: A prospective study in 121 patients. *Am J Med* 1993, 94:274–280.

38. Bisbe J, Miró JM, Moreno A, Mensa J: *Candida albicans* endocarditis possibly related to systemic candidiasis in a heroin addict. *Eur J Clin Microbiol Infect Dis* 1987, 6:657–658.

39. Mügge A, Daniel WG, Frank C, Lichtlen PR: Echocardiography in infective endocarditis: Reassessment of prognostic implications of vegetation size determined by the transthoracic and the transesophageal approach. *J Am Coll Cardiol* 1989, 14:631–638.

40. Daniel W, Müggue A, Martin R, *et al.*: Improvement in the diagnosis of abscesses associated with endocarditis by transesophageal echocardiography. *N Engl J Med* 1991, 324:795–803.

41. Manolis AS, Melita H: Echocardiographic and clinical correlates in drug addicts with infective endocarditis: Implications of vegetation size. *Arch Intern Med* 1988, 148:2461–2465.

42. Bayer AS, Blomquist IK, Bello E, *et al.*: Tricuspid valve endocarditis to *Staphylococcus aureus* correlation of two dimensional echocardiography with clinical outcome. *Chest* 1988, 93:247–253.

43. San Roman JA, Vilacosta I, Zamorano JL, *et al.*: Transesophageal echocardiography in right-sided endocarditis. *J Am Coll Cardiol* 1993, 21:1226–1230.

SELECTED BIBLIOGRAPHY

Arbulu A, Holmes RJ, Asfaw I: Surgical treatment of intractable right-sided endocarditis in drug addicts: 25 years' experience. *J Heart Valve Dis* 1993, 2:129–137.

Cherubin CE, Sapira JD: The medical complications of drug addiction and the medical assessment of the intravenous drug user: 25 years later. *Ann Intern Med* 1993, 119:1017–1028.

Hecht SR, Berger M: Right-sided endocarditis in intravenous drug users: Prognostic features in 102 episodes. *Ann Intern Med* 1992, 117:560–566.

Pulvirenti JJ, Kerns E, Benson C, *et al.*: Infective endocarditis in injection drug users: Importance of human immunodeficiency virus serostatus and degree of immunosuppression. *Clin Infect Dis* 1996, 22:40–45.

Sande MA, Lee BL, Millills J, Chambers HF: Endocarditis in intravenous drug users. In *Infective endocarditis*, 2nd ed. Edited by Kaye D. New York: Raven Press; 1992:345–359.

CHAPTER 2

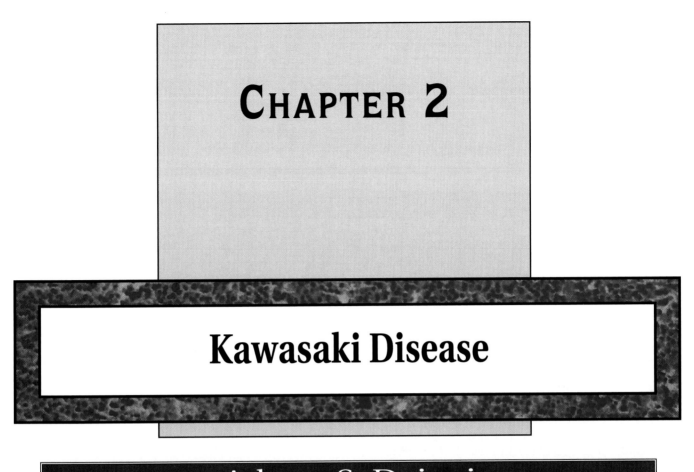

Kawasaki Disease

Adnan S. Dajani
Kathryn A. Taubert

KAWASAKI DISEASE (KD), a leading cause of acquired heart disease in children in the United States, is a generalized vasculitis of unknown etiology. Most affected children are under the age of 2 years, and 80% of cases occur in children under 5 years of age. There have been isolated reports of KD occurring in young adults, in whom it is more common in male than in female patients (1:1.5). Within the United States, the reported incidence of KD is 9.2 per 100,000 children younger than 5 years of age [1], and although the incidence of KD is higher in children of Asian ancestry, children of all racial backgrounds are affected. KD was first reported by Tomisaku Kawasaki in 1967 in Japan, and was originally referred to as "mucocutaneous lymph node syndrome" [2]. More than 116,000 cases have been reported in Japan through 1992 [3], and KD has been recorded worldwide [4]. Studies from Japan, Europe, and the United States indicate that epidemics of KD occur in approximate 3-year cycles.

Although the cause of KD remains unknown, its epidemiology and clinical presentation suggest a microbial agent. Speculated etiologic agents include rickettsiae, viruses, bacteria such as group A and other streptococci, propionibacteria, and candidae. One recent study has implicated superantigens—toxins produced by certain staphylococci and streptococci [5]. There has been no documentation of person-to-person transmission (even in day-care centers); cases among siblings are rare; and the recurrence rate is less than 2%.

Kawasaki disease can cause an arteritis of medium and large vessels, arterial aneurysms, valvulitis, and myocarditis. Coronary artery aneurysms may resolve or persist. These are of particular concern because they can lead to thrombosis, evolve into segmental stenosis, or, in very rare cases, rupture. Studies have shown that approximately 20% of untreated children develop coronary artery abnormalities. Coronary artery aneurysms are classified as small (<5 mm in internal diameter), medium (5 to 8 mm in internal diameter), or giant (>8 mm in internal diameter). Although approximately one half of all coronary artery aneurysms regress within 2 years, virtually none of the giant coronary artery aneurysms regress. Myocardial infarction can occur, typically in patients with giant coronary artery aneurysms. In the current era of diagnosis and treatment, the death rate is less than 1% for all patients with KD.

Because there is no specific diagnostic test for KD, a set of diagnostic criteria has been established by both the Japan Heart Foundation and the American Heart Association [6–9]. Despite the fact that the cause of KD is not currently known, treatment regimens have been developed. In the acute phase of the disease, treatment is directed particularly at reducing inflammation of the coronary arteries and the myocardium. This treatment includes aspirin and intravenous gammaglobulin.

Long-term follow-up of patients with KD is important. Natural history studies are not currently available, so some type of follow-up of all patients with cardiac involvement should be done. Guidelines for long-term management have been developed [9]. Patients are stratified into five risk levels based on their relative risk for cardiac ischemia. Recommendations for pharmacologic therapy, physical activity, follow-up and diagnostic testing, and invasive testing are included for each risk level.

EPIDEMIOLOGY

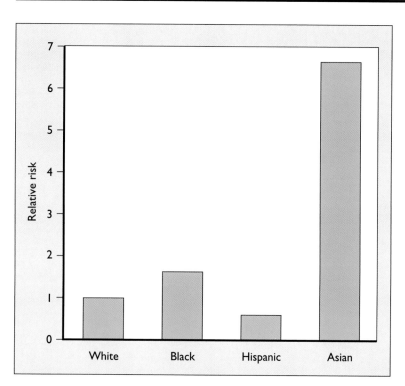

FIGURE 2-1 Relative risk for Kawasaki disease by race in US children younger than 5 years of age. Data are from a nationwide surveillance of Kawasaki disease by the Centers for Disease Control and Prevention for the years 1976 to 1984. Relative risk for whites is set at 1. Relative risk for blacks was about 1.5 times that of whites, whereas the relative risk in children of Asian ancestry was more than six times that of whites. Hispanic children had the lowest relative risk. (*Adapted from* Rauch [10].)

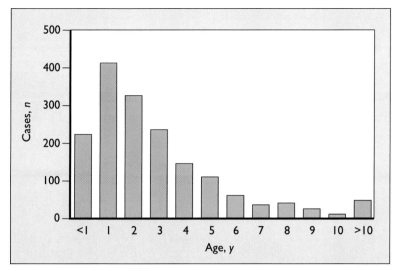

FIGURE 2-2 Kawasaki disease occurs predominantly in children younger than 5 years of age. For cases of Kawasaki disease reported to the Centers for Disease Control and Prevention between 1976 and 1984, peak incidence occurred in children between 1 and 2 years of age, and 80% of cases were reported in children less than 5 years of age. (*Adapted from* Rauch [10].)

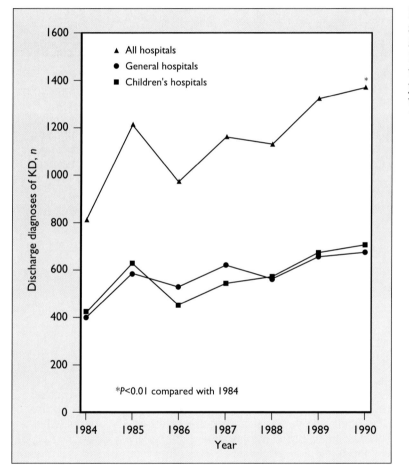

FIGURE 2-3 Discharge diagnoses of Kawasaki disease (KD) from a survey of 295 US hospitals, including 44 children's hospitals and 251 general hospitals with at least 400 beds and a pediatric ward. Hospitals were asked to report the number of discharge diagnoses for ICD.9CM diagnostic code 446.1 (Kawasaki disease) for the years 1984 to 1990. Yearly fluctuations were observed, and there was a significant increase in reported diagnoses between 1984 and 1990. (*Adapted from* Taubert *et al.* [1].)

PATHOLOGY

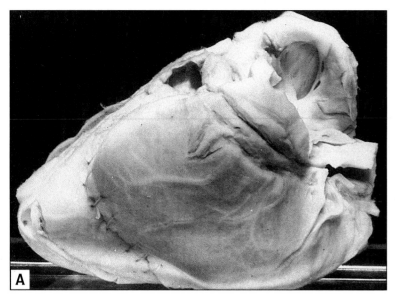

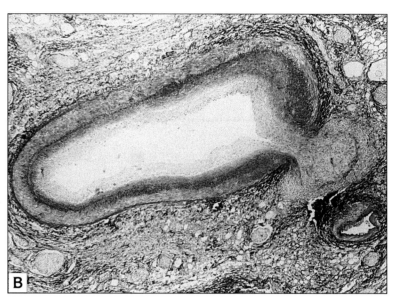

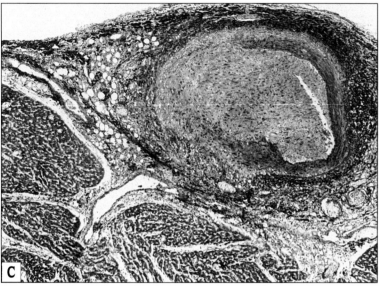

FIGURE 2-4 A, The heart of a boy aged 7 years who died in 1870 in London after "scarlatinal dropsy." Physicians preserved the heart in formalin, and it was found several years ago at St. Bartholomew's Hospital in London. Coronary aneurysms can be seen. The child's heart has been recently sectioned and photomicrographed. **B,** Endothelial proliferation. **C,** A thrombus totally occludes a coronary artery. The death of this child is consistent with the sequelae of Kawasaki disease. (*From* Shulman [11]; with permission.)

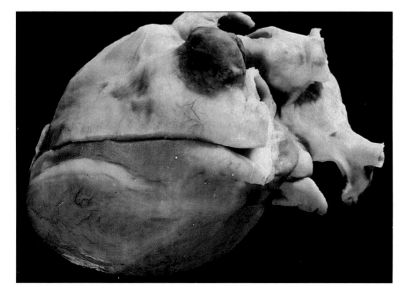

FIGURE 2-5 Complications of aneurysms secondary to Kawasaki disease. Kawasaki disease can lead (rarely) to aneurysm rupture. This figure shows one such case in a girl aged 16 months, when a saccular aneurysm in the proximal right coronary artery ruptured, leading to cardiac tamponade and death. (*From* Becker [12]; with permission.)

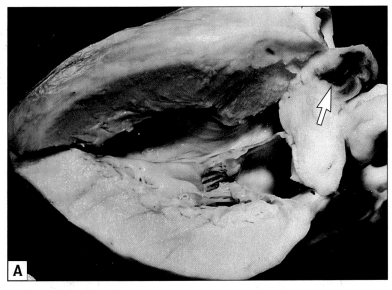

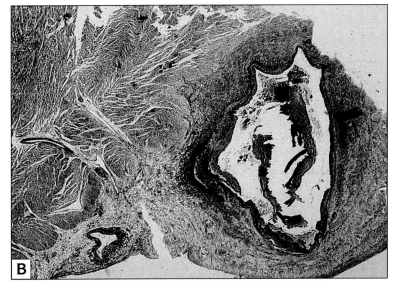

FIGURE 2-6 A, Dissection of the heart shown in Fig. 2-5 demonstrating a fusiform aneurysm (*arrow*) in the left coronary artery. **B,** An elastic tissue stain (×8) of this aneurysm, demonstrating massive inflammatory infiltration. Autopsy also revealed an arteritis of the principal muscular artery in the hilium of the left ovary. (*From* Becker [12]; with permission.)

DIAGNOSIS AND CLINICAL FEATURES

Diagnostic criteria of Kawasaki disease (principal clinical findings)

Generally high and spiking fever (often to ≥104°F) lasting at least 5 days; fever persists in untreated patients for 1–2 wk or longer

Presence of at least four of the following five principal features

Changes of peripheral extremities: distinctive changes that acutely include redness and swelling, and sometimes induration, of the hands and feet; after 1–3 wk, desquamation of the fingers and toes; after 1–2 mo, Beau's lines (white lines across the fingernails) may appear

Polymorphous exanthem rash: primarily truncal; can take several forms; and usually appears within 5 days after the onset of fever

Bilateral conjunctival injection: usually involves the bulbar conjunctivae; is not associated with an exudate; and is usually painless

Changes of the lips and oral cavity: including strawberry tongue, redness and cracking of the lips, and erythema of the oropharyngeal mucosa

Cervical lymphadenopathy if at least one lymph node is more than 1.5 cm in diameter: usually presents as unilateral lymphadenopathy, with firm and slightly tender nodes

Exclusion of other diseases with similar findings (*see* Fig. 2-8)

FIGURE 2-7 Diagnostic criteria. Many experts believe that, in the presence of classic features, the diagnosis of Kawasaki disease can be made by experienced observers prior to the fifth day of fever. The first four of the five principal clinical findings are seen in at least 90% of patients. Cervical lymphadenopathy is the least common of the five principal clinical features (observed in 50% to 75% of patients). (*Adapted from* Dajani *et al.* [8].)

Differential diagnosis of Kawasaki disease

Measles
Scarlet fever
Drug reactions
Stevens-Johnson syndrome
Other febrile viral exanthems
Rocky Mountain spotted fever
Staphylococcal scalded skin syndrome
Toxic shock syndrome
Juvenile rheumatoid arthritis
Leptospirosis
Mercury poisoning

FIGURE 2-8 Differential diagnosis of Kawasaki disease (KD). These diseases and disorders with similar clinical findings to those of KD should be ruled out. Careful consideration of measles in the differential diagnosis is especially important, particularly in light of recent outbreaks of measles in some urban US areas. Measles cases misdiagnosed as KD do not allow appropriate measles control measures to be promptly undertaken. Conversely, KD patients diagnosed with measles or other diseases or disorders will fail to receive prompt therapy that may prevent them from having long-term coronary artery disorders. (*From* Dajani *et al.* [8].)

Atypical KD

Manifestation	Atypical KD	Atypical KD in infants
Fever for ≥5 days	73%–90%	83%–93%
Mucositis	50%–80%	18%–66%
Rash	40%–100%	72%–100%
Cervical nodes ≥1.5 cm	0%–36%	0%–33%
Peripheral extremity edema or erythema*	15%–80%	17%–50%
Conjunctivitis	45%–78%	36%–67%
≤3 criteria	20%–75%	33%–79%
Coronary artery complications	21%–90%	86%–100%
Age		
Mean	16.4–26 mo	5.3–6.8 mo
Median	7–11 mo	4.5–8 mo
Male-to-female ratio	0.9:1–2.3:1	1:1–4.5:1
Mortality	10%–35%	17%–100%

*Includes desquamation as a peripheral extremity change.
KD—Kawasaki disease.

FIGURE 2-9 Atypical Kawasaki disease (KD). Atypical or incomplete cases of KD, in which patients have less than four of the five principal features, have been increasingly reported. Full diagnostic criteria are more often lacking in infants, especially those less than 6 months of age, than in older children. Patients with fever and less than four of the principal clinical features can be diagnosed as having KD when coronary artery disease is detected by two-dimensional echocardiography or coronary angiography. Several studies suggest that coronary arterial involvement is present in almost all infants with atypical KD. (*Adapted from* Kabani *et al.* [13]; with permission.)

Cardiac findings in acute Kawasaki disease

Pericardial effusion, echocardiographically documented in about 30% of patients with acute Kawasaki disease
Myocardial inflammation is common, with signs including:
  Tachycardia out of proportion to the degree of fever
  A gallop rhythm
  An electrocardiogram showing decreased R-wave voltage, ST-segment depression, T-wave flattening or inversion, and prolonged PR and/or QT intervals
  Ischemia-induced atrial or ventricular arrhythmias
  Congestive heart failure
Coronary artery abnormalities, usually beyond 10 days of onset of illness, including ectasia or aneurysms

FIGURE 2-10 Cardiac findings in acute Kawasaki disease (KD). Cardiovascular manifestations are often prominent in the acute phase of KD; some degree of myocarditis is virtually always present. Coronary artery aneurysms are the leading cause of both short- and long-term morbidity and mortality. These develop in approximately 20% of affected children with untreated KD. The aneurysms usually appear between 10 days and 4 weeks after the onset of symptoms. Certain factors increase the risk of development of coronary artery aneurysms (*see also* Fig. 2-11).

Factors associated with increased risk of developing coronary aneurysms

Male gender
Age <1 yr
Other signs and symptoms of pancarditis, including
  arrhythmias
Prolonged period of inflammation, including fever for
  >10 days
Recurrence of fever after an afebrile period of at least
  24 hr

FIGURE 2-11 Certain patient factors leading to an increased risk for the development of coronary arterial aneurysms. One should pay particular attention to patients with one or more of the factors listed in this figure.

Noncardiac clinical findings in acute Kawasaki disease

Musculoskeletal system
  Arthritis, arthralgia
Gastrointestinal tract
  Diarrhea, vomiting, abdominal pain
  Hepatic dysfunction
  Acute noncalculous distension (hydrops) of the gallbladder
Central nervous system
  Extreme irritability, especially in younger infants
  Aseptic meningitis
Respiratory tract
  Preceding respiratory illness
  Otitis media
  Pulmonary infiltrates
Other findings
  Erythema and induration at bacille Calmette-Guérin vaccine
    inoculation site
  Auditory abnormalities
  Testicular swelling
  Peripheral gangrene
  Aneurysms of medium-sized noncoronary arteries

FIGURE 2-12 Noncardiac findings in acute Kawasaki disease. Arthritis or arthralgia can occur in the first week of the illness and is usually polyarticular, involving the knees, ankles, and hands. A pauciarticular arthritis commonly appears during the second or third week of illness. Arthritis is more common in older girls. Lumbar puncture shows evidence of aseptic meningitis (presence of white blood cells, predominantly lymphocytes) in approximately one fourth of patients undergoing the procedure. Hydrops of the gallbladder, identified by abdominal ultrasound, is common during the first 2 weeks of the illness. Some other findings are less common. Patients who have giant coronary artery aneurysms are more likely than others to have noncoronary arterial involvement.

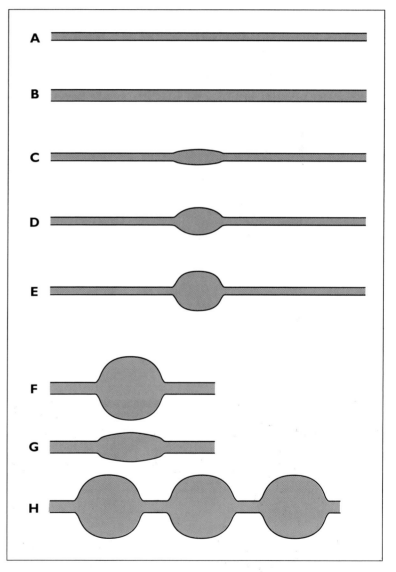

FIGURE 2-13 Types of coronary artery abnormalities in Kawasaki disease. **A,** A normal coronary artery 2 mm in internal diameter. (Normal coronary artery sizes range from 2 mm in infants and young children to 5 mm in teenagers [14].) **B,** An ectatic artery 3 mm in internal diameter (wider than normal but without aneurysms). **C,** A small aneurysm 4 mm in internal diameter (small aneurysms are <5 mm in internal diameter). **D,** A medium-sized aneurysm 7 mm in internal diameter (medium aneurysms are 5 to 8 mm in internal diameter). **E,** A giant aneurysm 10 mm in internal diameter (giant aneurysms are >8 mm in internal diameter). **F–H,** Aneurysms can be saccular (circular-appearing; *panel 13F*), fusiform (cigar-shaped; *panel 13G*), or segmental (*panel 13H*).

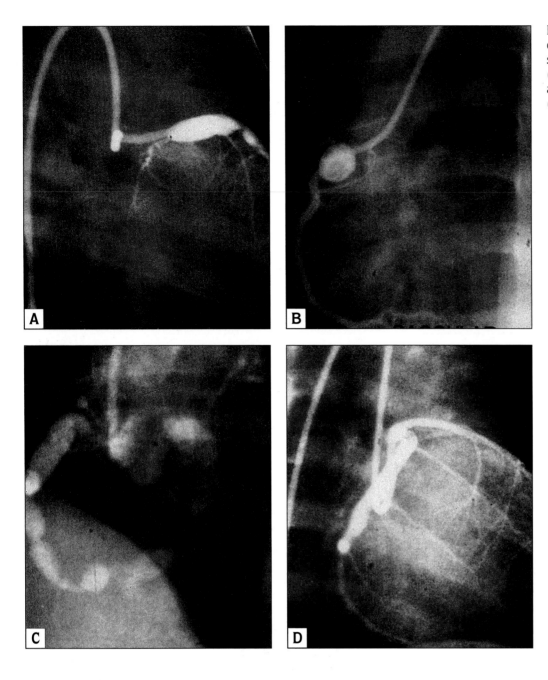

FIGURE 2-14 A–D, Coronary angiograms of patients with Kawasaki disease demonstrating fusiform (*panel 14A*), saccular (*panel 14B*), and segmental (*panel 14C*) aneurysms and an ectatic coronary artery (*panel 14D*).

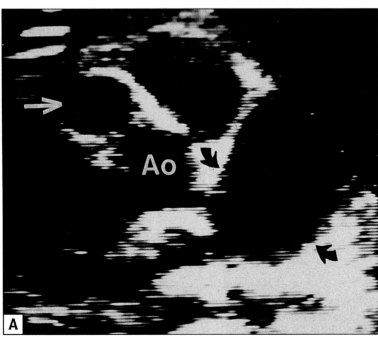

FIGURE 2-15 Two-dimensional echocardiograms in a boy aged 2 years, 11 months with acute Kawasaki disease. **A,** Left parasternal short-axis view demonstrating a giant left proximal coronary artery aneurysm (35 × 25 mm; *black arrows*) and an aneurysm in the right coronary artery (*white arrow*). (*continued*)

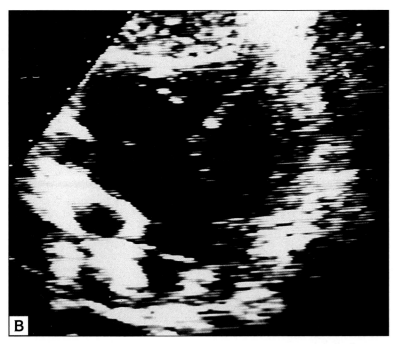

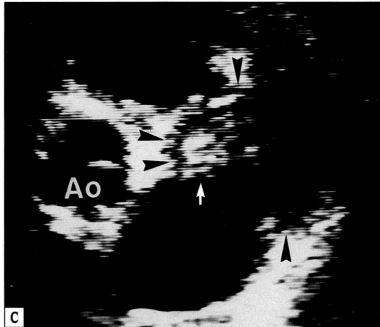

FIGURE 2-15 (*continued*) **B,** The subcostal view reveals two giant aneurysms in the right coronary artery. The proximal one is 18 × 18 mm, and the distal one is 10 × 10 mm. **C,** A thrombus (*white arrow*) partially occupying the left coronary artery giant aneurysm. The *arrowheads* define the lumen of the aneurysm. Ao—aorta. (*From* Lima *et al.* [15]; with permission.)

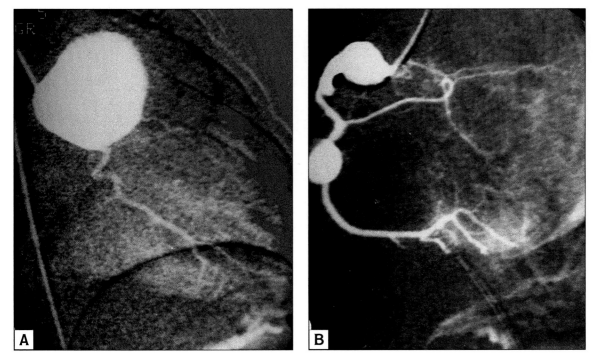

FIGURE 2-16 Coronary arteriograms demonstrating the aneurysms shown in Fig. 2-15. **A,** The giant left proximal coronary artery aneurysm. **B,** The two giant aneurysms in the right coronary artery. Right coronary artery ectasia is seen between the two aneurysms. (*From* Lima *et al.* [15]; with permission.)

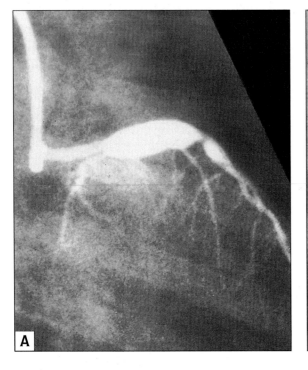

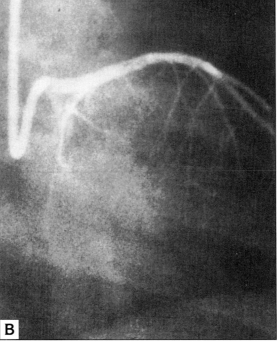

FIGURE 2-17 Left coronary arteriograms from a male infant who contracted Kawasaki disease at age 6 months. **A,** Arteriogram 1 month after onset of Kawasaki disease. Fusiform aneurysms are observed in the left anterior descending coronary artery. **B,** Arteriogram 16 months later, showing regression of the aneurysm. (Panel 17A *from* Takahashi *et al.* [16]; with permission.)

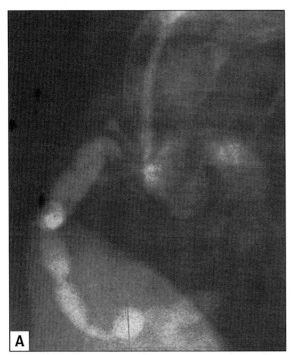

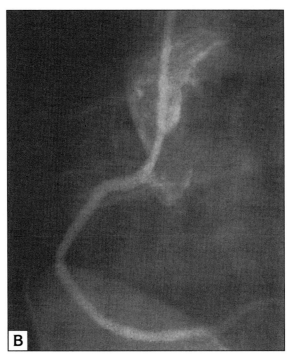

FIGURE 2-18 Right coronary arteriograms from a male infant who contracted Kawasaki disease at age 6 months (same patient as in Fig. 2-17). **A,** Multiple aneurysms can be seen 1 month after onset of the disease. **B,** Regression of the aneurysms 16 months later (17 months after onset of disease).

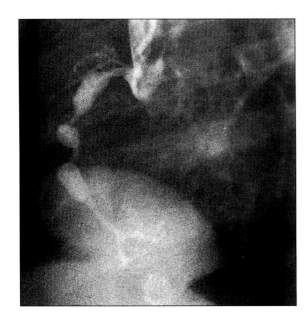

FIGURE 2-19 Right coronary arteriogram from a girl aged 17 months who was diagnosed with Kawasaki disease at age 15 months. Two months after onset of disease, three aneurysms are present, with possible discrete stenoses between aneurysmal segments. (*From* Takahashi *et al.* [16]; with permission.)

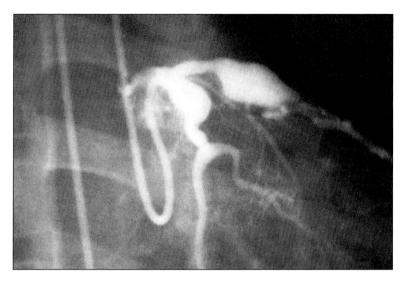

FIGURE 2-20 Aneurysms of the left anterior descending and the left circumflex coronary arteries in a 6-year-old boy who was diagnosed with Kawasaki disease and giant aneurysms 5 years earlier, at age 13 months. Giant coronary artery aneurysms (internal diameter of at least 8 mm) rarely regress. These patients have a worse prognosis than patients without giant aneurysms, and have the greatest risk for development of stenosis, thrombosis, or myocardial infarction.

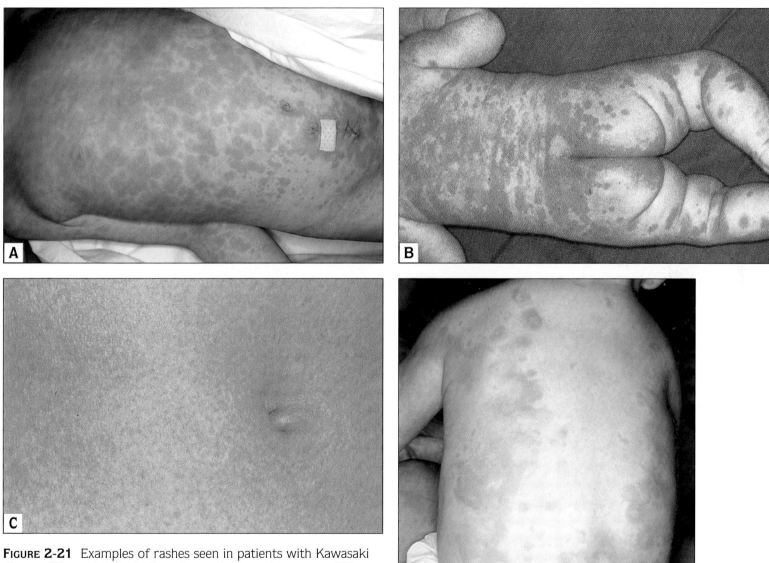

FIGURE 2-21 Examples of rashes seen in patients with Kawasaki disease. The rash is typically polymorphous and appears within 5 days of the onset of fever. **A–D,** Such rashes may take various forms including an urticarial exanthem (*panel 21A*), a maculo-papular morbilliform eruption (*panel 21B*), a scarlatiniform derma (*panel 21C*), or an erythema-multiforme–like rash (*panel 21D*). Bullous eruptions have not been described. (*continued*)

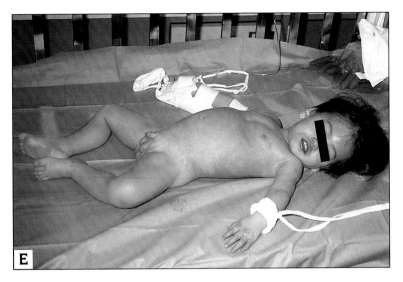

E

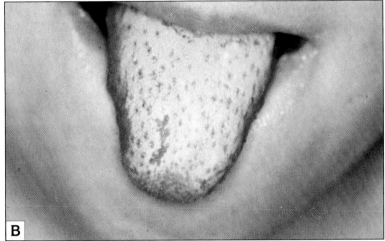

FIGURE 2-21 (*continued*) **E,** The rash is usually extensive, involving the trunk and extremities with accentuation in the perineal region. (Panel 21B *from* Dajani *et al.* [7]; with permission.)

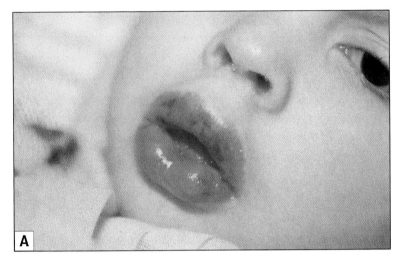

A

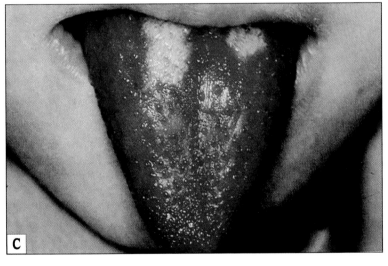

C

FIGURE 2-22 **A–C,** Mucous membrane changes in Kawasaki disease involve the conjunctivae, oral cavity and lips (*panels 22A–22C*), and the urethra. Bilateral conjunctival injection usually begins shortly after the onset of fever. It typically involves the bulbar conjunctivae much more than the palpebral or tarsal conjunctivae, is not associated with an exudate, and is usually painless. Changes in the lips and oral cavity include erythema and cracking of the lips, strawberry tongue, and erythema of the oropharyngeal mucosa. No ulcerations are seen. (Panel 22A *from* Dajani *et al.* [7]; with permission.)

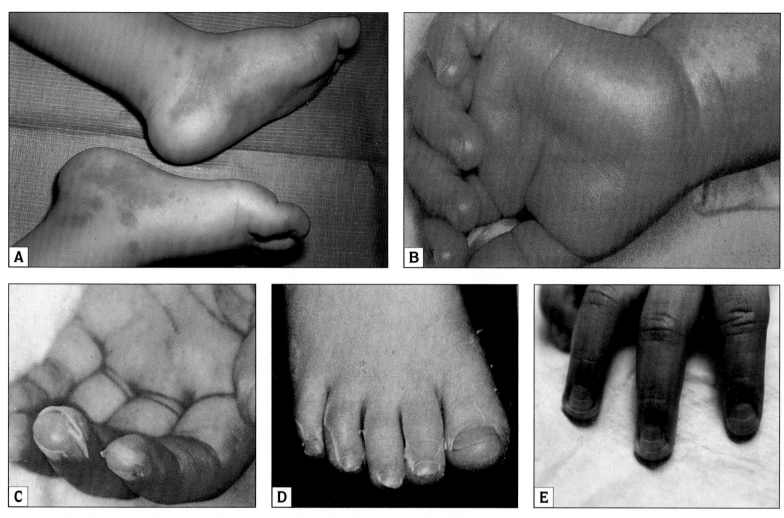

FIGURE 2-23 Changes in the extremities are distinctive. **A** and **B,** Erythema of the palms and soles and/or firm, sometimes painful induration of the hands or feet often occurs in the early phase of the disease. **C** and **D,** Desquamation of the fingers and toes usually begins 1 to 3 weeks after onset of fever in the periungual region and may extend to the palms and toes. **E,** Approximately 1 to 2 months after the onset of fever, deep transverse grooves across the nails (Beau's lines) may appear. (Panels 23B and 23C *from* Dajani *et al.* [7]; with permission.)

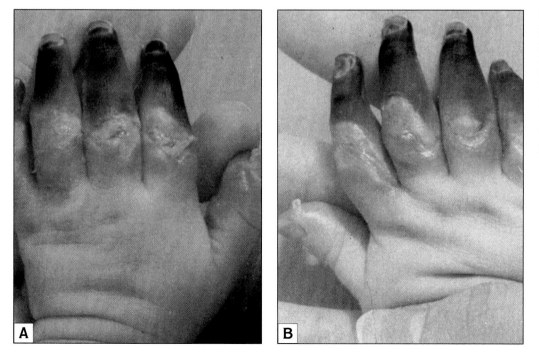

FIGURE 2-24 A and **B,** Peripheral gangrene secondary to arterial involvement in an infant aged 2 months with Kawasaki disease. This is a rare complication of the disease that occurs in young infants (all reported cases have been 7 months of age or younger at onset of disease [17]). Frequently associated findings include giant coronary and peripheral aneurysms.

LABORATORY FINDINGS

Laboratory findings in Kawasaki disease

Neutrophilia with immature forms
Elevated erythrocyte sedimentation rate
Positive C-reactive protein
Elevated serum α_1-antitrypsin
Anemia
Hypoalbuminemia
Elevated serum IgE
Thrombocytosis
Proteinuria
Sterile pyuria
Elevated serum transaminases

FIGURE 2-25 Laboratory findings in Kawasaki disease. Laboratory findings are nondiagnostic for Kawasaki disease, but may assist in diagnosis. The elevated platelet count usually appears after the first week of illness. The proteinuria is probably secondary to fever. The erythrocyte sedimentation rate and C-reactive protein are almost invariably elevated.

Immune system irregularities in Kawasaki disease

Activation of monocytes/macrophages
Increased activated T-helper cells
Decreased T-suppressor cells
Increased activated B cells
Cytokine secretion, including:
  Interleukin-1
  Interleukin-2
  Interleukin-6
  Tumor necrosis factor-a
  Interferon-g
Appearance of circulating antibodies cytotoxic to vascular
  endothelial cells

FIGURE 2-26 Immune system irregularities in Kawasaki disease. In response to an unknown triggering process, immunoregulatory abnormalities are observed in Kawasaki disease. It is postulated that the various secreted cytokines target vascular endothelial cells, producing cell-surface antigens. Antibodies produced against these antigens then target the vascular endothelium, resulting in a cascade of events leading to vascular damage.

Association of KD with toxin-producing bacteria

Toxin	Patients with KD, n (n=16)	Controls, n (n=15)
TSST-1		
Staphylococcus aureus (white)	11	0
TSST-secreting		
S. aureus (gold)	0	1
SPEB and SPEC		
Group A streptococci	2	0
Total	13*	1*

*P<0.0001 (Fisher's exact test).

KD—Kawasaki disease; SPEB—streptococcal pyrogenic exotoxin B; SPEC—streptococcal pyrogenic exotoxin C; TSST—toxic shock syndrome toxin.

FIGURE 2-27 Association of Kawasaki disease (KD) with toxin-producing bacteria. Bacteria from 16 patients with acute, untreated KD and from 15 control subjects were cultured. Bacteria were obtained from the throat, rectum, axilla, and groin. Thirteen of the 16 cultures from the patients with KD were positive for bacteria-producing toxins, whereas only one of the 15 control cultures was positive. Breakdown of the isolates is listed in the figure. These data suggest that KD may be caused by a superantigen. (*Adapted from* Leung *et al.* [5].)

THERAPY AND LONG-TERM FOLLOW-UP

Recommended therapy during the acute stage of Kawasaki disease

IVGG
(2 g/kg as single infusion over 12 hr [preferred])
or
(400 mg/kg/d for 4 days; each dose infused over 2 hr [alternate])
plus
Aspirin
(80–100 mg/kg/d orally in four equally divided doses until
    patient is afebrile [some clinicians recommend high-dose
    aspirin until the 14th day of illness])
    then
(3–5 mg/kg orally once daily up to 6–8 wk)

IVGG—intravenous gammaglobulin.

FIGURE 2-28 Recommended therapy during the acute stage of Kawasaki disease. In the absence of an etiologic agent, initial therapy for Kawasaki disease is currently targeted toward reducing inflammation of the myocardium and coronary artery walls and reducing fever. Intravenous gammaglobulin (IVGG) given in addition to aspirin has been shown to be superior to aspirin alone in reducing inflammation and preventing the development of coronary artery aneurysms [18–20], especially giant aneurysms [21]. Some patients come to the physician within 10 days of the onset of illness but already have coronary artery ectasia or aneurysms. These patients should receive the above aspirin and IVGG regimen, although current data are lacking on the long-term benefits of such therapy. Aspirin is reduced to a lower dose after the febrile period. This is done for its antithrombotic effect. It should be discontinued 6 to 8 weeks after the onset of illness if no coronary arterial abnormalities are present by echocardiography. Aspirin is continued indefinitely if there are coronary arterial abnormalities. (*From* Dajani *et al.* [8].)

Risk levels used in stratification

Risk level	Criteria
I	Patients with no coronary artery changes demonstrated by echocardiography at any stage of illness
II	Patients with transient coronary ectasia on echocardiography, which disappears during the acute illness
III	Patients with a small to medium solitary coronary aneurysm demonstrated by echocardiography or angiography
IV	Patients with one or more giant coronary artery aneurysms or multiple small to medium aneurysms, without obstruction on echocardiography, preferably confirmed by coronary angiography
V	Patients with coronary artery obstruction confirmed by angiography

FIGURE 2-29 Clinical experience allows patients with Kawasaki disease to be stratified into risk levels based on their relative risk of myocardial ischemia. The risk level for a patient can change over time when there is a change in coronary artery morphology. A patient could move to a lower risk level (with regression of aneurysms) or to a higher risk level (with development of thrombosis or stenosis).

Recommendations for risk level I

Pharmacologic therapy: None beyond initial 6–8 wk

Physical activity: No restrictions beyond initial 6–8 wk

Follow-up and diagnostic testing: None beyond 1st yr unless evidence of cardiac disease suspected

Invasive testing: None recommended

FIGURE 2-30 Recommendations for risk level I. These patients have no demonstrated coronary artery changes at any stage of their illness. Pharmacologic therapy during the initial 6 to 8 weeks is listed in Fig 2-28. Three recent studies have indicated abnormal convalescent serum lipid profiles in some children after the febrile stage of Kawasaki disease; these abnormalities usually returned to normal by a year after the onset of the disease [22–24]. Counseling of these patients and their parents should adhere to the standard dietary recommendations for children and adolescents [25], and the physician may choose to remeasure the lipids a year later. All patients in this risk level should be directed to follow the usual practice of well-child care.

Recommendations for risk level II

Pharmacologic therapy: None beyond initial 6–8 wk

Physical activity: No restrictions beyond initial 6–8 wk

Follow-up and diagnostic testing: None beyond 1st yr
unless evidence of cardiac disease suspected; physician
may choose to see patients at 3- to 5-yr intervals

Invasive testing: None recommended

FIGURE 2-31 Recommendations for risk level II. These patients demonstrate transient coronary ectasia on echocardiography, which disappears during the acute illness. Pharmacologic therapy during the initial 6 to 8 weeks is listed in Fig. 2-28. Because long-term natural history data are not available, some pediatric cardiologists choose to see these patients at 3- to 5-year intervals to monitor their cardiovascular status. For comments on lipid profiles and routine follow-up care, *see* Fig. 2-30.

Recommendations for risk level III

Pharmacologic therapy: Aspirin (3–5 mg/kg/d) at least until
abnormalities resolve

Physical activity: In 1st decade of life, no restriction beyond
initial 6–8 wk; in 2nd decade, physical activity guided
by stress testing every other year; competitive contact
athletics with endurance training discouraged

Follow-up and diagnostic testing: Annual follow-up with
echocardiogram ± electrocardiogram in 1st decade of life

Invasive testing: Angiography, if stress testing or echocardiogram suggests stenosis

FIGURE 2-32 Recommendations for risk level III. These patients demonstrate a small- to medium-sized solitary coronary artery aneurysm on echocardiography. Antithrombotic doses of aspirin are recommended while coronary artery abnormalities are present. If a patient is exposed to varicella or influenza, the risk of Reye's syndrome increases and aspirin should be discontinued temporarily. Alternate therapy is dipyridamole (2 to 3 mg/kg two or three times a day) for approximately 2 weeks. Administration of influenza vaccine is recommended in these patients on long-term aspirin therapy.

Recommendations for risk level IV

Pharmacologic therapy: Long-term aspirin (3–5 mg/kg/d) ± warfarin sodium

Physical activity: In 1st decade of life, no restriction beyond initial 6–8 wk; in 2nd
decade, annual stress testing guides recommendations; strenuous athletics strongly
discouraged; if stress test rules out ischemia, noncontact recreational sports allowed

Follow-up and diagnostic testing: Annual follow-up with echocardiogram ± ECG ±
chest radiography ± additional ECG at 6-month intervals; in 1st decade of life,
consider pharmacologic stress testing; annual stress testing in patients over age
10 yr should include evaluation of myocardial perfusion

Invasive testing: Angiography, if stress testing or echocardiogram suggests stenosis;
elective catheterization in the absence of noninvasive evidence of myocardial
ischemia may be useful to conclusively rule out subclinical major coronary artery
obstructions in certain situations, such as when a patient has atypical chest pain,
ability to perform dynamic stress testing is limited by age, or unique activity restrictions or insurability recommendations are needed

ECG—electrocardiogram.

FIGURE 2-33 Recommendations for risk level IV. These patients demonstrate one or more giant coronary artery aneurysms, or multiple small to medium aneurysms, without obstruction by echocardiography, preferably confirmed by angiography. If warfarin is used as an adjunct to aspirin therapy, an International Normalized Ratio of 2.0 to 3.0 should be maintained. If a patient is exposed to varicella or influenza, the risk of Reye's syndrome increases and aspirin should be discontinued temporarily. Alternate therapy is dipyridamole (2 to 3 mg/kg two or three times a day) for approximately 2 weeks. Administration of influenza vaccine is recommended in these patients on long-term aspirin therapy.

Recommendations for risk level V

Pharmacologic therapy: Long-term aspirin (3–5 mg/kg/d) ± warfarin sodium; calcium channel blockers should be considered to reduce myocardial oxygen consumption

Physical activity: Contact sports, isometrics, and weight training should be avoided; other recommendations for noncompetitive, noncontact low to moderate physical activity is guided by outcome of stress testing or myocardial perfusion scan

Follow-up and diagnostic testing: Echocardiogram + electrocardiogram at 6-month intervals and annual Holter monitor test + annual stress testing with evaluation of myocardial perfusion; in younger patients or patients not able to perform dynamic exercise, pharmacologic stress testing with myocardial perfusion can be done

Invasive testing: Cardiac catheterization with selective angiography recommended to aid therapeutic options and identify extent of collateral perfusion; repeat angiography with new-onset or worsening ischemia suggested by noninvasive diagnostic testing or clinical presentation

FIGURE 2-34 Recommendations for risk level V. These patients demonstrate coronary artery obstruction confirmed by angiography. If warfarin is used as an adjunct to aspirin therapy, an International Normalized Ratio of 2.0 to 3.0 should be maintained. If a patient is exposed to varicella or influenza, the risk of Reye's syndrome increases and aspirin should be discontinued temporarily. Alternate therapy is dipyridamole (2 to 3 mg/kg two or three times a day) for approximately 2 weeks. Administration of influenza vaccine is recommended in these patients on long-term aspirin therapy. Therapeutic options for patients with severe coronary artery obstruction include coronary artery bypass graft surgery and percutaneous transluminal coronary angioplasty, although data on the use of angioplasty are limited and have not shown consistent improvement. Some patients may experience an acute myocardial infarction, and rapid thrombolytic therapy is indicated.

Fate of myocardial infarction in KD

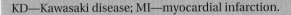

In a retrospective study of 195 patients with MI:

142 of 195 had the MI within 1 yr after KD onset
77 of 142 had the MI within 3 mo after KD onset
Mortality rate for first MI was 22% (43 deaths)
Of the 152 survivors of the first MI: 24 had a second MI (16%); mortality was 63% (15 deaths)
Of the 9 survivors (from 24 victims) of the second MI: 6 had a third MI, and only 1 survived

KD—Kawasaki disease; MI—myocardial infarction.

FIGURE 2-35 Fate of myocardial infarction in Kawasaki disease (KD). Kato and coworkers [26] conducted a nationwide survey in Japan in the mid-1980s. Data were collected on 195 patients with myocardial infarction due to KD. Seventy-three percent had the infarction within 1 year of the diagnosis of KD, with about half of these first-year infarctions occurring within the first 3 months of KD diagnosis. Data from this study and other reports indicate that most patients do not have a history of chest pain prior to the myocardial infarction. In Kato *et al.*'s study, only 3 (1.5%) patients had a history of chest pain. (*Adapted from* Kato *et al.* [26].)

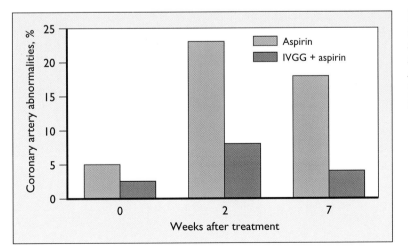

FIGURE 2-36 Prevalence of coronary artery abnormalities as detected by echocardiography in 84 children who received aspirin alone, 100 mg/kg/d for 14 days, and 84 children who received aspirin with intravenous gammaglobulin (IVGG), 400 mg/kg/d for 4 days. The differences between the two groups were significant ($P=0.01$ at 2 weeks and $P=0.005$ at 7 weeks). (*Adapted from* Newburger *et al.* [18].)

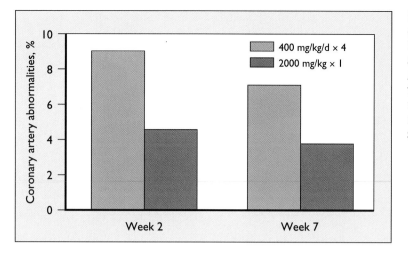

FIGURE 2-37 Prevalence of coronary artery abnormalities as detected by echocardiography in 263 patients who received intravenous gammaglobulin (IVGG), 400 mg/kg/d for 4 days, and 260 patients who received IVGG, 2000 mg/kg infused once. At 2 weeks, differences were significant ($P=0.045$). At 7 weeks, there were fewer coronary artery abnormalities in patients who received the 2000-mg/kg dose than in those who received 400 mg/kg/d for 4 days. However, the differences were not statistically significant ($P=0.099$). (*Adapted from* Newburger *et al.* [19].)

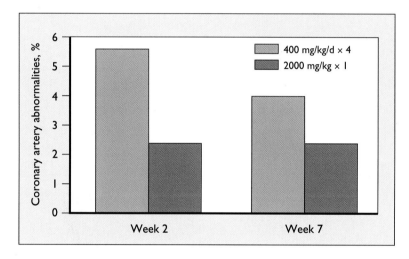

FIGURE 2-38 Prevalence of coronary artery abnormalities as detected by echocardiography in 252 patients who received intravenous gammaglobulin (IVGG), 400 mg/kg/d for 4 days, and 254 patients who received IVGG, 2000 mg/kg infused once. Data shown here are identical to that in Fig. 2-37 except that patients with coronary artery abnormalities on enrollment were excluded from analysis. Although there was a trend for less frequent coronary artery abnormalities in patients who received IVGG at 2000 mg/kg/d, the differences were not statistically significant ($P=0.067$ at 2 weeks and $P=0.307$ at 7 weeks). (*Adapted from* Newburger *et al.* [19].)

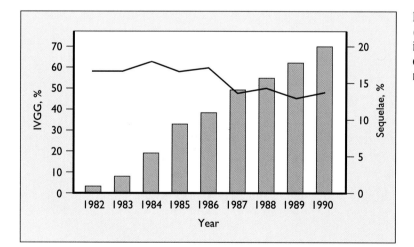

FIGURE 2-39 Yearly proportions of cases with cardiac sequelae (*line*) and cases that received intravenous gammaglobulin (IVGG) in Japan. Although there has been a substantial increase in the use of IVGG, the decrease in frequency of cardiac abnormalities is only modest. (*Adapted from* Yanagawa [27].)

REFERENCES

1. Taubert KA, Rowley AH, Shulman ST: Seven-year national survey of Kawasaki disease and acute rheumatic fever. *Pediatr Infect Dis J* 1994, 13:704–708.

2. Kawasaki T: Acute febrile mucocutaneous syndrome with lymphoid involvement with specific desquamation of the fingers and toes in children (in Japanese). *Jpn J Allergy* 1967, 16:178–222.

3. Yanagawa H, Yashiro M, Nakamura Y, *et al.*: Epidemiologic pictures of Kawasaki disease in Japan: From the nationwide incidence survey in 1991 and 1992. *Pediatrics* 1995, 95:475–479.

4. Taubert KA: Epidemiology of Kawasaki disease in the United States and worldwide. *Prog Pediatr Cardiol* 1997, 6:181–185.

5. Leung DYM, Meissner HC, Fulton DR, *et al.*: Toxic shock syndrome toxin-secreting *Staphylococcus aureus* in Kawasaki syndrome. *Lancet* 1993, 342:1385–1388.

6. Japan Kawasaki Disease Research Committee: *Diagnostic Guidelines of Kawasaki Disease*. Tokyo: Japan Kawasaki Disease Research Committee; 1984.

7. Dajani AS, Bisno AL, Chung KJ, *et al.* for the Committee on Rheumatic Fever, Endocarditis, and Kawasaki Disease: *Diagnostic Guidelines for Kawasaki Disease*. Dallas, TX: American Heart Association; 1989.

8. Dajani AS, Taubert KA, Gerber MA, *et al.*: Diagnosis and therapy of Kawasaki disease in children. *Circulation* 1993, 87:1776–1780.

9. Dajani AS, Taubert KA, Takahashi M, *et al.*: Guidelines for long-term management of patients with Kawasaki disease. *Circulation* 1994, 89:918–922.

10. Rauch AM: Kawasaki syndrome: Critical review of U.S. epidemiology. In *Kawasaki Disease*. Edited by Shulman ST. New York: Alan R. Liss, Inc; 1987; 33–44.

11. Shulman ST: A commentary on disease mechanism. In *Proceedings of the Fourth International Symposium on Kawasaki Disease*. Edited by Takahashi M, Taubert K. Dallas, TX: American Heart Association; 1993:223–225.

12. Becker AE: Kawasaki disease: Reflections on pathological observations. In *Proceedings of the Fourth International Symposium on Kawasaki Disease*. Edited by Takahashi M, Taubert K. Dallas, TX: American Heart Association; 1993:226–230.

13. Kabani A, Joffe A, Jadavji T: Recognition of atypical Kawasaki disease. In *Proceedings of the Fourth International Symposium on Kawasaki Disease*. Edited by Takahashi M, Taubert K. Dallas, TX: American Heart Association; 1993:42–47.

14. Arjunan K, Daniels SR, Meyer RA, *et al.*: Coronary artery caliber in normal children and patients with Kawasaki disease but without aneurysms: An echocardiographic and angiocardiographic study. *J Am Coll Cardiol* 1986, 8:1119–1124.

15. Lima M, Kaku S, Macedo A, *et al.*: Echocardiographic diagnosis and surgical treatment of giant coronary arterial aneurysms. In *Proceedings of the Fourth International Symposium on Kawasaki Disease*. Edited by Takahashi M, Taubert K. Dallas, TX: American Heart Association; 1993:404–407.

16. Takahashi M, Schieber RA, Wishner SH, *et al.*: Selective coronary arteriography in infants and children. *Circulation* 1983, 68:1021–1028.

17. Tomita S, Chung K, Mas M, *et al.*: Peripheral gangrene associated with Kawasaki disease. In *Proceedings of the Fourth International Symposium on Kawasaki Disease*. Edited by Takahashi M, Taubert K. Dallas, TX: American Heart Association; 1993:27–31.

18. Newburger JW, Takahashi M, Burns JC, *et al.*: The treatment of Kawasaki syndrome with intravenous gammaglobulin. *N Engl J Med* 1986, 315:341–347.

19. Newburger JW, Takahashi M, Beiser AS, *et al.*: A single infusion of intravenous gammaglobulin compared to four daily doses in the treatment of acute Kawasaki syndrome. *N Engl J Med* 1991, 324:1633–1639.

20. Furusho K, Kamiya T, Kaano H, *et al.*: High-dose intravenous gammaglobulin for Kawasaki disease. *Lancet* 1984, 2:1055–1058.

21. Rowley AH, Duffy CE, Shulman ST: Prevention of giant coronary artery aneurysms in Kawasaki disease by intravenous gammaglobulin therapy. *J Pediatr* 1988, 113:290–294.

22. Newburger JW, Burns JC, Beiser AS, Loscalzo J: Altered lipid profile after Kawasaki syndrome. *Circulation* 1991, 84:625–631.

23. Inoue O, Sugimura T, Kato H: Long-term lipid profiles in patients with Kawasaki disease. In *Proceedings of the Fourth International Symposium on Kawasaki Disease*. Edited by Takahashi M, Taubert K. Dallas, TX: American Heart Association; 1993:305–309.

24. Salo EPI, Pesonen EJ, Viikari JSA: Serum cholesterol during and after Kawasaki disease. *J Pediatr* 1991, 119:557–561.

25. National Cholesterol Education Program: *Report of the Expert Panel on Blood Cholesterol Levels in Children and Adolescents*. Bethesda, MD: National Heart, Lung, and Blood Institute; 1991. (NIH publication #91-2732, 1991.)

26. Kato H, Ichinose E, Kawasaki T: Myocardial infarction in Kawasaki disease: Clinical analyses in 195 cases. *J Pediatr* 1986, 108:923–927.

27. Yanagawa H: Epidemiological pictures of Kawasaki disease in Japan. In *Proceedings of the Fourth International Symposium on Kawasaki Disease*. Edited by Takahashi M, Taubert K. Dallas, TX: American Heart Association; 1993:1–5.

SELECTED BIBLIOGRAPHY

Dajani AS, Taubert KA, Gerber MA, *et al.*: Diagnosis and therapy of Kawasaki disease in children. *Circulation* 1993, 87:1776–1780.

Dajani AS, Taubert KA, Takahashi M, *et al.*: Guidelines for long-term management of patients with Kawasaki disease. *Circulation* 1994, 89:918–922.

Kawasaki T: Acute febrile mucocutaneous syndrome with lymphoid involvement with specific desquamation of the fingers and toes in children (in Japanese). *Jpn J Allergy* 1967, 16:178–222.

Newburger JW, Takahashi M, Beiser AS, *et al.*: A single infusion of intravenous gammaglobulin compared to four daily doses in the treatment of acute Kawasaki syndrome. *N Engl J Med* 1991, 324:1633–1639.

CHAPTER 3

Pathology: Anatomy and Predisposing Cardiac Lesions

Cathal O'Sullivan
C. Glenn Cobbs

THE PURPOSE OF THIS CHAPTER is to illustrate the characteristics of infectious endocarditis using figures and text. This condition continues to intrigue both physicians and surgeons. Before the introduction of antimicrobial chemotherapy it was almost universally fatal. Today, successful management requires detailed knowledge of microbiology, antimicrobial therapy, cardiac pathophysiology, and cardiovascular surgery. Introduction of the echocardiogram has greatly facilitated precise identification of gross cardiac pathology.

There has been a striking change in the epidemiology of infectious endocarditis in developed countries.

Reduction in rheumatic fever incidence has markedly decreased the number of patients with rheumatic valvular disease. Congenital and acquired valvular lesions now comprise the primary underlying disorders in developed countries. Prosthetic valve endocarditis is an especially important topic.

We also attempt to illustrate current thoughts regarding the pathogenesis of infectious endocarditis, and some examples of animal model data are included. We have included several illustrations that describe important cardiac abnormalities. Finally, we address briefly cardiac infections in immunocompromised patients.

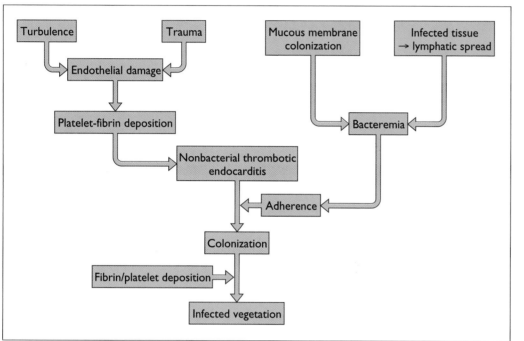

FIGURE 3-1 A proposed pathogenesis of infective endocarditis (IE). Much of the data on pathogenesis of IE has been derived from catheter-induced valvular trauma in rabbits and rodents; however, its precise relevance to the pathogenesis of IE in humans is debatable.

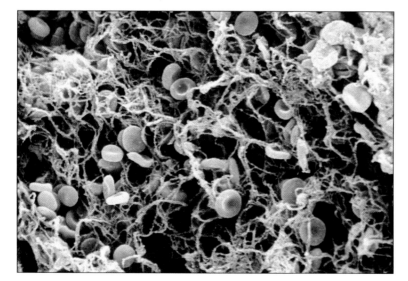

FIGURE 3-2 Scanning electron micrograph of fibrin/platelet collection (nonbacterial thrombotic endocarditis) on rabbit cardiac valve (lesion induced by catheter). Numerous red cells are visible among the network of fibrin and platelets.

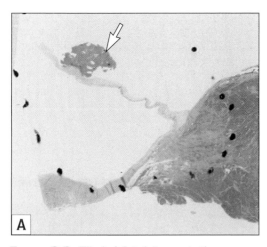

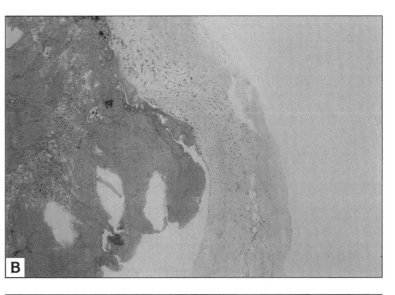

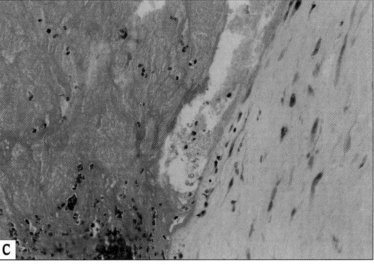

FIGURE 3-3 Fibrin/platelet vegetation.
A, Low-power view of sterile fibrin/platelet vegetation (*arrow*) on the ventricular aspect of the aortic valve leaflet. The patient had marantic endocarditis secondary to mucin-producing adenocarcinoma of the breast. **B** and **C**, Higher-power microscopic views of fibrin/platelet vegetation. The deeply staining tissue is the fibrin/platelet thrombus, whereas the valvular fibroelastic tissue stains pale. Inflammatory cells are rare. Some red cells are evident. There is relatively little evidence of organization of the thrombus suggesting recent occurrence. The patient had numerous cerebral, splenic, and renal infarcts secondary to emboli.

Clinical conditions associated with nonbacterial thrombotic endocarditis

Malignancy: adenocarcinoma of pancreas, lung, stomach, etc
Connective tissue diseases, *eg*, polyarteritis nodosa
Intracardiac catheters
Endocardial trauma of any cause

FIGURE 3-4 Clinical conditions associated with the development of sterile vegetations or nonbacterial thrombotic endocarditis. The term *marantic endocarditis* is associated with malignancy and wasting conditions. The vegetations of marantic endocarditis are sterile and are not associated with destruction of the underlying valve. Portions of marantic vegetations may embolize. These embolic phenomena may be the first sign of an underlying malignancy. In contrast, the sterile vegetations seen in patients with lupus erythematosus do not embolize. These vegetations may be widely disseminated on the endocardium, including nonvalvular sites.

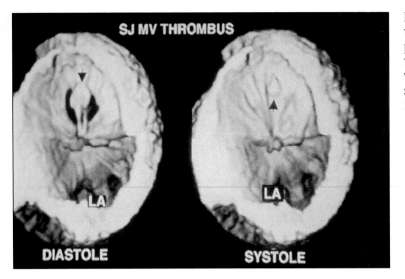

FIGURE 3-5 Three-dimensional echocardiographic image of thrombus (*arrowheads*) involving a St. Jude mitral valve (SJMV) prosthesis in both the open and closed positions. The high resolution of this recently developed digital imaging technique is noteworthy. Computer software reconstructs digitized two-dimensional transesophageal images into a three-dimensional image. LA—left atrium. (*From* Nanda *et al.* [1]; with permission.)

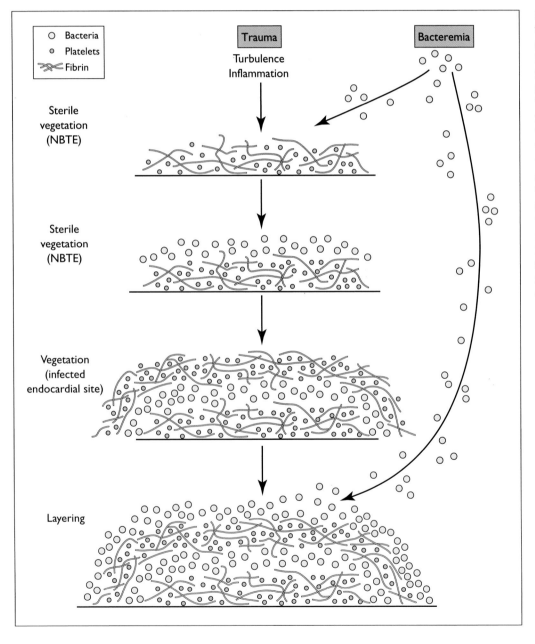

FIGURE 3-6 Pathogenesis of an infected vegetation. Damage to the endothelial surface of the valve exposes collagen, leading to the deposition of platelets and fibrin. In the event of bacteremia, this sterile thrombus may become infected. The bacteremia may result from extension from tissue sites via the lymphatics or through direct capillary inoculation, as in the case of dental/genitourinary manipulation. The seeding of the thrombus with organisms complexed with antibody triggers the further deposition of fibrin and platelets. In this way a "layering" of the vegetation occurs. The bacteremia of infective endocarditis is continuous, the result of the persistent embolization of small fragments of the vegetation as shown. (NBTE—nonbacterial thrombotic endocarditis.)

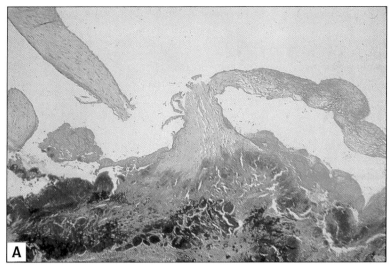

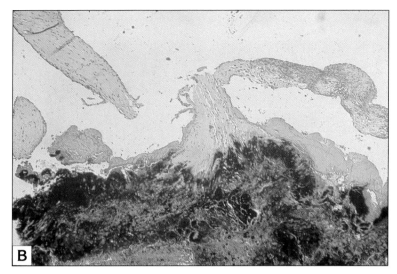

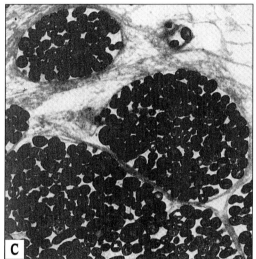

FIGURE 3-7 Microscopic views of infected vegetations. **A,** Light microscopic view of a vegetation stained by hematoxylin-eosin. **B,** Light microscopic view of the same vegetation stained by tissue Gram stain demonstrates gram-positive organisms in the dense dark staining layer. **C,** Electron micrograph of experimentally induced rabbit vegetation. The layering of fibrin around colonies of *Streptococcus sanguis* is apparent. The layers of fibrin serve to protect the nidus of infection from the host's immune response. (Panel 7C *from* Durack [2]; with permission.)

HEMODYNAMIC FACTORS

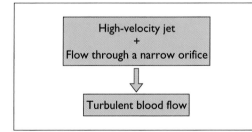

FIGURE 3-8 Hemodynamic factors associated with nonbacterial thrombotic endocarditis. Turbulent blood flow is the major factor causing endocardial damage and platelet/fibrin deposition (nonbacterial thrombotic endocarditis). This event occurs when a high-velocity jet stream together with flow through a narrow orifice produces a significant pressure gradient. It is believed that the turbulent flow denudes the involved endothelium, exposing collagen fibers and resulting in platelet/fibrin deposition.

Intracardiac location of vegetations

Cardiac valve affected	Patients with endocarditis, %	Normal resting pressure on closed valve, *mm Hg*
Mitral	86.0	116
Aortic	55.0	72
Tricuspid	19.6	24
Pulmonic	1.1	5

FIGURE 3-9 Correlation of intracardiac location of vegetations with resting pressure of cardiac valves. This correlation probably reflects the occurrence of turbulent blood flow rather than the actual pressure exerted on the valve, as surmised by Lepeschkin [3]. (*Adapted from* Lepeschkin [3].)

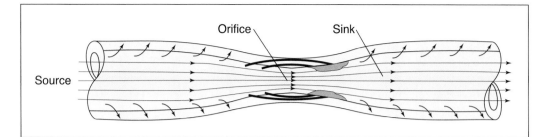

FIGURE 3-10 In vitro model of turbulent cardiac blood flow. A Venturi effect is produced when blood flows from a high-pressure source through a narrow orifice into a low-pressure sink. Rodbard [4] injected nebulized suspensions of *Serratia marcescens* into an airstream passing through Venturi-shaped agar tubes. He showed that maximal position occurred immediately beyond the orifice. Pathologic findings in patients with endocarditis revealed a similar distribution, *ie*, the major site of deposition was in the region just beyond the orifice (*eg*, ventricular surface of aortic valve leaflets in aortic valve endocarditis). This area represents the area of lowest lateral pressure. Rodbard surmised that the intima in this region would be "despoiled of its oxygen and nutrients and surcharged with accumulated metabolic end products." Although it is unlikely that ischemia is the dominant factor in the distribution of sterile vegetations, it does appear that this area is the most frequently affected. Reductions in the high-pressure system (*eg*, congestive cardiac failure) or increases in the orifice size (*eg*, large ventricular septal defects) result in a reduction in the degree of turbulence. Patients with these disorders are less likely to develop infective endocarditis. (*Adapted from* Rodbard [4].)

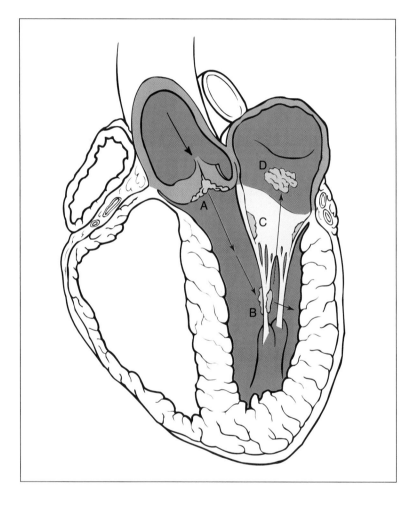

FIGURE 3-11 Distribution of sterile vegetations. The sites of sterile vegetations are shown as they relate to hemodynamic factors, as first outlined by Rodbard [4]. The *arrows* illustrate the direction of the abnormal blood flow in aortic incompetence (*left*) and mitral regurgitation (*right*). *A* denotes the ventricular surface of the aortic valve; *B*, a vegetation on the chordae tendineae of the aortic leaf of the mitral valve; *C*, the atrial surface of the mitral valve; and *D*, the atrial endocardium (MacCallum's patch). Although not shown, the distribution of vegetations in tricuspid insufficiency, ventricular septal defect, patent ductus arteriosus, and arteriovenous fistulae follow the same principles. (*Adapted from* Rodbard [4].)

Distribution of vegetations in infective endocarditis

Condition	High-pressure source	Orifice	Low-pressure sink	Location of vegetation	Satellite lesions
Aortic insufficiency	Aorta	Incompetent valve	Left ventricle	Ventricular surface of aortic valve	Mitral chordae
Mitral regurgitation	Left ventricle	Incompetent mitral valve	Left atrium	Atrial surface of mitral valve	Atrium
Tricuspid regurgitation	Right ventricle	Incompetent tricuspid valve	Right atrium	Atrial surface of tricuspid valve	—
Ventricular septal defect	Left ventricle	Septal defect	Right ventricle	Right ventricular surface of defect	Pulmonary artery
Coarctation of aorta	Central aorta	Coarctation	Distal aorta	Downstream aortic wall	—

FIGURE 3-12 Distribution of vegetations in infective endocarditis. Frequently patients have more than one isolated cardiac lesion resulting in multiple vegetations. (*Adapted from* Rodbard [4].)

MICROBIAL CHARACTERISTICS IN INFECTIVE ENDOCARDITIS

A. In vitro adhesion of selected bacteria to canine aortic valve leaflets

Organism (strains, *n*)	Adherence ratio $\times 10^{5*}$
Enterococci (3)	1300–1750
Viridans streptococci (3)	350–700
Staphylococcus aureus (1)	530–580
Staphylococcus epidermidis (2)	450
Pseudomonas aeruginosa (2)	300–380
Escherichia coli (2)	2
Klebsiella pneumoniae (2)	4.5

*Adherence ratio = $\dfrac{\text{colony-forming units adherent bacteria}}{\text{colony-forming units inoculum}}$

FIGURE 3-13 A, In vitro adhesion of selected bacteria to canine aortic valve leaflets. This investigation revealed that adhesion rates were characteristic of bacterial species. The observed epidemiology of infective endocarditis, *ie*, the predominance of gram-positive organisms as causative agents, was supported by this study, which demonstrated that bacterial adherence to cardiac valve surfaces is species specific [5]. **B,** Microbial isolates in patients with native valve infective endocarditis. The predominant streptococcal species isolated are members of the viridans group. The percentage of cases classified as culture-negative endocarditis has decreased with the introduction of more-sensitive blood culture techniques. (Panel 13A *adapted from* Gould *et al.* [5]; panel 13B *from* Korzeniowski and Kaye [6]; with permission.)

B. Microbial isolates in patients with native valve infective endocarditis

	Children, %		Adults, %			
	Neonates	Older children	Age <65 y	Age >65 y	Pregnant patients	IVDAs
Streptococci	20	40–50	50–70	30	60	6–12
Enterococci	—	4	10	15	6	8
Staphylococci	60	30	25	45	18	60
Staphylococcus aureus	(80)	(80)	(90)	(65)	(90)	(99)
Coagulase-negative	(20)	(20)	(10)	(35)	(10)	(1)
Gram-negative bacilli	10	5	<1	5	2	10
Fungal	10	1	<1	—	—	5
Polymicrobial	4	—	—	4	—	5
Culture negative	4	0–15	5–10	5	4	4–10

IVDAs—intravenous drug abusers.

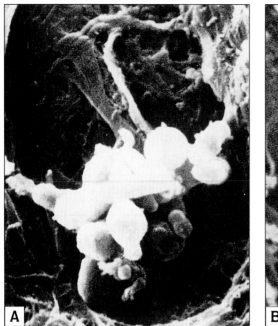
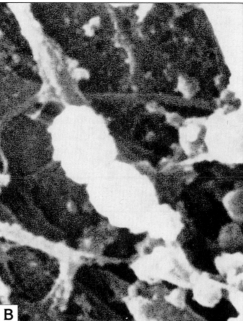

FIGURE 3-14 A and **B**, Scanning electron micrographs of experimental rabbit endocarditis with two species of viridans streptococci. *Panel 14A* shows the production of glycocalyx (also called *dextran*, *exopolysaccharide*, or *slime*); whereas panel 14B does not. This material is believed to act by blocking host defenses and impairing antimicrobial activity, thereby allowing the bacteria to persist. Glycocalyx also plays a role in adhesion of the organism to sterile vegetations and foreign bodies such as prosthetic valves and intravenous catheters. (*From* Mills *et al.* [7]; with permission.)

Microbial virulence factors implicated in the pathogenesis of infective endocarditis	
Factor	**Microorganism**
Adhesion	
Glycocalyx (*eg*, dextran, exopolysaccharide)	Streptococci
	Staphylococci, yeast
Laminin-binding proteins	Streptococci
Fibronectin-binding ligand	*Staphylococcus aureus*
	Streptococcus pneumoniae
	Candida albicans
Platelet-binding potential, class I	—
antigen—adh$^+$ phenotype	
Platelet aggregation	
Class II antigen—agg$^+$ phenotype	Staphylococci
	Streptococci
Platelet microbicidal proteins or	
thrombodefensins	
Resistance to their cidal action	Staphylococci
Tissue factor induction	
Increased production → thrombus formation	*S. aureus*
	Enterococcus spp

FIGURE 3-15 Some proposed microbial virulence factors implicated in the pathogenesis of infective endocarditis. These data are predominantly derived from animal studies using genetically altered bacterial mutants. The relative role played by each of these microbial factors (and presumably others as yet unidentified) in the causation of infective endocarditis in a given patient remains uncertain. Therefore, care must be taken in extrapolating the data to humans.

PREDISPOSING VALVULAR LESIONS

Incidence of infective endocarditis in patients with selected cardiac malformations

Cardiac abnormality	Endocarditis, %	Incidence per 1000 patient years, *n*
Tetralogy of Fallot	—	18.0
Ventricular septal defect		
Simple	—	1.0–1.8
With aortic regurgitation	12	23.0
Patent ductus arteriosus	20	3.3
Pulmonary stenosis	—	0.2
Aortic stenosis		
Valvular	10–15	1.8–2.0
Subaortic, hypertrophic	5	—
Coarctation of aorta	20–25	4.0
Coronary artery fistula	10	—

FIGURE 3-16 Incidence of infective endocarditis in patients with selected cardiac malformations. The underlying congenital heart defects among children with infective endocarditis are shown. The relative risk of developing infective endocarditis for each lesion also is presented. The likelihood that a particular lesion becomes infected is related to the degree of turbulence produced. Technical advances in terms of more aggressive management of cyanotic heart disease have led to a relative decrease in the number of children with cyanotic congenital heart disease and a concomitant decline in the incidence of endocarditis in patients with left-to-right shunts such as ventricular septal defects and patent ductus arteriosus. (*Adapted from* Rosenthal and Nadas [8]; with permission.)

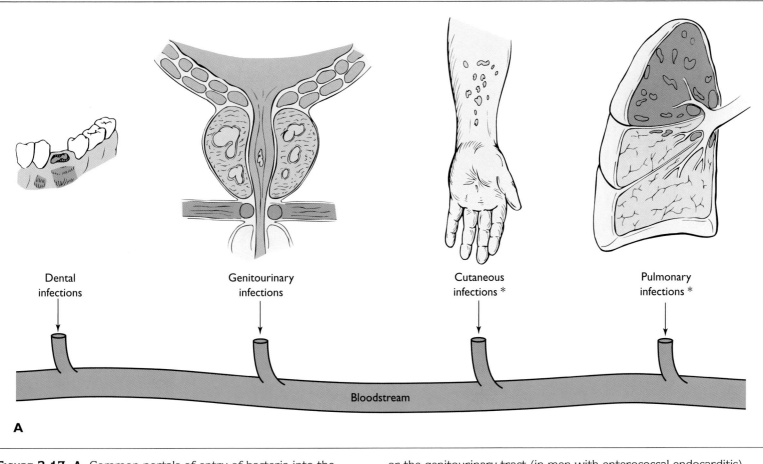

Dental infections

Genitourinary infections

Cutaneous infections *

Pulmonary infections *

Bloodstream

A

FIGURE 3-17 A, Common portals of entry of bacteria into the bloodstream. The source of bacteremia, when apparent, varies with the population studied. In most tertiary-care facilities, the source of bacteremia is the gums and teeth (in cases of viridans streptococci) or the genitourinary tract (in men with enterococcal endocarditis). In intravenous drug users, the portal of entry is the skin. *Asterisks* indicate that bloodstream invasion occurs via the lymphatic system, *ie,* indirectly. (*continued*)

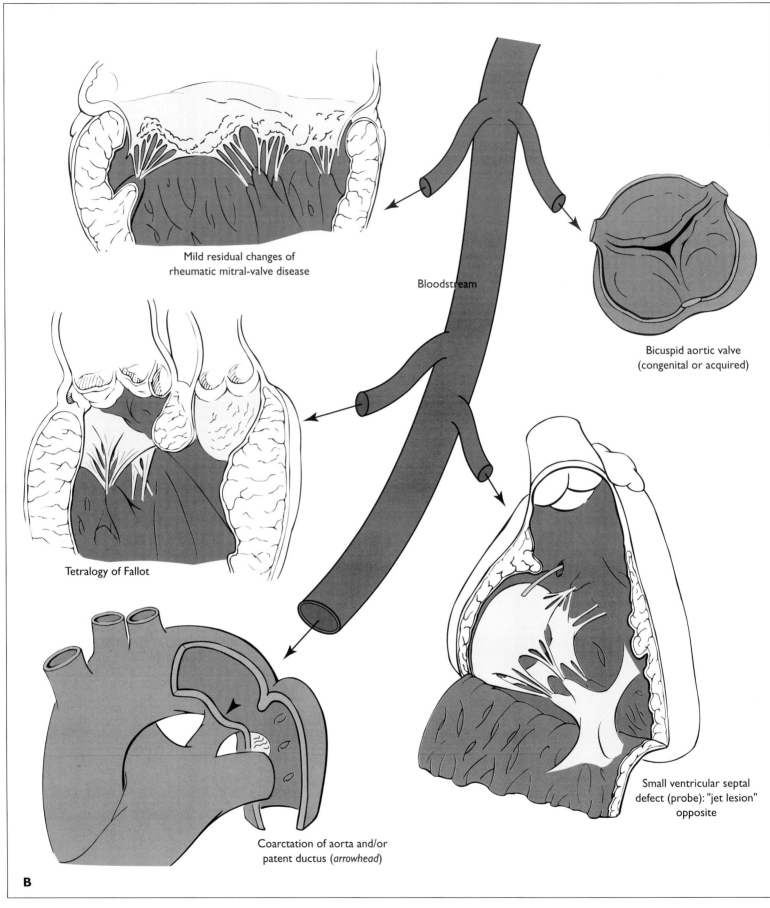

Mild residual changes of
rheumatic mitral-valve disease

Bloodstream

Bicuspid aortic valve
(congenital or acquired)

Tetralogy of Fallot

Coarctation of aorta and/or
patent ductus (*arrowhead*)

Small ventricular septal
defect (probe): "jet lesion"
opposite

B

FIGURE 3-17 (*continued*) **B,** Five different underlying cardiac abnor-malities. Tetralogy of Fallot, a cause of right-sided endocarditis, is shown. Note that the area under the pulmonary valve, *ie,* the pulmonary infundibulum (*arrowhead*), is the area susceptible to infection. Also illustrated is a small ventricular septal defect. Here, the jet lesion affects the tricuspid valve and right ventricle. (*Adapted from* Netter [9].)

Incidence of predisposing valvular lesions in adult patients with native valve endocarditis

	Age <60 y, %	Age >65 y, %	IVDAs, %
Mitral valve prolapse	20–50	10	—
Congenital heart disease	10–20	2	10
Degenerative heart disease	—	30	—
Rheumatic heart disease	25–30	8	—
None (*ie*, "normal valves")	25–50	40	90 (?)
Other*	10–15	10	—

*Includes idiopathic hypertrophic cardiomyopathy, Marfan's syndrome, etc.

IVDAs—intravenous drug abusers.

FIGURE 3-18 Incidence of predisposing valvular lesions in adult patients with native valve endocarditis. The number of patients with rheumatic heart disease continues to decline in line with the decline (with notable exceptions) in the incidence of rheumatic fever in industrialized nations, although it remains a major cause of valvular heart disease in the developing world. The variation between different studies also reflects differences in classification by different authors. (*Adapted from* Korzeniowski and Kaye [6]; with permission.)

Heart valves affected in infective endocarditis

Valve	%
Aortic	5–36
Mitral	28–45
Aortic and mitral	0–35
Tricuspid	0–6
Pulmonary	<1
Right- and left-sided	0–4

FIGURE 3-19 Heart valves affected in infective endocarditis. These figures reflect the differences among the various studies and the different populations studied. In particular, the rates quoted reflect differences in the population demographics, economic status of the population, and proportion of urban to rural cases (*eg*, the reduction in the prevalence of rheumatic heart disease and an increase in intravenous drug use alters the relative frequency of mitral and tricuspid valve endocarditis, respectively).

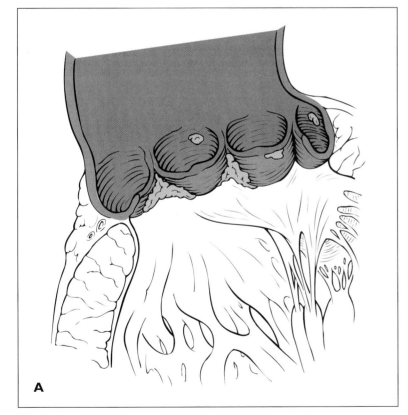

A

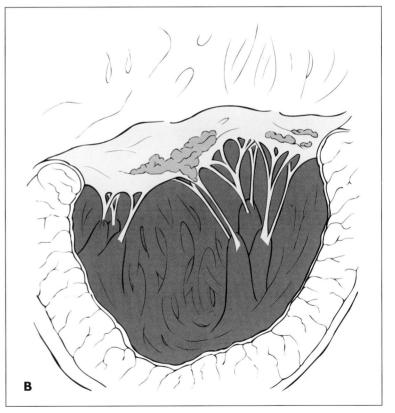

B

FIGURE 3-20 Early vegetations of bacterial endocarditis on the aortic and mitral valves. **A**, The vegetation on the aortic valve involves the area of fusion of commissures. **B**, In mitral valve endocarditis, the vegetations characteristically commence on the atrial surface of the valve, along the contact line of closure. (*Adapted from* Netter [9].)

AORTIC VALVE ENDOCARDITIS

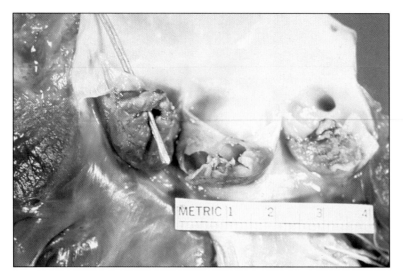

FIGURE 3-21 Pneumococcal aortic valve endocarditis. Marked tissue destruction of all three cusps and macroscopic necrosis of the left coronary cusp is shown. Although pneumococcal endocarditis was a relatively common cause of infective endocarditis in the preantibiotic era, it is now estimated that only one patient (frequently a patient suffering from alcoholism) with pneumococcal endocarditis will present to a large tertiary referral center every 2 years. When such a case does occur, however, it is a virulent infection with an acute course that may occur on previously normal valves. In this way the infection resembles *Staphylococcus aureus*, group A streptococcal, and gonococcal infective endocarditis. (*Courtesy of* W.E. Dismukes, MD.)

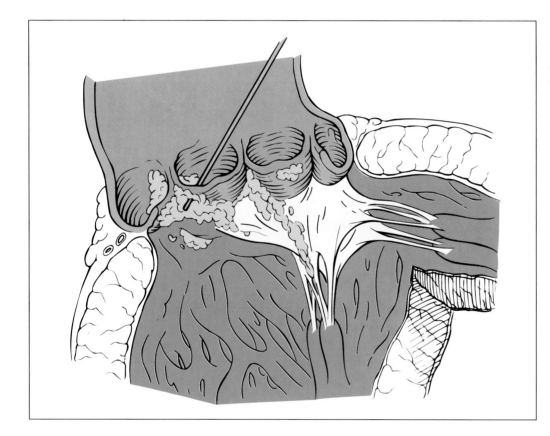

FIGURE 3-22 Advanced aortic valve endocarditis. Perforation of the noncoronary cusp is shown with resultant jet lesion on the septal wall. Clearly shown is the ease with which the advanced infection can extend from the aortic valve onto the anterior cusp of the mitral valve and chordae tendineae. (*Adapted from* Netter [9].)

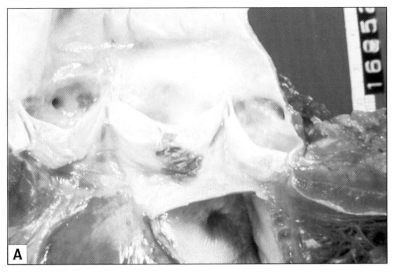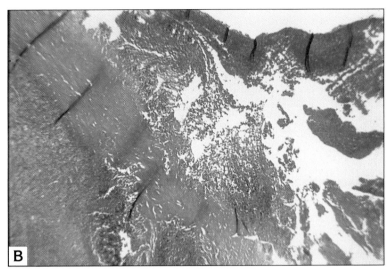

FIGURE 3-23 *Staphylococcus aureus* endocarditis. **A,** The infection involved predominantly the noncoronary cusp of the aortic valve, and the clinical course was subacute in nature. **B,** Hematoxylin- eosin stain of the excised valve shows the vegetation and a suben- docardial abscess. (*Courtesy of* W.E. Dismukes, MD.)

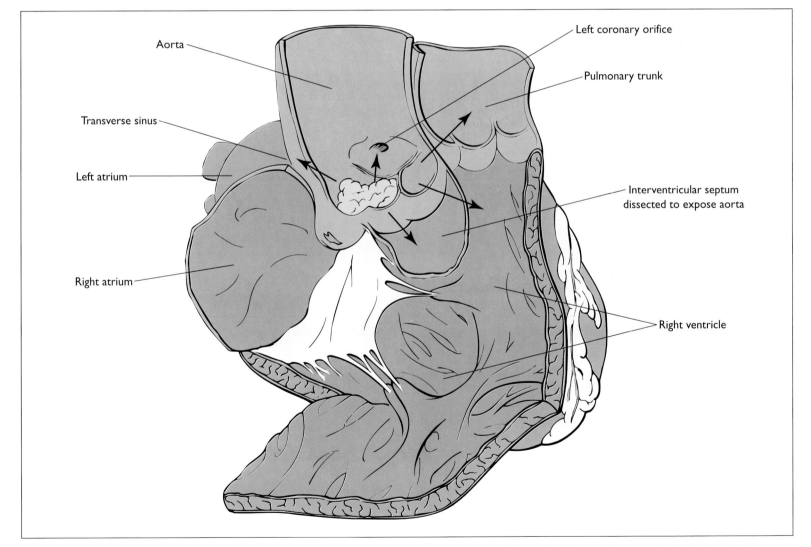

FIGURE 3-24 Advanced bacterial endocarditis of the aortic valve. The schematic shows the aortic valve/outflow tract together with a cutaway of the right side of the heart. The local complica- tions of aortic valve infective endocarditis are highlighted. The vegetation has caused a mycotic aneurysm of the posterior sinus, which is shown bulging and rupturing into the right atrium. The five *arrows* illustrate the other structures that can be involved by direct rupture or bulging of a mycotic aneurysm secondary to aortic valve endocarditis. (*Adapted from* Netter [9].)

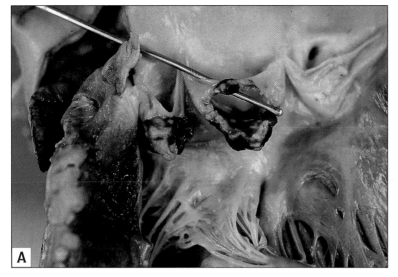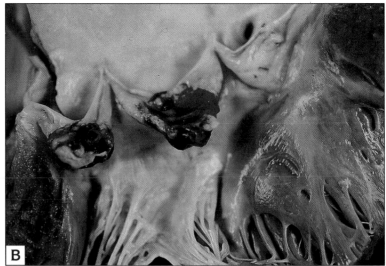

FIGURE 3-25 Aortic valve with large hemorrhagic vegetations on both the left and noncoronary cusps. **A**, The metal probe highlights the large perforation of the noncoronary cusp on removal

of the thrombus. **B**, A similar perforation was present on the left coronary cusp. Small areas of calcification can be seen in the right coronary leaflet. (*Courtesy of* W.E. Dismukes, MD.)

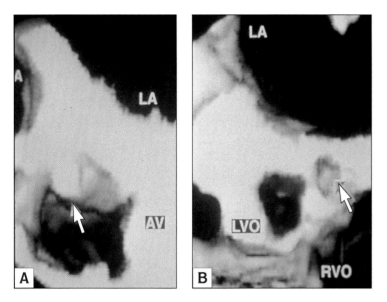

FIGURE 3-26 A and **B**, Three-dimensional echocardiograms of patient with complicated aortic valve endocarditis. A large vegetation (*panel 26A; arrow*) is visible on the aortic valve together with an abscess (*panel 26B; arrow*) involving the mitral-aortic intervalvular fibrosa. AV—aortic valve; LA—left atrium; LVO—left ventricular outflow tract; RVO—right ventricular outflow tract. (*From* Nanda *et al.* [1]; with permission.)

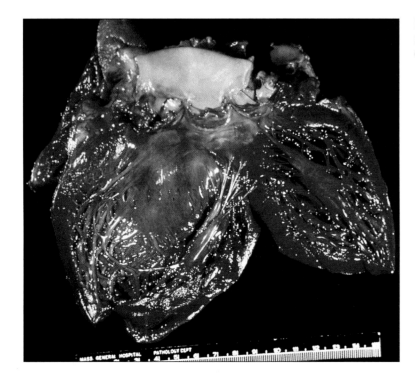

FIGURE 3-27 Aortic valve endocarditis. The fungating, hemorrhagic vegetation was caused by *Staphylococcus aureus* and has destroyed the coronary cusp. (*Courtesy of* W.E. Dismukes, MD.)

MITRAL VALVE ENDOCARDITIS

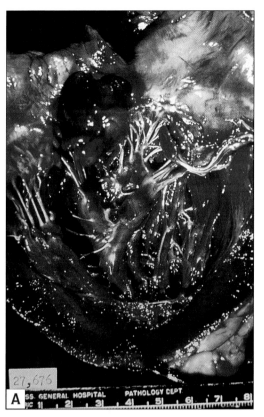

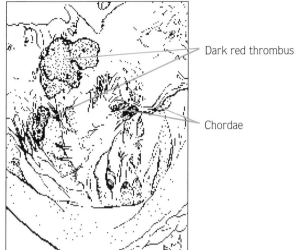

Dark red thrombus

Chordae

FIGURE 3-28 Mitral valve infective endocarditis. **A**, A large hemorrhagic vegetation
is present on the anterior leaflet of the
valve. Rupture of a number of chordae
tendineae is visible. **B**, Unlike *panel 28A*,
here the major finding at autopsy was
destruction of the underlying valve leaflet
by the vegetation. (*Courtesy of* W.E.
Dismukes, MD.)

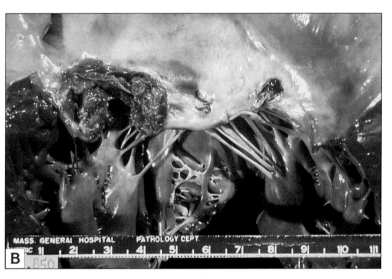

TRICUSPID VALVE ENDOCARDITIS

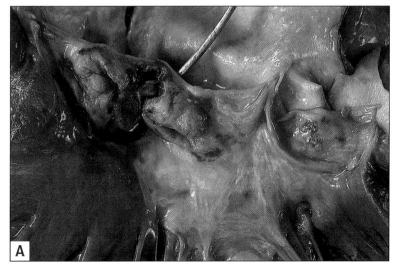

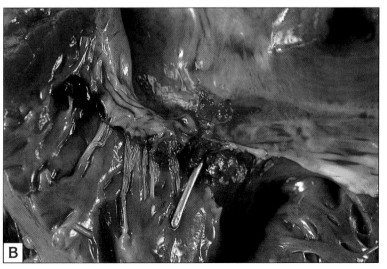

FIGURE 3-29 *Staphylococcus aureus* aortic and tricuspid valve
endocarditis in a patient with endstage renal disease. **A** and **B**, A
fistula extends from the base of the right coronary cusp (*panel
29A*) to the right ventricle just below the septal cusp of the tricuspid valve (*panel 29B*). This infection arose in an arteriovenous
shunt used for dialysis. Tricuspid valve endocarditis most
frequently occurs in intravenous drug users, and *Staphylococcus
aureus* is the most frequently isolated pathogen.

Right-sided endocarditis secondary to Swan-Ganz catheterization	
	Consecutively autopsied patients, *n(%)*
Patients with Swan-Ganz catheter	142
>1 subendocardial right-sided lesion	55
Subendocardial hemorrhage	29 (53)
Sterile thrombus	12 (22)
Hemorrhage	11 (20)
Infective endocarditis	2 (4)
Pulmonary valve 3, right atrium 1	
Patients without Swan-Ganz catheter	87
>1 subendocardial right-sided lesion	3 (3.4)

FIGURE 3-30 Right-sided endocarditis secondary to Swan-Ganz catheterization. This study assessed both infectious and noninfectious local complications of Swan-Ganz catheter use, *eg*, hemorrhage, thrombus formation, and infection. These data mirror those of experimental infective endocarditis in animals and strongly support the pathophysiologic mechanisms outlined in the figure. It is noteworthy that no cases of tricuspid valve infection were found. (*Adapted from* Rowley *et al.* [10].)

PROSTHETIC VALVE ENDOCARDITIS

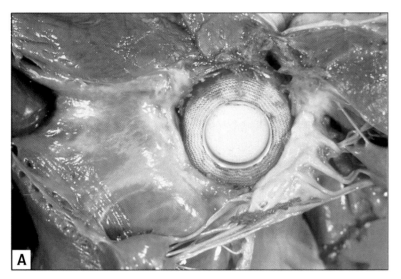
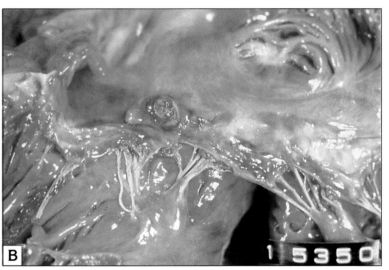

FIGURE 3-31 Prosthetic valve endocarditis caused by *Enterococcus* species. The autopsy findings revealed that the infection had extended from the prosthetic valve to the noncoronary cusp and right atrium. **A**, The closed valve from the left ventricular aspect with perivalvular dehiscence at its superior aspect is shown. **B**, The end of the fistulous tract entering the right atrium above the tricuspid valve is shown.

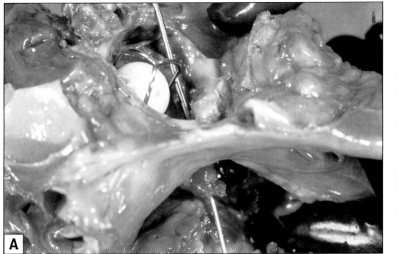

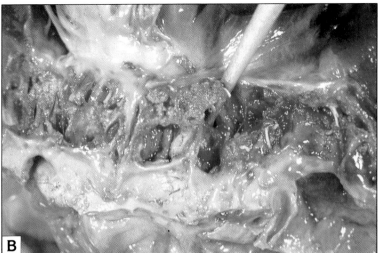

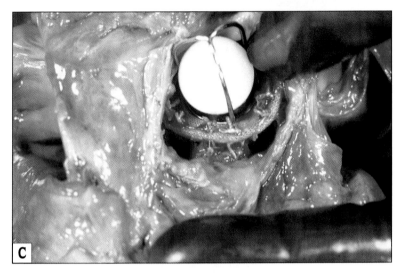

Figure 3-32 Prosthetic valve endocarditis in a patient with a Starr-Edwards mitral valve prosthesis. **A,** The metal probe extends from the left ventricular through the noncoronary cusp into the right atrium. **B,** The atrioventricular annulus is shown following removal of the prosthetic valve. Note the probe at the site of densely clustered vegetations. **C,** Dehiscence of the prosthetic mitral valve is shown from the ventricular aspect. There appears to be little inflammation on the valve itself. The infection and secondary valve dehiscence begins at the suture line of the valve to the annulus. With this degree of valve dehiscence it is not surprising that this patient had rocking of his valve on echocardiogram. (*Courtesy of* W.E. Dismukes, MD.)

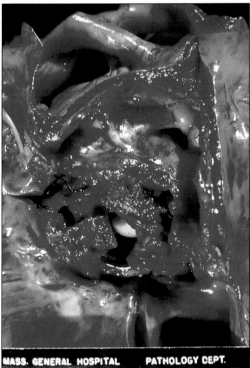

Figure 3-33 Prosthetic valve endocarditis of a mitral prosthesis. Viewed from the atrial aspect of the valve, the overlying vegetation adherent to the metal support of the valve can be seen. (*Courtesy of* W.E. Dismukes, MD.)

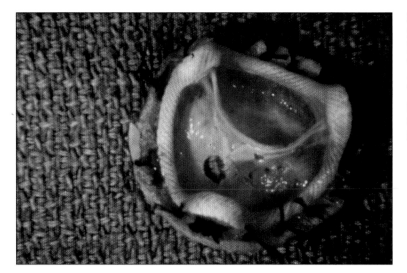

FIGURE 3-34 Bioprosthetic aortic valve from a patient with Q fever endocarditis. Valve leaflet perforation is shown. Endocarditis is the major clinical manifestation of chronic Q fever. Prosthetic valves are well recognized as a risk factor for the development of *Coxiella burnetii* infective endocarditis. Fever is frequently absent. The vegetations in Q fever endocarditis differ in both gross and microscopic appearance; microscopically there is a subacute and chronic inflammatory cell infiltrate associated with large foamy macrophages.

REFERENCES

1. Nanda NC, Abd-Rahman SM, Khatri G: Incremental value of three-dimensional echocardiography over transesophageal multiplane two-dimensional echocardiography in qualitative and quantitative assessment of cardiac masses and defects. *Echocardiography* 1995, 12:619–628.

2. Durack DT: Experimental bacterial endocarditis: IV structure and evolution of very early lesions. *J Pathol* 1975, 115:81–89.

3. Lepeschkin E: On the relation between the site of valvular involvement in endocarditis and the blood pressure resting on the valve. *Am J Med Sci* 1952, 224:318–319.

4. Rodbard S: Blood velocity and endocarditis. *Circulation* 1963, XXVIII:18–28.

5. Gould K, Ramirez-Ronda C, Holmes R, *et al.*: Adherence of bacteria to heart valves in vitro. *J Clin Invest* 1975, 56:1364–1370.

6. Korzeniowski O, Kaye D: Endocarditis. In *Infectious Diseases*. Edited by Gorbach S, Bartlett J, Blacklow N. Philadelphia: WB Saunders; 1992:548–557.

7. Mills J, Pulliam L, Dall L, *et al.*: Exopolysaccharide production by viridans streptococci in experimental endocarditis. *Infect Immun* 1984, 43:359–367.

8. Rosenthal A, Nadas A: Infective endocarditis in infancy and childhood. In *Infective Endocarditis*. Edited by Rahimtoola SH. New York: Grune and Stratton; 1978:149–178.

9. Netter FH: *The Ciba Collection of Medical Illustrations*, vol 5. Edited by Yonkman FF. Summit, NJ: Ciba Pharmaceutical Products; 1969.

10. Rowley K, Clubb S, Smith W, *et al.*: Right-sided infective endocarditis as a consequence of flow-directed pulmonary-artery catheterization. *New Engl J Med* 1984, 311:1152–1156.

SELECTED BIBLIOGRAPHY

Feigin RD, Cherry JC: *Textbook of Pediatric Infectious Diseases*, 4th ed. Philadelphia: WB Saunders, 1992.

Gorbach S, Bartlett J, Blacklow N: *Infectious Diseases*. Philadelphia: WB Saunders, 1992.

Kaye D: *Infective Endocarditis*. New York: Raven Press, 1992.

Mandell G, Bennett J, Dolin R: *Principles and Practice of Infectious Diseases*, 4th ed. New York: Churchill Livingstone, 1995.

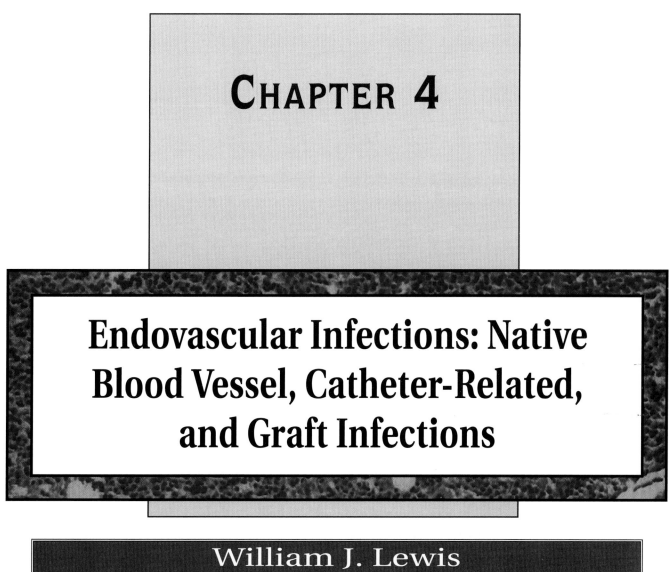

CHAPTER 4

Endovascular Infections: Native Blood Vessel, Catheter-Related, and Graft Infections

William J. Lewis
Robert J. Sherertz

ENDOVASCULAR INFECTIONS are infections inside the vascular system. They can involve arteries, capillaries, veins, or the heart. Infections involving the heart will be discussed in other chapters. Infections involving the arteries, capillaries, or veins occur most commonly by one of two routes: 1) hematogenous seeding from another site or 2) contiguous spread from an adjacent infection. Hematogenous seeding was much more common in the preantibiotic era. In recent years, device-related infections associated with vascular catheters and vascular grafts have become more frequent as more and more patients undergo these medical interventions. This chapter provides a visual overview of the spectrum of endovascular infections.

Epidemiology of suppurative thrombophlebitis

Superficial veins
  Peripheral catheter related
  Non–catheter related
    Secondary to venous trauma (*eg*, intravenous drug abuse)
    Secondary to dermal infection (rare)
Central veins
  Central venous catheter related
  Noncatheter related
    Pelvic veins (postpartum)
    Intracranial venous sinuses (meningitis, sinusitis)
    Portal veins (intra-abdominal infections)

FIGURE 4-1 Epidemiology of suppurative thrombophlebitis. Suppurative thrombophlebitis implies infection and inflammation of a vein in association with thrombus formation. Generally, the problem of suppurative thrombophlebitis can be broadly categorized by location such as that occurring in superficial veins and central veins. Because suppurative thrombophlebitis is now largely a problem that affects commonly cannulated veins, the problem can be further broken down into catheter-related and non–catheter-related infections. Catheter-related infections occur in a variety of clinical settings and range from colonization of the catheter material with minimal evidence of local or systemic inflammation to more overt clinical infection such as suppurative thrombophlebitis or catheter-related bacteremia (or fungemia) and sepsis syndrome. Non–catheter-related suppurative thrombophlebitis has become relatively uncommon since the advent of antibiotics, but recognition of the clinical entities remains important.

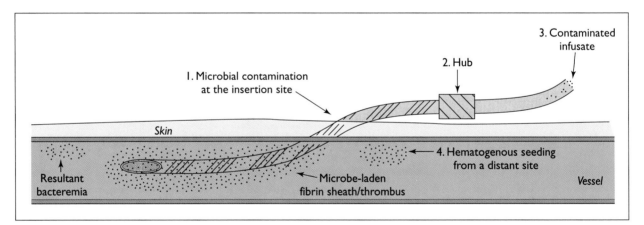

FIGURE 4-2 Pathogenesis of catheter-related venous infection. Intravenous catheters are the most common source of device-related infections. In general, either (or both) of two mechanisms are considered to be the original source of the vast majority of catheter-related bloodstream infections: contamination at the insertion site (*1*), which usually occurs *during* the first week of catheterization, and contamination of the catheter hub (*2*) or from any of the various connections along the infusion line, which usually occurs *after* the first week of catheterization. Generally, microbes colonizing the patient's skin or attending healthcare worker's skin or gloves are responsible for contamination at the insertion site or the hub. Rarely, contaminated skin preparations or local wounds can cause contamination at the insertion site. Less common sources of catheter-related bloodstream infection include the infusate (*3*), such as large-volume parenteral solutions, blood products, total parenteral nutrition, and intravenous medicines, which may be associated with outbreaks of infusion-related bloodstream infections, and hematogenous seeding (*4*) of catheters, which occurs most commonly in patients in the intensive care unit. When a catheter-related thrombus becomes infected (suppurative thrombophlebitis), whether in a great central or peripheral vein, the vein can become a source of bacteremia or fungemia even though the insertion site might lack any sign of infection or inflammation in more than half the cases [1].

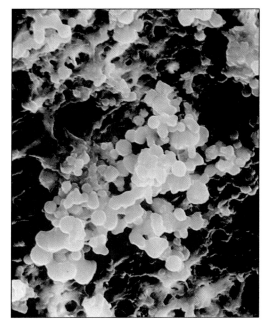

FIGURE 4-3 Electron microscopy of catheter-related biofilm formation. It is generally believed that catheter-related infections begin with colonization of the catheter. The process of colonization is a complex one that is yet to be fully understood. The initial step for most short-term catheters is the association of organisms on the skin of the patient with the external surface of the catheter. It appears that the organisms specifically bind to adherent host proteins such as fibronectin and fibrinogen as well as to adherent platelets. By the time of their removal, approximately 5% to 25% of intravenous cannulas are colonized by bacteria or fungus when determined by quantitative or semiquantitative methods. For longer duration catheters, colonization is more commonly associated with the catheter lumen, usually due to hub contamination. In either case, when examined by electron microscopy, both the internal and external surfaces of central venous catheters removed from patients have been universally shown to have some degree of biofilm formation. (*Courtesy of* I. Raad, MD.)

SUPERFICIAL SUPPURATIVE VENOUS THROMBOPHLEBITIS

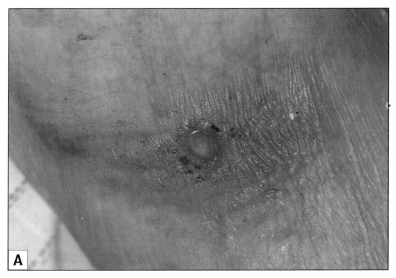

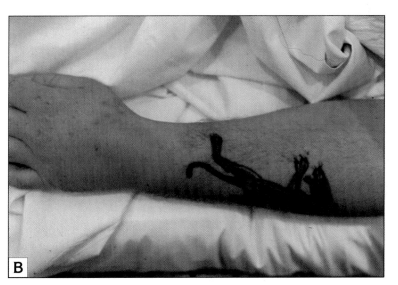

A

B

FIGURE 4-4 Clinical manifestations of peripheral catheter-related suppurative thrombophlebitis. **A,** Intravenous site in the antecubital fossa of a patient with local pain, erythema, and tenderness. In addition to local signs of inflammation and purulence at the intravenous site, systemic signs and symptoms such as fever, chills, and malaise were present. Blood cultures and cultures of the excised vein grew *Staphylococcus aureus*. **B,** Infusion phlebitis. Inflammation without infection surrounding a cannulated, peripheral vein is seen in approximately two thirds of peripheral intravenous catheters by the fourth day. Signs and symptoms of infusion phlebitis include local pain, erythema, tenderness, and frequently a palpable cord. Although conflicting studies exist, many studies show a correlation between infusion phlebitis and catheter-related infection [1]. Infusion phlebitis may mimic infection, as in this patient with phlebitis secondary to receiving intravenous cephalothin, and vice versa. (Panel 4B *courtesy of* D.G. Maki, MD.)

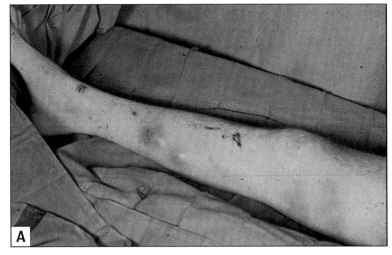

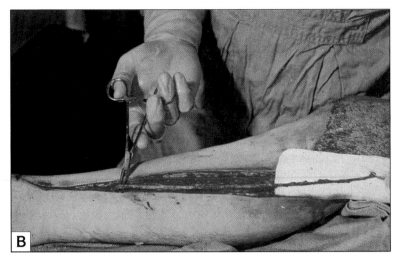

FIGURE 4-5 Management of peripheral catheter-related thrombophlebitis. In patients with superficial vein suppurative thrombophlebitis, the treatment of choice is surgical excision of the vein and administration of antibiotics. This burn victim developed a persistent bacteremia, which was attributed to a suppurative

thrombophlebitis at an old intravenous site in a lower extremity. **A,** Two areas of focal swelling are shown overlying an infected saphenous vein. **B,** Surgical excision of the vein shown in *panel 5A.* (*Courtesy of* the Department of Surgery, Bowman Gray School of Medicine of Wake Forest University.)

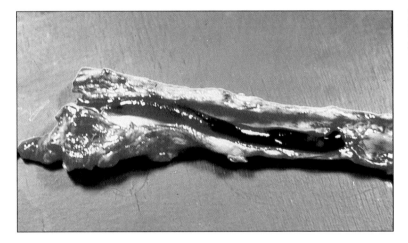

FIGURE 4-6 Pathology of peripheral catheter-related thrombophlebitis. An excised infected vein, with surrounding tissue, is opened to reveal the intravascular thrombus. (*From* Lambert and Farrar [2]; with permission.)

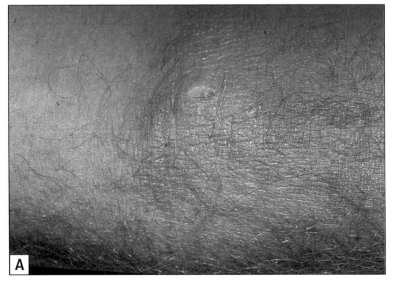

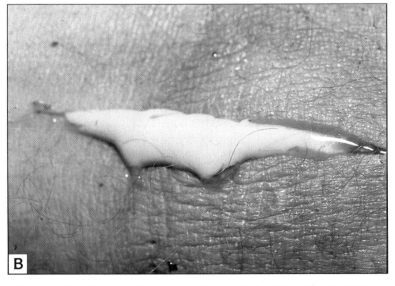

FIGURE 4-7 Pathogenesis of noncatheter-related venous infection: venous infections in intravenous drug abuse. This intravenous drug abuser had *Staphylococcus aureus* suppurative thrombophlebitis in an antecubital vein. **A,** There were few signs of

infection directly over the involved vein at the time of presentation. **B,** However, on incision of the vein, it is obvious that the vein is full of purulent material. (*continued*)

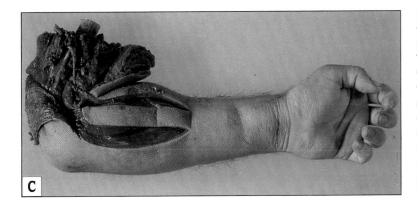

FIGURE 4-7 (*continued*) **C**, Associated fasciitis necessitated amputation of the arm. Venous infections after injection of nonsterile, illicit drugs with nonsterile equipment are commonly encountered. Typically, these infections occur in the smaller peripheral veins of the extremities (more often in the upper than the lower extremities). But with repeated injection of chemical irritants, these veins can become sclerosed, often forcing the user to resort to the use of atypical locations for their injections. Thus, clinicians may encounter unusual venous infections, such as those involving the external jugular vessels or femoral veins. Although extremely rare in the antibiotic era, superficial suppurative thrombophlebitis can also complicate dermal infections by spread of the infection in a contiguous fashion. (*Courtesy of* P. Lance, MD.)

CENTRAL VENOUS CATHETER-RELATED INFECTIONS

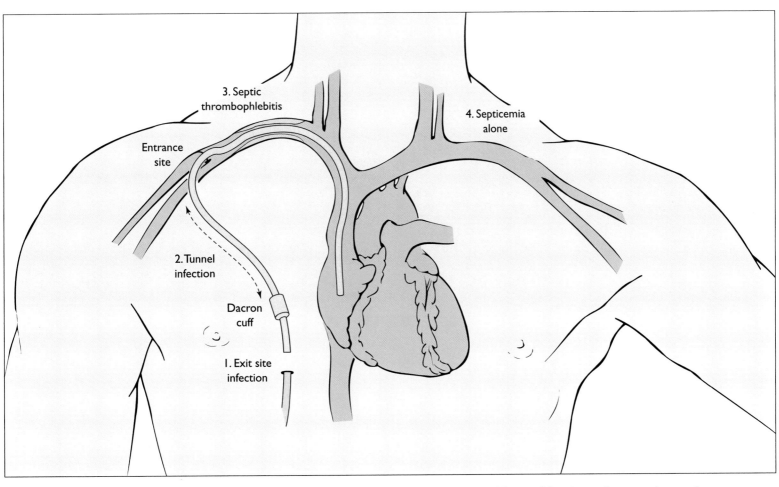

FIGURE 4-8 Clinical manifestations of central venous catheter infections. Signs and symptoms associated with central venous catheter infections are quite varied. The most common manifestation is unexplained fever secondary to catheter lumen or tip infection (*4*). Less commonly, patients may get exit site infections (*1*) with erythema with or without purulence and, even less frequently, septic thrombophlebitis (*3*). In patients with tunneled catheters, a tunnel tract infection (*2*) may develop, which is associated with overlying tenderness, erythema, or cellulitis. (*Adapted from* Press *et al.* [3].)

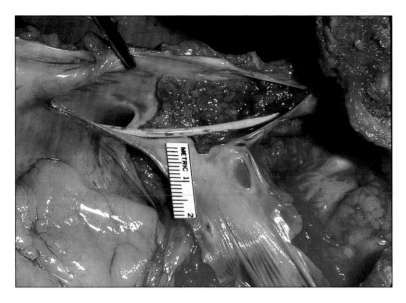

FIGURE 4-9 Internal manifestations of central venous catheter-related infections. Central venous catheter infections typically have few external manifestations with the exception of systemic signs such as fever and chill. Internally, these infections may be associated with a variety of findings. This patient had a large infected thrombus associated with a pulmonary artery catheter. (*Courtesy of* P. Lance, MD.)

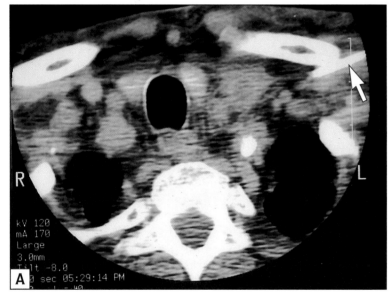

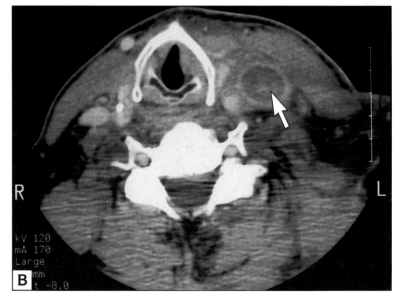

FIGURE 4-10 A, Computed tomographic scan of a patient, hospitalized for an unrelated condition, who developed fever, chills, and a swollen, painful neck 8 days after placement of a left subclavian central venous catheter (*arrow*). **B**, Enhanced computed tomography scan of the same patient showing the catheter-related infection that resulted in a thrombosed, infected left internal jugular vein (*arrow*).

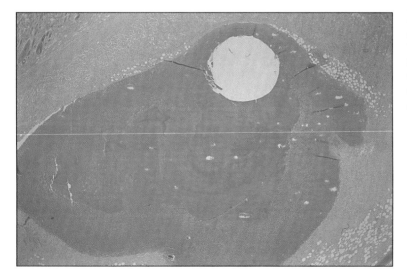

FIGURE 4-11 Subcutaneous catheter-related infections. In an attempt to decrease infections associated with long-term central venous catheters, a portion of the catheter is often tunneled subcutaneously. However, the tunneled portion of the catheter can become infected, necessitating device removal (*ie*, removal of the foreign body). In this figure, the tunnel once occupied by a catheter is shown with surrounding necrosis and suppuration.

Microbiology of catheter-related infections

Peripheral IV catheter	Central IV catheter	Contaminated IV infusate
Coagulase-negative staphylococci	Coagulase-negative staphylococci	*Enterobacter cloacae*
Staphylococcus aureus	*S. aureus*	*Enterobacter agglomerans*
Candida spp	*Candida* spp	*Serratia marcescens*
	Klebsiella and *Enterobacter* spp	*Klebsiella* spp
	Corynebacterium spp	*Pseudomonas* spp
	Rarely:	*Xanthomonas maltophilia*
	Trichophyton beiglii	*Citrobacter freundii*
	Fusarium spp	*Flavobacterium* spp
	Malassezia furfur	*Candida tropicalis*
	Mycobacterium spp	

IV—intravenous.

FIGURE 4-12 Microbiology of catheter-related infections. The organisms causing three major categories of catheter-related infection are shown in descending order of frequency. (*Adapted from* Maki [1].)

NON–CATHETER-RELATED CENTRAL VENOUS INFECTIONS

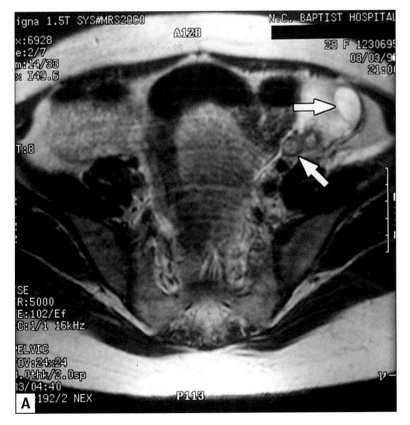

FIGURE 4-13 Puerperal ovarian vein thrombophlebitis. A woman aged 24 years developed slowly progressive lower abdominal pain, fever, and chills 6 days after an uneventful vaginal delivery. Initially, outpatient oral antibiotics were given as empiric treatment of possible endometritis. She was admitted for reevaluation after her temperature reached 106°F. Puerperal ovarian vein thrombophlebitis was suspected by the infectious diseases consultant, and a magnetic resonance image (MRI) was obtained. **A**, The MRI demonstrates a thrombus in the tortuous left ovarian vein (*lower arrow*), as well as a slightly edematous ovary (*upper arrow*). (*continued*)

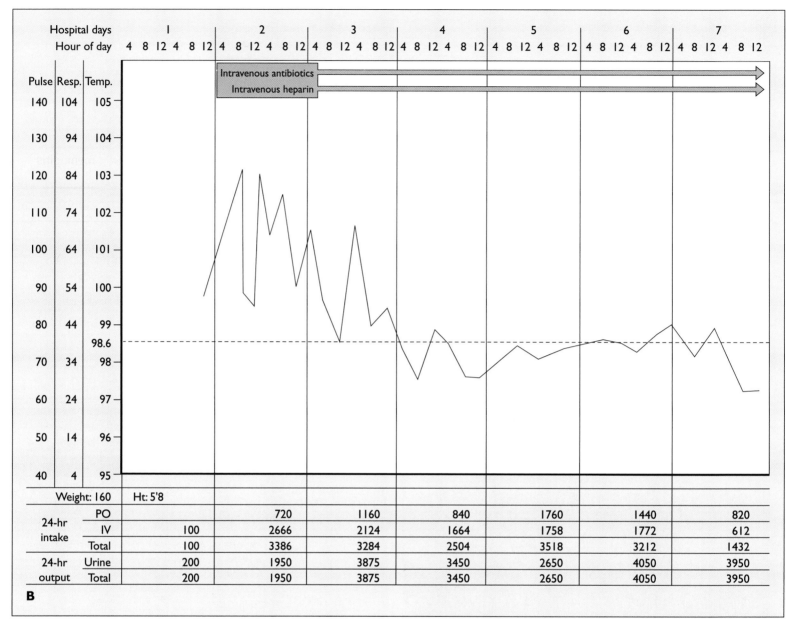

Hospital days		1		2		3		4		5		6		7	

Weight: 160	Ht: 5'8						
24-hr intake	PO		720	1160	840	1760	1440	820
	IV	100	2666	2124	1664	1758	1772	612
	Total	100	3386	3284	2504	3518	3212	1432
24-hr output	Urine	200	1950	3875	3450	2650	4050	3950
	Total	200	1950	3875	3450	2650	4050	3950

B

FIGURE 4-13 (*continued*) **B**, Her fever declined rapidly after initiation of heparin therapy and intravenous antibiotics. Septic pelvic venous thrombophlebitis generally occurs following childbirth, but it can occur following abortion and gynecologic surgery and in conjunction with severe pelvic infection. This condition has a reported prevalence of 0.04% to 0.18% in the postpartum patient and usually occurs in association with puerperal endometritis. A proposed mechanism for this disorder following childbirth has large numbers of bacteria entering the endometrial cavity from the genital tract. After entering the uterus, the bacteria evade host defenses with the help of virulence factors (*eg*, group B streptococcal capsule), then enter and colonize the pelvic venous drainage by way of uterine veins. Endovascular damage can follow, and, in conjunction with pregnancy-related hypercoaguable state and venous stasis, thrombogenesis can result in septic pelvic thrombophlebitis. The right ovarian vein is most commonly involved. This pelvic vein is the most stasis prone because it is more anatomically susceptible to uterine compression and has a more horizontal course in the pelvis as compared with the left ovarian vein [4].

Intracranial venous infection
Cavernous sinus thrombosis   Lateral sinus thrombosis   Superior sagittal sinus thrombosis

FIGURE 4-14 Intracranial venous infection. Infection involving the major dural venous sinuses has become relatively rare since the advent of antibiotics. In the preantibiotic era, septic thrombosis of the cavernous sinus was largely a complication associated with infections involving the medial one third of the face (nose, orbits, tonsils, and soft palate). By entering the facial veins or the pterygoid plexus, bacteria could reach the cavernous sinuses by way of the superior or inferior ophthalmic veins. Alternatively, as a complication of ear infection, bacteria could enter emissary veins from the mastoid air cells, move into the sigmoid sinuses, then enter the cavernous sinus by way of the inferior petrosal sinuses. In the antibiotic era, infection involving the sphenoid and/or ethmoid sinus has become the most common cause of septic cavernous sinus thrombosis due to direct spread or by way of small emissary veins. When reviewed, septic lateral sinus thrombosis has been found to almost always be associated with spread from the mastoid air cells, usually complicating acute or chronic otitis media. Spread of the bacteria from the mastoid air cells to the lateral and sigmoid sinus occurs either by direct spread or by way of emissary veins. Septic thrombosis of the superior sagittal sinus was almost always a complication of bacterial meningitis in the preantibiotic era. Spread of bacteria occurred by way of diploic veins or by direct spread from the meninges to the sinus. In the antibiotic era, about one half of the cases of septic thrombosis of the superior sagittal sinus are secondary to meningitis. Infection involving air sinuses is now the second most common cause of this complication. Infection involving the ethmoid and maxillary sinuses can spread to the superior sagittal sinus by way of ethmoidal veins. Infection of the frontal sinuses can involve the superior sagittal sinus after first involving nearby cortical veins. Additionally, sagittal sinus thrombosis can occur as an extension of septic thrombosis from the lateral dural sinus [5].

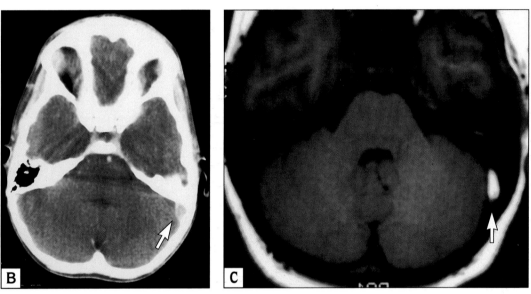

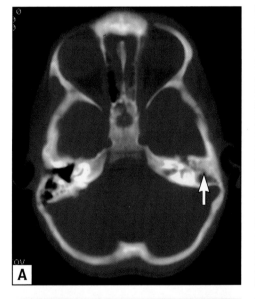

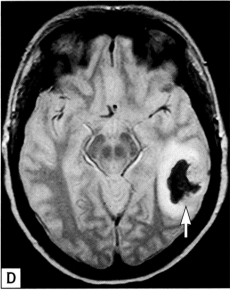

FIGURE 4-15 Venous sinus thrombosis in the antibiotic era. **A,** A bone window computed tomographic scan demonstrated left mastoiditis (*arrow*) in a patient who presented with left-sided headache. **B,** With contrast, the same computed tomographic scan showed an area of enhancement adjacent to a thrombosed left sigmoid dural sinus (*arrow*). **C,** With magnetic resonance imaging scans, lateral sinus thrombosis (*arrow*) will appear as a bright enhancing area with T1-weighted imaging. **D,** Lateral sinus thrombosis can be complicated by intracranial hemorrhage (*arrow*) as shown on this T2-weighted image. (*continued*)

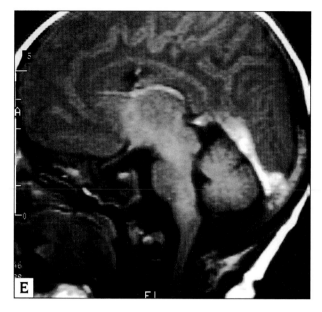

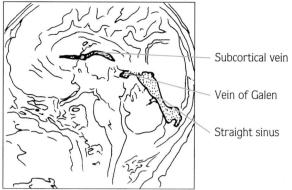

Subcortical vein

Vein of Galen

Straight sinus

FIGURE 4-15 (*continued*) **E,** In this unusual case, a child developed meningoencephalitis complicated by thrombosis of a subcortical vein, vein of Galen, and the straight sinus, as is shown in this T1-weighted magnetic resonance image.

VASCULAR GRAFT INFECTIONS

Modes of vascular graft infections

Endogenous skin flora
Break in sterile technique
Improperly sterilized equipment
Clean-contaminated surgery
Infected lymph node or lymphatic drainage of an infected distal site
Organisms from diseased arterial walls or thrombus
Extension from a postoperative infectious process to involve the graft
Bacteremia

FIGURE 4-16 Modes of vascular graft infections. Contamination of prosthetic grafts usually occurs by one of the modes listed in the figure at the time of implantation. The incidence of prosthetic graft infections is difficult to ascertain because a long delay often occurs between the original procedure and the onset of symptoms. Reported incidences vary with regard to the location of the graft and the series reviewed, but overall they range from 0% to 3.5%, mostly in retrospective studies. Although the incidence of upper extremity infections involving prosthetic materials (excluding dialysis access grafts) is very low, grafts involving the lower extremities and extra-anatomic bypass grafts become infected in 2% to 5% of cases. However, under certain circumstances the incidence of prosthetic graft infections can be much higher. For example, studies in patients undergoing clean, elective vascular procedures found subsequent graft infections in 2% of primary cases but in 28% of reoperative cases [6].

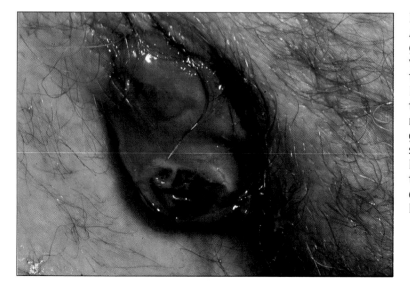

FIGURE 4-17 Clinical presentation of early vascular graft infection. A patient presented with an infected femoropopliteal graft in the groin 6 weeks after surgery. Approximately 50% of all cases of vascular graft infections present with local signs including pain, tenderness, exposed graft material, or an open draining sinus. Infections that occur early (generally within 4 months after implantation) are more commonly due to *Staphylococcus aureus* or gram-negative organisms. Compared with late-onset infections, early graft infections present more often with systemic signs and symptoms as well as wound infection and anastomotic bleeding. Femoropopliteal, iliofemoral, and aortofemoral vascular graft infections are characteristically associated with surgical site infections, especially in the groin. (*Courtesy of* the Department of Surgery, Bowman Gray School of Medicine of Wake Forest University.)

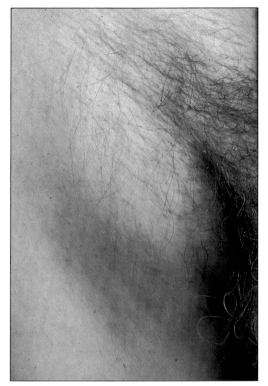

FIGURE 4-18 Vascular graft infection presenting with subtle findings. This patient presented with a swollen and slightly tender groin 6 months (late-appearing infection) after aortofemoral graft placement. Systemic signs and symptoms are generally absent, and blood cultures are typically negative with late-appearing infections. However, one half of patients will have evidence of anastomotic false aneurysm, and the overlying skin may be erythematous and warm. Coagulase-negative staphylococcus is a common pathogen in late-appearing vascular graft infections. Fungal pathogens (*eg, Candida albicans*) are also causes of late infection. (*Courtesy of* the Department of Surgery, Bowman Gray School of Medicine of Wake Forest University.)

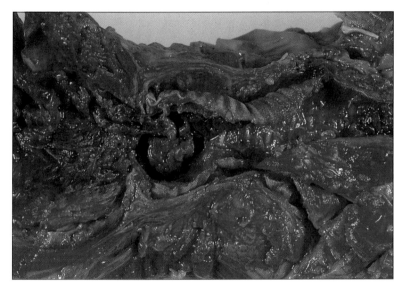

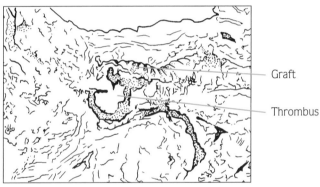

FIGURE 4-19 Autopsy specimen of an infected vascular graft. (*Courtesy of* the Department of Surgery, Bowman Gray School of Medicine of Wake Forest University.)

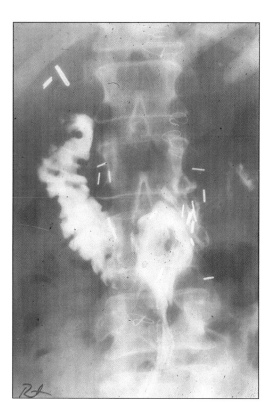

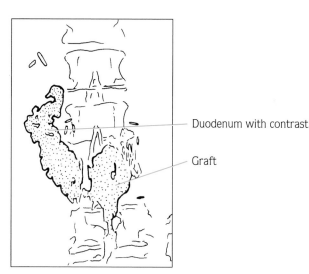

Duodenum with contrast

Graft

FIGURE 4-20 Aortogram of an aortoduodenal fistula in a patient with an aortic vascular graft infection who presented with fever and gastrointestinal bleeding. A complication of the use of vascular grafts in the abdominal aorta is infection with erosion into the gastrointestinal tract associated with gastrointestinal bleeding and bacteremia. Infection of an intra-abdominal aortic graft, when it occurs in the early postoperative period, is often not recognized due to lack of specific symptoms. Such patients may have unexplained sepsis or have only a prolonged ileus. At times, erosion of an aortic graft infection into the gastrointestinal tract occurs, resulting in an aortoenteric fistula. Resultant gastrointestinal bleeding can be either subtle or acutely devastating. (*Courtesy of* the Department of Surgery, Bowman Gray School of Medicine of Wake Forest University.)

DIAGNOSIS OF VASCULAR GRAFT INFECTIONS

Diagnosis of vascular graft infections
Duplex ultrasound
Computed tomography
Magnetic resonance imaging
Radionuclide scans
Arteriography
Culture data
Gastrointestinal endoscopy

FIGURE 4-21 Diagnosis of vascular graft infections. Timely diagnosis of vascular graft infections is essential. At times the patient will present with signs and symptoms that would require emergency surgery (*eg*, a rapidly bleeding graft-enteric fistula), thus establishing a diagnosis visually. Usually, due to the lack of specific symptoms, imaging studies such as ultrasonography, computed tomography, magnetic resonance imaging, or arteriography can aid in establishing the diagnosis. These studies help to establish the adequacy of graft incorporation and the anastomoses and the presence of local inflammation. Microbiologic testing is necessary to confirm the diagnosis and can be obtained through computed tomography or ultrasound-guided aspiration as well as intraoperatively. Gastrointestinal endoscopy is often used in the evaluation of gastrointestinal bleeding. The visualization of graft material during endoscopy establishes the diagnosis [6].

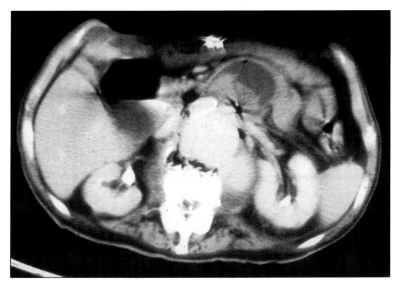

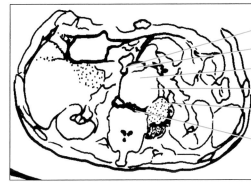

- Perigraft air
- Aortic graft
- Aortoenteric fistula
- Aortic aneurysm
- Perigraft fluid collection
- Perigraft air and vertebral body erosion

FIGURE 4-22 Computed tomographic (CT) scan demonstrating a large aneurysm adjacent to the graft with associated air in the soft tissues and vertebral bone destruction. The CT scan also shows adherent bowel with thickened walls and with what turned out to be an aortoenteric fistula. Contrasted CT is best for detecting perigraft healing abnormalities and determining the extent of involvement. CT criteria include perigraft fluid collections, focal bowel wall thickening, and pseudoaneurysm formation. Presence of air in the perigraft tissue can be normal up to 6 weeks after surgery but is more likely to be associated with infection thereafter. CT-guided aspiration of perigraft fluid collections can aid in the diagnosis. Magnetic resonance imaging can provide better definition of soft tissues and can provide additional information in the form of magnetic resonance imaging angiography. (*Courtesy of* the Department of Surgery, Bowman Gray School of Medicine of Wake Forest University.)

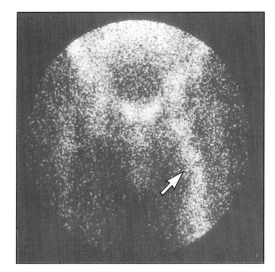

FIGURE 4-23 Indium-111–labeled white blood cell study showing increased uptake (*arrow*) in a person who presented with fever and leukocytosis weeks after femoropopliteal grafting. Radionuclide scanning can be very useful at times but can be falsely positive in the early postoperative period due to graft healing. Later, scanning may be falsely negative due to the low virulence of some organisms such as coagulase-negative staphylococcus. (*Courtesy of* the Department of Surgery, Bowman Gray School of Medicine of Wake Forest University.)

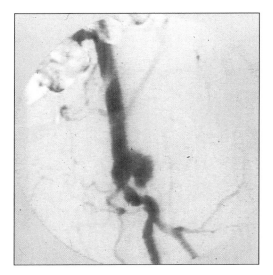

FIGURE 4-24 Arteriogram demonstrating the presence of an aneurysm at the distal anastomosis of an infected iliofemoral graft. Arteriography helps to guide surgical intervention but is not used to establish a diagnosis. Arteriography has the ability to demonstrate aneurysms, sites of anastomoses, and patency of circulation. (*Courtesy of* the Department of Surgery, Bowman Gray School of Medicine of Wake Forest University.)

INFECTIVE ENDARTERITIS AND "MYCOTIC ANEURYSMS"

Etiology of mycotic aneurysms

Infected normal arteries
Infected aneurysms
  Atherosclerotic
  Nonatherosclerotic
    Cystic medial necrosis
    Pseudoaneurysm
Infected atherosclerotic plaques
Syphilitic

FIGURE 4-25 Etiology of "mycotic aneurysms." The terminology of infections involving arteries can be confusing due to imprecision in the way the terms are applied. The term *mycotic aneurysm* was originally used by Osler to describe the mushroom-shaped aneurysms found in persons with endocarditis. The use of this term to describe infection in a preexisting aneurysm or pseudo-aneurysm strays from Osler's original description. Nonetheless, "mycotic" aneurysm is used broadly to describe all aneurysms of infectious etiology. If one considers the preexistant state of the vessel, further distinctions can be made in the description of arterial infections. The source of the invading organisms can be intravascular (embolic or bacteremic) or extravascular (contiguous site or iatrogenic) [7].

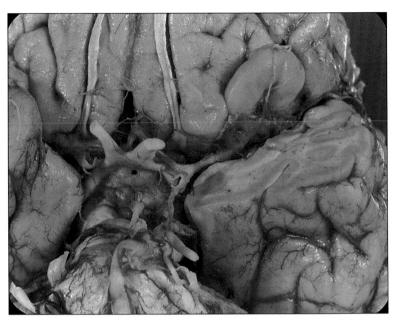

FIGURE 4-26 Autopsy specimen revealing a mycotic aneurysm in the left middle cerebral artery of a patient who died of *Staphylococcus aureus* infective endocarditis. In infective endocarditis, the majority (70%) of mycotic aneurysms form in the sinus of Valsalva or in the supravalvular proximal thoracic aorta. When these aneurysms form in intracranial arteries, the middle cerebral artery is most commonly affected. Multiple aneurysms are not unusual. The arteries involved in aneurysm formation secondary to infective endocarditis are often normal prior to involvement. Patients with these aneurysms are generally without symptoms with the exception of severe headaches, which are often seen. (*Courtesy of* P. Lance, MD.)

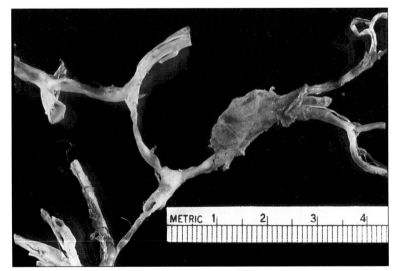

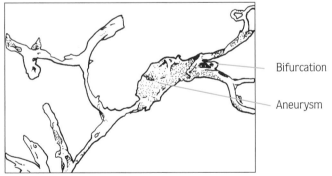

FIGURE 4-27 Autopsy specimen showing the excised aneurysmal artery from a patient who died of infective endocarditis. As is characteristic, this aneurysm formed at a bifurcation point. (*Courtesy of* P. Lance, MD.)

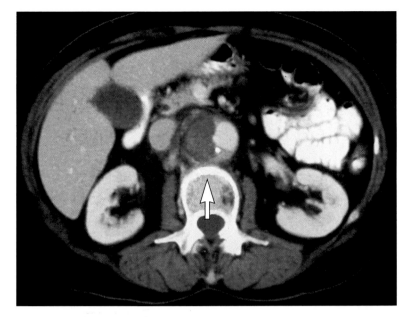

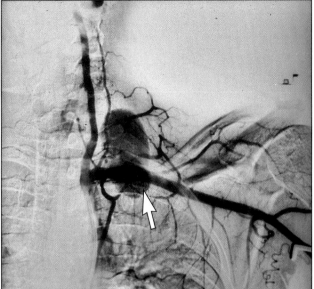

FIGURE 4-28 Computed tomographic scan showing an infected aneurysmal dilatation of the abdominal aorta (*arrow*). The patient presented with a flulike illness and back pain. Symptoms continued and an abdominal computed tomographic scan was obtained after abdominal pain began and fever worsened. Note the presence of an aortic calcification, which may denote an atherosclerotic plaque. Blood cultures and operative cultures grew *Streptococcus pneumoniae*. In this patient it was believed that an atherosclerotic plaque was infected during a bacteremia. Four mechanisms have been proposed to result in infection of arterial walls: 1) septic emboli of the vasa vasorum, 2) hematogenous seeding of the intima from a distant source, 3) extension from a contiguous focus, and 4) trauma [7].

FIGURE 4-29 Angiogram showing an aneurysm (*arrow*) of the subclavian artery. Pseudoaneurysms arise from trauma or from iatrogenic causes and can become infected. This patient developed a traumatized subclavian artery during subclavian central line placement. Fever, chills, and leukocytosis developed days after line placement. Blood and operative cultures grew *Staphylococcus aureus*. (*Courtesy of* the Department of Surgery, Bowman Gray School of Medicine of Wake Forest University.)

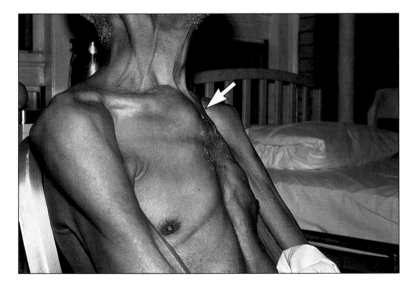

FIGURE 4-30 Endarteritis involving the vasa vasorum. This otherwise asymptomatic man was found to have a chest wall mass (*arrow*) and an aortic regurgitation murmur as well as dilation of the ascending aorta on chest radiograph. Laboratory studies revealed positive nontreponemal and treponemal tests diagnosing syphilis. The underlying pathology is an endarteritis involving the vasa vasorum, which resulted in medial necrosis, destruction of elastic tissue, and aneurysm formation. (*Courtesy of* S. Pegram, MD.)

REFERENCES

1. Maki DG: Infections due to infusion therapy. In *Hospital Infections*, 3rd ed. Edited by Bennett JV, Brachman PS. Boston: Little, Brown and Company; 1992:849–898.

2. Lambert HP, Farrar WE, eds.: *Slide Atlas of Infectious Diseases*. London: Gower Medical Publications; 1982.

3. Press OW, Ramsey PG, Larson EB, *et al.*: Hickman catheter infections in patients with malignancies. *Medicine* 1984, 63:189–200.

4. Duff P: Septic pelvic thrombophlebitis. In *Obstetric and Perinatal Infections*. Edited by Charles D. St. Louis: Mosby–Year Book; 1993:104–108.

5. Southwick FS, Richardson EP, Swartz MN: Septic thrombosis of the dural venous sinuses. *Medicine* 1986, 65:82–106.

6. Bandyk DF, Esses GE: Prosthetic graft infections. *Surg Clin North Am* 1994, 74:571–590.

7. Scheld WM, Sande MA: Endocarditis and intravascular infections. In *Principles and Practice of Infectious Diseases*, 4th ed. Edited by Mandell GL, Bennett JE, Dolin R. New York: Churchill Livingstone; 1995:740–783.

SELECTED BIBLIOGRAPHY

Bandyk DF, Esses GE: Prosthetic graft infections. *Surg Clin North Am* 1994, 74:571–590.

Duff P: Septic pelvic thrombophlebitis. In *Obstetric and Perinatal Infections*. Edited by Charles D. St. Louis: Mosby–Year Book; 1993:104–108.

Maki DG: Infections due to infusion therapy. In *Hospital Infections*, 3rd ed. Edited by Bennett JV, Brachman PS. Boston: Little, Brown and Company; 1992:849–898.

Scheld WM, Sande MA: Endocarditis and intravascular infections. In *Principles and Practice of Infectious Diseases*, 4th ed. Edited by Mandell GL, Bennett JE, Dolin R. New York: Churchill Livingstone; 1995:740–783.

Southwick FS, Richardson EP, Swartz MN: Septic thrombosis of the dural venous sinuses. *Medicine* 1986, 65:82–106.

CHAPTER 5

Infections of Prosthetic Heart Valves

Adolf W. Karchmer

PROSTHETIC VALVE ENDOCARDITIS (PVE) is now a common clinical variant of infective endocarditis and accounts for 15% or more of all cases of endocarditis reported in medical centers with active cardiac surgery programs. Recent studies suggest that 1.5% to 3.0% of patients undergoing valve replacement develop PVE within the initial 12 months after surgery and that the cumulative percent experiencing PVE rises to 3.2% to 5.7% at the end of 5 years.

The pathogenesis of PVE involves a complex series of biochemical, biophysical, and biologic interactions between microorganisms, prosthetic devices, and patients. These interactions influence not only the microbiology of PVE (*eg*, facilitating the adherence of some organisms to foreign material), but ultimately the strategies for treatment and treatment outcome. For example, staphylococci infecting foreign materials are extremely resistant to antibiotics, unless combination therapy including rifampin is used. Blunted host defense mechanisms in the immediate area (microlocale) of the infected device also compromise the elimination of infection unless the foreign material is removed.

The clinical events that give rise to valve seeding and the time at which these events occur influence the microbiology of PVE and the pathologic consequences. Many of the cases developing during the initial year after valve placement represent intraoperative or perioperative contamination or early postoperative nosocomial infection. The microbiology of these early-onset cases of PVE reflects their nosocomial nature and differs notably from later-onset cases that are acquired as a consequence of transient bacteremia occurring in the community setting. Early-onset cases begin at the valve sewing ring–annulus interface and as a result are complicated by a high incidence of invasive perivalvular infection, necrosis of the valve annulus, and dehiscence and dysfunction of the prosthetic valve.

The antibiotic regimens used to treat PVE caused by specific microorganisms are similar, albeit usually administered for a longer time, to those regimens used in the treatment of native valve infection caused by the analogous organisms. The regimens are reasonably effective when used to treat uncomplicated PVE (noninvasive infection) caused by highly susceptible organisms. In contrast, destructive or invasive infection often results in valve dysfunction and hemodynamic compromise with a resultant need for valve replacement surgery. More antibiotic-resistant organisms are also extremely difficult to eradicate from foreign devices, providing further need for valve replacement to eliminate infection. Only with optimal antimicrobial therapy and aggressive surgical intervention (when indicated) can maximal cure rates for PVE be obtained.

INCIDENCE OF PROSTHETIC VALVE ENDOCARDITIS

Cumulative incidence of PVE		Patients with PVE by months after surgery, %		
Study	Valve replacement patients, *n*	12 mo	48 mo	60 mo
Rutledge *et al.* [1] (1956–1981)*	1598	1.4	—	3.2
Ivert *et al.* [2] (1975–1979)	1465	3.0	4.1	—
Calderwood *et al.* [3] (1975–1982)	2608	3.1	5.4	5.7
Arvay and Lengyel [4] (1981–1985)	912	—	—	4.9

*Years during which surgery was performed.

PVE—prosthetic valve endocarditis.

FIGURE 5-1 Cumulative incidence of prosthetic valve endocarditis. Studies using thorough case finding strategies reveal that 1.5% to 3.0% of valve recipients develop prosthetic valve endocarditis during the initial year after surgery. By 4 to 5 years later the cumulative incidence of prosthetic valve endocarditis ranges from 3.2% to 5.7% [1–4].

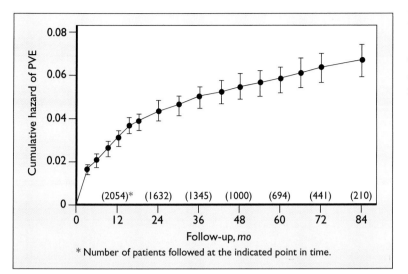

FIGURE 5-2 Cumulative hazard of prosthetic valve endocarditis (PVE). The slope of the curve depicting the cumulative hazard for PVE is steepest during the initial year, reflecting the greatest risk for infection during this period. Thereafter, the slope of the curve, although less steep, remains positive, reflecting a continued risk for developing PVE [3].

MICROBIOLOGY

Microbiology of prosthetic valve endocarditis occurring since 1975

Organism	Cases, n (%)		
	<2 mo after cardiac surgery (n=73)	2–12 mo after cardiac surgery (n=38)	>12 mo after cardiac surgery (n=94)
Coagulase-negative staphylococci	28 (38)	19 (50)	14 (15)
Staphylococcus aureus	10 (14)	4 (11)	12 (13)
Gram-negative bacilli	8 (11)	2 (5)	1 (1)
Streptococci	0	1 (3)	31 (33)
Enterococci	5 (7)	2 (5)	10 (11)
Diphtheroids	9 (12)	1 (3)	2 (2)
HACEK group*	0	1 (3)	11 (12)
Fungi	7 (10)	2 (5)	3 (3)
Miscellaneous	3 (4)	2 (5)	1 (1)
Culture negative	3 (4)	4 (11)	9 (10)

*Includes *Haemophilus aphrophilus/parainfluenzae*, *Actinobacillus actinomycetemcomitans*, *Cardiobacterium hominis*, *Eikenella corrodens*, and *Kingella kingae*.

FIGURE 5-3 Microbiology of prosthetic valve endocarditis (PVE) occurring since 1975. PVE may arise as a nosocomial complication of valve replacement surgery or as a consequence of bacteremia, with or without an apparent portal of entry, which occurs after discharge from the hospital. Nosocomial cases occur during the initial weeks and months after valve surgery. In some nosocomial cases caused by coagulase-negative staphylococci, the onset of clinical endocarditis may be significantly delayed (2 to 12 months) [5,6]. Cases presenting 1 or more years after valve replacement are typically community acquired and result from transient bacteremia. The microbiology of PVE reflects this pattern of acquisition; coagulase-negative staphylococci are the predominant pathogens during the initial year after valve replacement and organisms typical of native valve endocarditis are prominent among the causes of later-onset PVE. More than 80% of the coagulase-negative staphylococci causing PVE during the initial year after valve replacement are methicillin resistant. In contrast, less than 30% of the coagulase-negative staphylococci causing endocarditis 1 or more years after surgery are resistant to methicillin [7].

RISK FACTORS

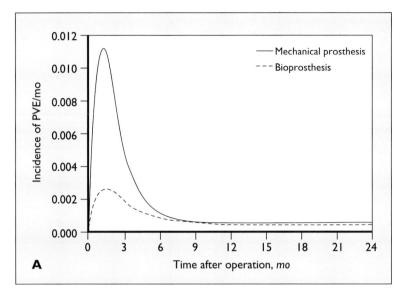

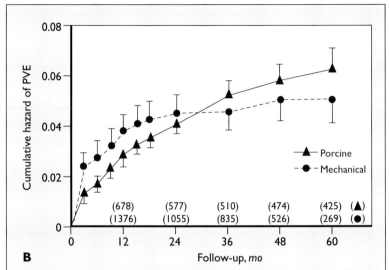

FIGURE 5-4 Risk factors for developing prosthetic valve endocarditis (PVE). The factors associated with an increased risk of developing PVE have not been fully elucidated. In studies that utilize both thorough case finding and sophisticated multivariate analyses, the risk of infection is not associated with valve position (aortic vs mitral). In addition, the overall risk of endocarditis is similar for mechanical and bioprosthetic valves. Nevertheless, there are indications that the risk of infection for these two generic types of prosthetic valves differ over time. **A,** This curve depicting the cumulative hazard for PVE among patients with porcine bioprosthetic valves and mechanical valves indicates a significantly higher risk for PVE developing in recipients of mechanical valves during the first 3 months after valve implantation [2]. **B,** In a large study, the risk of PVE developing in recipients of porcine bioprosthetic valves was greater than that for recipients of mechanical valves when the period 12 months or more

after surgery was examined [3]. In addition, in examining patients 1 year or more after surgery, Arvay and Lengyel [4] also noted that recipients of bioprosthetic valves were at greater risk for developing PVE compared with mechanical valve recipients. In addition, observations in some studies suggest that the risk of PVE is increased with more prolonged or complex surgery, *eg*, insertion of multiple prosthetic valves or longer periods on cardiopulmonary bypass. However, other studies do not confirm this hypothesis. Further clarification of the risk for developing PVE will undoubtedly require studies of larger populations and techniques whereby nosocomial infection can be clearly distinguished from community-acquired endocarditis. The latter is particularly important given the likelihood that there are different mechanisms for seeding prosthetic valves operative in these two epidemiologic settings. (Panel 4B *adapted from* Calderwood *et al.* [3]; with permission.)

PATHOLOGY AND CLINICAL FEATURES

Intracardiac pathology associated with endocarditis involving mechanical prosthetic valves				
	Total patients, *n*	Annulus invasion, *n* (%)	Myocardial abscess, *n* (%)	Orifice occlusion, *n* (%)
Autopsy pathology	74	63 (85)	24 (32)	14 (19)
Surgical and autopsy pathology	85*	36 (42)	12 (14)	3 (4)

*Total number of all patients in report, including those surviving without surgery.

FIGURE 5-5 Intracardiac pathology associated with endocarditis involving mechanical prosthetic valves. The pathology of prosthetic valve endocarditis (PVE) differs notably from that associated with native valve endocarditis. Native valve endocarditis is largely confined to the valve leaflets, whereas PVE commonly extends into the valve annulus or adjacent myocardial tissue. PVE involving mechanical prostheses is often complicated by annulus invasion, myocardial abscess, extension of infection from the aortic site into the pericardial space, or bulky vegetations that may occlude the valve orifice [8–12].

Intracardiac pathology of endocarditis involving porcine bioprosthetic valves				
Onset after surgery, *mo*	Total patients, *n*	Invasive infection, *n* (%)	Leaflet infection only, *n* (%)	Site not examined, *n*
≤12	49	29 (59)	2 (4)	18
>12	36	9 (25)	9 (25)	18

FIGURE 5-6 Intracardiac pathology of endocarditis involving porcine bioprosthetic valves. Invasive infection, similar to that associated with infection of mechanical prosthetic valves, is noted commonly when porcine bioprosthetic valves become infected during the initial year after valve placement. Extension of infection into the annulus and adjacent tissue occurs less frequently when porcine prosthetic valve endocarditis develops 1 or more years after surgery [13]. (*Adapted from* Karchmer and Gibbons [14].)

Clinical features of PVE		
	Patients with feature by time of onset of PVE after cardiac surgery, %	
Feature	≤2 mo (*n*=36)	>2 mo (*n*=93)
Fever	97	99
Regurgitant murmur	47	54
Splenomegaly	36	32
Petechiae (skin/conjunctivae)	56	53
Peripheral signs	14	28
Congestive heart failure	36	49
Central nervous system embolus/hemorrhage	11	27
Anemia (hematocrit <35%)	89	72
Leukocytosis (>12,000 leukocytes/mm^3)	78	51
Hematuria	NE	65

NE—not evaluable; PVE—prosthetic valve endocarditis.

FIGURE 5-7 Clinical features of prosthetic valve endocarditis (PVE). The symptoms and signs associated with PVE (especially in those cases with onset more than 1 year after surgery) are similar to those encountered among patients with native valve endocarditis. Symptoms and signs of PVE are rarely diagnostic in themselves. In contrast to patients with native valve endocarditis, those with PVE have a higher frequency of clinical findings related to perivalvular invasion and destructive infection. These findings include new regurgitant murmurs of valve dysfunction, symptoms of congestive heart failure due to valvular dysfunction, and cardiac rhythm disturbances. Among patients with the onset of PVE before discharge from the hospital after cardiac surgery, the symptoms and signs of endocarditis may be obscured by the impact of recent surgery or postoperative complications. (*Adapted from* Karchmer and Gibbons [14] and Leport *et al.* [15].)

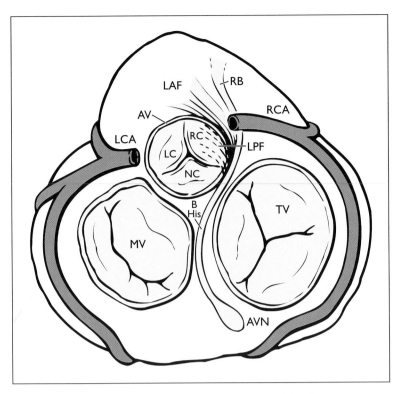

subsequent development of paravalvular regurgitant flow. If this valve dysfunction is hemodynamically significant or if a paravalvular abscess results from invasive infection, surgical intervention is required as part of therapy. Accordingly, it is important that patients who are at risk for these complications be recognized and that invasive infection be identified promptly. Invasive infection is more likely when prosthetic valve endocarditis occurs within the year after valve replacement and when the infected prosthesis is in the aortic position [16]. Invasive infection is suggested by the development of new murmurs of valve dysfunction, fever persisting more than 9 or 10 days despite appropriate antimicrobial therapy, and the development of new electrocardiographic conduction disturbances. Because of the proximity of the conduction system to the aortic valve annulus in the area of the noncoronary and right coronary cusps, infection extending into paravalvular tissue may interrupt the cardiac conduction and result in various rhythm disturbances. Conduction abnormalities are seen less frequently during mitral valve infection. This lower frequency of conduction disturbances relates in part to a lower frequency of invasion complicating mitral valve infection and to a greater separation of the mitral annulus from the proximal conduction system as compared with the analogous relationship of the aortic valve. AV—aortic valve; AVN—atrioventricular mode; B His—common bundle of His; LAF—left anterior fascicle of left bundle branch; LC—left coronary cusp; LCA—left coronary artery; LPF—left posterior fascicle of left bundle branch; MV—mitral valve; NC—noncoronary cusp; RB—right bundle branch; RC—right coronary cusp; RCA—right coronary artery; TV—tricuspid valve. (*Adapted from* Hutter and Moellering [17].)

FIGURE 5-8 Superior view of anatomic relationships between cardiac valves and conduction system. Invasive infection may be associated with the dehiscence of anchoring sutures and the

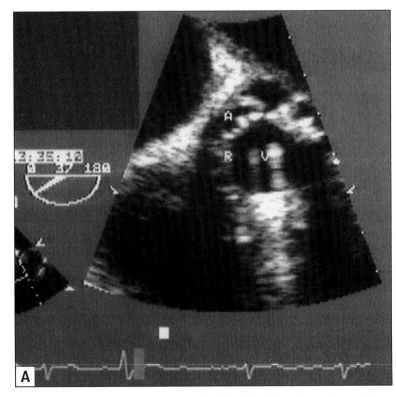

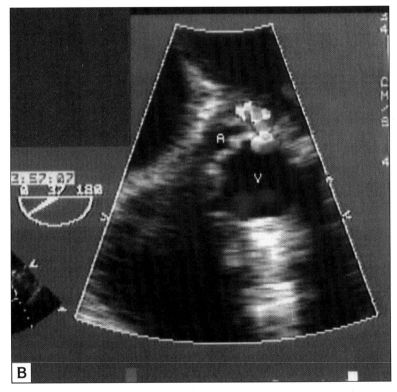

FIGURE 5-9 Two-dimensional and color-flow Doppler echocardiography detecting an abscess around the aortic valve annulus. In assessing prosthetic valves, particularly those in the mitral position, transesophageal echocardiograms are markedly more sensitive than are transthoracic studies for detecting vegetations, paravalvular infection and abscesses, valve dysfunction, and flow through fistulae [18,19]. **A,** Transesophageal short axis view at the level of the St. Jude aortic valve reveals an extensive abscess (A) surrounding the valve ring (R). **B,** Identical echocardiogram from the same patient. However, this projection uses color-flow Doppler to demonstrate the blood flow through part of the abscess cavity. V—mechanical valve leaflets.

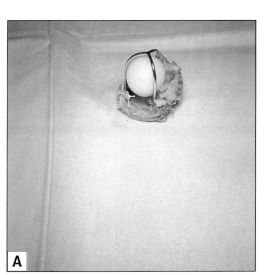

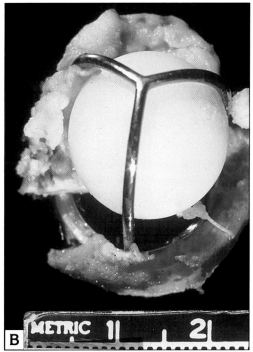

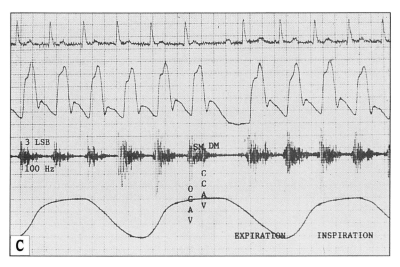

FIGURE 5-10 *Aspergillus* prosthetic valve endocarditis. **A** and **B**, The large *Aspergillus*-infected vegetation of this Starr-Edwards aortic prosthetic valve prevented the poppet from seating during diastole and thus caused hemodynamically significant aortic regurgitation. **C**, In addition, infection extended into the paravalvular tissue and disrupted the conduction system. This disruption resulted in Wenckebach phenomenon (*top line*), which is seen on the electrocardiogram tracing. The simultaneous phonocardiogram (*third line*) tracing displays the systolic murmur (SM) due to the large vegetation in the valve orifice and the decrescendo diastolic murmur (DM) that occurred because the poppet could not seat in the valve ring during diastole. The closing click (CCAV) of the valve is diminished to absent due to the poppet's restricted mobility [20]. The *second line* is the carotid artery pulse tracing. (Panels 10B and 10C *from* Scully *et al.* [20]; with permission.)

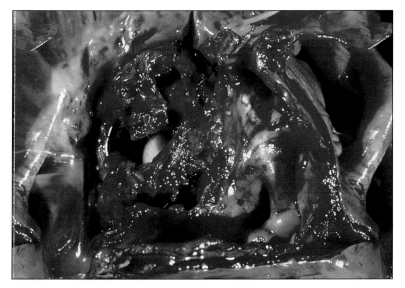

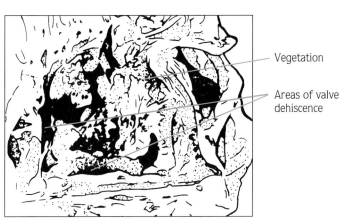

FIGURE 5-11 Starr-Edwards valve in the aortic position infected by *Staphylococcus epidermidis*. The valve orifice is obstructed by the large vegetation. Additionally, the valve has dehisced from the annulus in 50% of its circumference, resulting in hemodynamically significant aortic regurgitation.

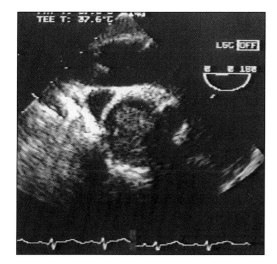

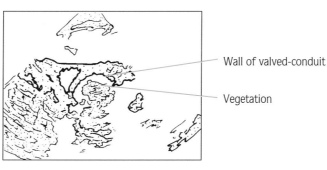

Wall of valved-conduit

Vegetation

FIGURE 5-16 Infected valved-ascending aorta conduit. This transesophageal echocardio-gram reveals a valved-conduit at the aortic position that has become infected by staphylo-cocci. This image, just distal to the aortic valve, shows a large vegetation that virtually fills the aortic outflow track during systole. Typically, infection of this device is associated with disruption of suture line and false aneurysm (abscess) formation where the conduit is sown to the aortic root.

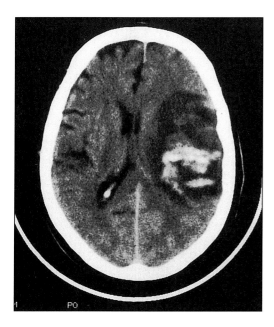

FIGURE 5-17 Hemorrhagic infarction following a left middle cerebral artery embolus. This contrast-enhanced computed tomographic scan illustrates a devastating septic embolic infarct involving the left temporoparietal area (middle cerebral artery), which has become complicated by hemorrhage and marked cerebral edema. The frequency of neurologic complications of prosthetic valve endocarditis (PVE), primarily embolic stroke and intracranial hemorrhage, ranges from 20% to 35% and is comparable to that noted among patients with native valve endocarditis. Available data suggest that continuing careful anticoagulation therapy during PVE involving mechanical valves is associated with a reduced frequency of embolic strokes compared with no anticoagulation in this patient group (16 of 133 [12%] vs 32 of 76 [42%]). Furthermore, neither the frequency of death nor intracranial hemorrhage is increased by anticoagulant therapy. Data are insufficient to draw conclusions regarding the impact of anticoagulant therapy on the frequency of central nervous system complications in patients with PVE involving bioprosthetic valves. It is recommended that patients who develop PVE on a valve that requires antico-agulant therapy (or who require anticoagulation for illnesses unrelated to endocarditis) be carefully continued on such therapy during antibiotic treatment of PVE. Anticoagulation should be reversed if PVE is complicated by intracranial hemorrhage. As in patients with native valve endocarditis, effective antibiotic therapy appears to reduce the risks of systemic embolization [21].

TREATMENT

Conditions warranting consideration of cardiac surgical treatment of PVE

Moderate to severe heart failure due to prosthesis dysfunction (incompetence or obstruction)
Invasive destructive paravalvular infection
    Partial valve dehiscence
    New or progressive conduction system disturbances
    Fever persisting ≥10 days during appropriate antibiotic therapy
    Purulent pericarditis
    Sinus of Valsalva aneurysm or intracardiac fistula
    Myocardial invasion demonstrated by echocardiography
Uncontrolled bacteremic infection despite optimal antimicrobial therapy
Infection caused by selected organisms
    Fungi
    Staphylococcus aureus
    Coagulase-negative staphylococci
    Pseudomonas aeruginosa
Relapse after appropriate antimicrobial therapy
Persistent temperature during therapy for culture-negative PVE in absence of other causes of fever
Recurrent arterial emboli

PVE—prosthetic valve endocarditis.

FIGURE 5-18 Conditions warranting consideration of cardiac surgical treatment of prosthetic valve endocarditis (PVE). Despite treatment with increasingly potent antimicrobial regimens, the outcome of PVE did not significantly improve during the early 1970s. Subsequently, overall survival rates increased to 70% to 75%, and the rates for patients with late-onset PVE caused by less virulent, antibiotic-susceptible organisms (viridans streptococci, fastidious gram-negative coccobacillary organisms, and enterococci) approached 85%. Undoubtedly, outcomes have improved for many reasons: the recognition of methicillin resistance among coagulase-negative staphylococci and the development of appropriate therapy, improved antimicrobial regimens, earlier diagnosis of PVE, new techniques for noninvasive evaluation of intracardiac complications, and increased ability to support critically ill patients through major surgical procedures and the immediate postoperative recovery period. A major contribution to higher cure rates, however, was the recognition of the invasive and destructive nature of PVE and the feasibility of the surgical replacement of an actively infected prosthetic valve without inevitable recrudescent endocarditis on the new prosthesis. In addition, the development of complex, creative surgical techniques for the replacement of dysfunctional infected prostheses and the repair of destroyed cardiac structures was critical. The conditions warranting careful consideration of surgical treatment of patients with PVE are not the result of controlled experiments but rather have evolved over time as a result of the careful study of this infection and its response to treatment. Some of these clinical conditions are not absolute indications for surgery (*eg*, specific causative organisms, recurrent arterial emboli), whereas other conditions virtually require surgical intervention for successful outcome (*eg*, heart failure resulting from valve dysfunction, uncontrolled infection). Recent studies suggest that as many as 65% of patients with PVE have conditions rendering them candidates for surgical intervention. The timing of surgical intervention must be individualized. Survival rates are inversely related to the severity of heart failure and cardiac dysfunction at the time of surgery. Thus, although it is desirable to control infection prior to surgical intervention and the implantation of a new prosthetic valve, prolonged antibiotic therapy in an attempt to achieve this control in the face of worsening heart failure or continued uncontrolled infection is counterproductive and associated with increased mortality [14,22,23].

REFERENCES

1. Rutledge R, Kim J, Applebaum RE: Actuarial analysis of the risk of prosthetic valve endocarditis in 1,598 patients with mechanical and bioprosthetic valves. *Arch Surg* 1985, 120:469–472.

2. Ivert TSA, Dismukes WE, Cobbs CG, *et al.*: Prosthetic valve endocarditis. *Circulation* 1984, 69:223–232.

3. Calderwood SB, Swinski LA, Waternaux CM, *et al.*: Risk factors for the development of prosthetic valve endocarditis. *Circulation* 1985, 72:31–37.

4. Arvay A, Lengyel M: Incidence and risk factors of prosthetic valve endocarditis. *Eur J Cardiothorac Surg* 1988, 2:340–346.

5. Archer GL, Vishniavsky N, Stiver HG: Plasmid pattern analysis of *Staphylococcus epidermidis* isolates from patients with prosthetic valve endocarditis. *Infect Immunol* 1982, 35:627–632.

6. van den Broek PJ, Lampe AS, Berbee GAM, *et al.*: Epidemic of prosthetic valve endocarditis caused by *Staphylococcus epidermidis*. *Br Med J* 1985, 291:949–950.

7. Karchmer AW, Archer GL, Dismukes WE: *Staphylococcus epidermidis* causing prosthetic valve endocarditis: Microbiologic and clinical observations as guides to therapy. *Ann Intern Med* 1983, 98:447–455.

8. Arnett EN, Roberts WC: Prosthetic valve endocarditis: Clinicopathologic analysis of 22 necropsy patients with comparison of observations in 74 necropsy patients with active infective endocarditis involving natural left-sided cardiac valves. *Am J Cardiol* 1976, 38:281–291.

9. Richardson JV, Karp RB, Kirklin JW, Dismukes WE: Treatment of infective endocarditis: A 10-year comparative analysis. *Circulation* 1978, 58:589–597.

10. Lieberman JR, Callaway GH, Salvati EA, *et al.*: Treatment of the infected total hip arthroplasty with a two-stage reimplantation protocol. *Clin Orthop* 1994, 301:205–212.

11. Cherry JJ Jr, Roland CF, Pairolero PC, *et al.*: Infected femorodistal bypass: Is graft removal mandatory? *J Vasc Surg* 1992, 15:295–305.

12. Rose AG: Prosthetic valve endocarditis: A clinicopathological study of 31 cases. *S Afr Med J* 1986, 69:441–445.

13. Fernicola DJ, Roberts WC: Frequency of ring abscess and cuspal infection in active infective endocarditis involving bioprosthetic valves. *Am J Cardiol* 1993, 72:314–323.

14. Karchmer AW, Gibbons GW: Infections of prosthetic heart valves and vascular grafts. In *Infections Associated With Indwelling Devices*. Edited by Bisno AL, Waldvogel FA. Washington, DC: American Society for Microbiology; 1994:213–249.

15. Leport C, Vilde JL, Bricaire F, *et al.*: Fifty cases of late prosthetic valve endocarditis: Improvement in prognosis over a 15-year period. *Br Heart J* 1987, 58:66–71.

16. Calderwood SB, Swinski LA, Karchmer AW, *et al.*: Prosthetic valve endocarditis: Analysis of factors affecting outcome of therapy. *J Thorac Cardiovasc Surg* 1986, 92:776–783.

17. Hutter AM Jr, Moellering RC: Assessment of the patient with suspected endocarditis. *JAMA* 1976, 235:1603–1605.

18. Daniel WG, Mügge A, Martin RP, *et al.*: Improvement in the diagnosis of abscesses associated with endocarditis by transesophageal echocardiography. *N Engl J Med* 1991, 324:795–800.

19. Daniel WG, Mügge A, Grote J, *et al.*: Comparison of transthoracic and transesophageal echocardiography for detection of abnormalities of prosthetic and bioprosthetic valves in the mitral and aortic positions. *Am J Cardiol* 1993, 71:210–215.

20. Scully RE, Galdabini JJ, McNeely BU: Case records of the Massachusetts General Hospital: Case 39-1976. *N Engl J Med* 1976, 295:718–724.

21. Davenport J, Hart RG: Prosthetic valve endocarditis 1976–1987: Antibiotics, anticoagulation, and stroke. *Stroke* 1990, 21:993–999.

22. Baumgartner WA, Miller DC, Reitz BA, *et al.*: Surgical treatment of prosthetic valve endocarditis. *Ann Thorac Surg* 1983, 35:87–102.

23. Boyd AD, Spencer FC, Isom OW, *et al.*: Infective endocarditis: An analysis of 54 surgically treated patients. *J Thorac Cardiovasc Surg* 1977, 73:23–30.

SELECTED BIBLIOGRAPHY

Douglas JL, Cobbs CG: Prosthetic valve endocarditis. In *Infective Endocarditis*. Edited by Kaye D. New York: Raven Press; 1992:375–396.

Karchmer AW, Gibbons GW: Infections of prosthetic heart valves and vascular grafts. In *Infections Associated With Indwelling Devices*. Edited by Bisno AL, Waldvogel FA. Washington, DC: American Society for Microbiology; 1994:213–249.

Nataf P, Jault F, Dorent R, *et al.*: Extra-annular procedures in the surgical management of prosthetic valve endocarditis. *Eur Heart J* 1995, 16(Suppl B):99–102.

Vered Z, Mossinson D, Peleg E, *et al.*: Echocardiographic assessment of prosthetic valve endocarditis. *Eur Heart J* 1995, 16(Suppl B):63–67.

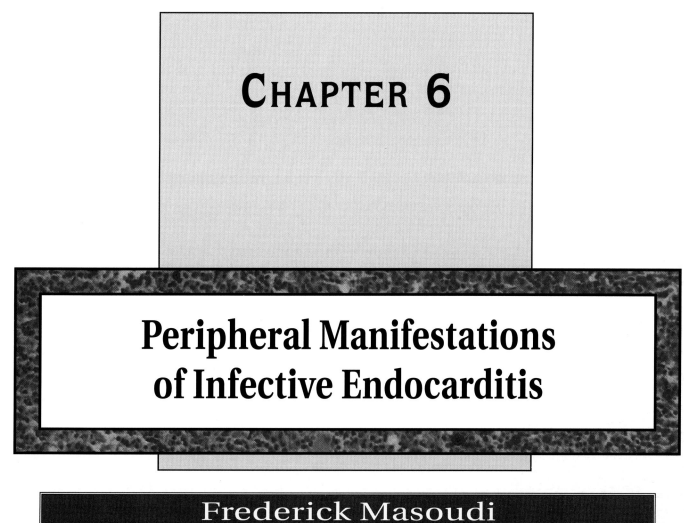

CHAPTER 6

Peripheral Manifestations of Infective Endocarditis

Frederick Masoudi
Henry F. Chambers

ERIPHERAL MANIFESTATIONS of endocarditis are due to the intravascular, principally valvular, location of the primary lesion, *ie*, the infected vegetation, and the immune stimulation that the continuous presentation of bacterial antigens provokes. Classically, peripheral manifestations often were attributed to immune-mediated phenomena, such as vasculitis due to immune-complex deposition. Embolization of infected fragments that have broken off from the friable vegetation and lodged in large, medium, and small vessels, perhaps accompanied by a secondary vasculitis, is the more likely explanation for most peripheral manifestations of endocarditis, with the

exception of glomerulonephritis. Embolic events, strokes in particular, are an important cause of morbidity in patients with endocarditis.

Although understanding of the mechanisms responsible for the evolution of the vegetation and embolization has improved greatly, there still are no reliable and accurate means of predicting or preventing these events. Recognition of these peripheral manifestations as indicative of underlying endocarditis is important for prompt diagnosis of the disease so that appropriate antimicrobial therapy, which remains the most effective method of reducing the risk of embolization, can be instituted.

PATHOGENESIS

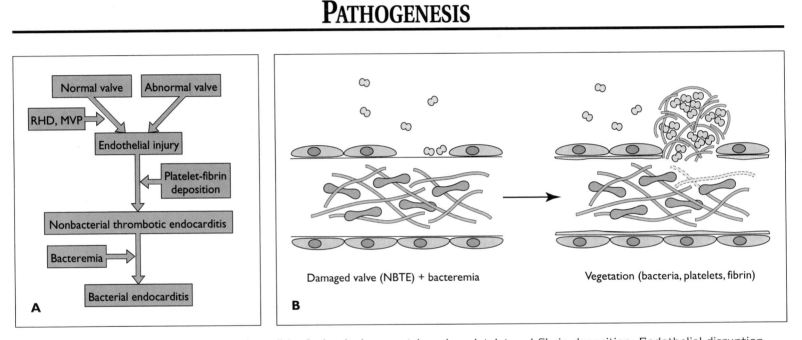

FIGURE 6-1 Pathogenesis of infective endocarditis. **A**, A valvular abnormality, either congenital or acquired, is the proposed essential element for initiation of endocardial infection. Infection of an apparently normal valve is probably explained by the presence of a clinically undetectable abnormality (*ie*, no murmur is heard) or a transient alteration in valvular endothelium that predisposes to adherence of bacteria to its surface. In grossly injured or damaged valves, the single cell layer of the endothelial surface is disrupted, exposing collagen and other basement membrane proteins and triggering platelet and fibrin deposition. Endothelial disruption leads to the formation of a sterile platelet-fibrin thrombus. **B**, Bacteria expressing the appropriate receptors can bind to the damaged endothelial surface of the platelet-fibrin thrombus. In the absence of adequate host defenses, the bacteria rapidly multiply, propagating further platelet-fibrin deposition and evolution of a mature, infected vegetation. MVP—mitral valve prolapse; NBTE—nonbacterial thrombotic endocarditis; RHD—rheumatic heart disease.

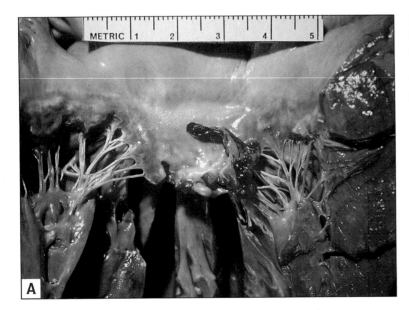

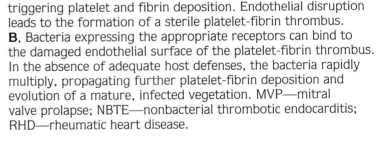

FIGURE 6-2 A, Infected vegetations on rheumatic mitral valve. The infected vegetation plays a central role in all clinical manifestations of infective endocarditis. Vegetations can be quite large, reaching 1 cm or more in size. The vegetations are teeming with bacteria, which can reach densities of 10^8 to 10^9 colony-forming units per gram of infected tissue. (*continued*)

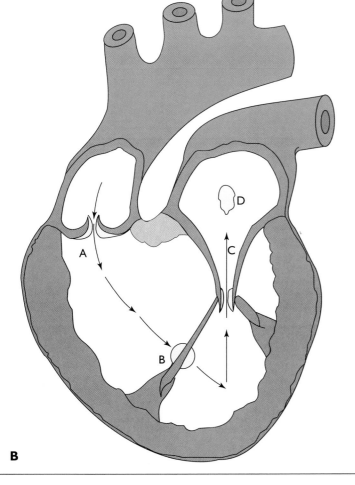

B

C. Frequency of peripheral manifestations of endocarditis

Any embolic phenomenon	>50%
Stroke	25%
Osler nodes	10%–25%
Splinter hemorrhages	15%–20%
Petechiae	25%–40%
Janeway lesions	<10%
Roth spots	5%–10%
Mycotic aneurysms	20%
Septic complications (*eg*, pneumonia, meningitis)*	20%

*Pneumonia or pulmonary radiographic findings are present in 50% to 75% of patients with tricuspid valve endocarditis.

FIGURE 6-2 (*continued*) **B**, Characteristic sites of formation of vegetations in the heart. Regurgitant flow and jets produce endothelial injury on the ventricular surface of aortic valve leaflets (*A*) or on chordae tendineae or papillary muscles (*B*) in aortic insufficiency. In mitral insufficiency, lesions are located on the atrial surface of the valve (*C*) or in the atrial wall (*D*). **C**, Frequency of peripheral manifestations of endocarditis. (Panel 2B *from* Scheld [1].)

Mechanisms of injury in endocarditis

Valve destruction
Bacterial seeding leading to metastatic infection at extracardiac sites
Embolization of systemic and pulmonary vasculature
Immune-complex disease

FIGURE 6-3 Mechanisms of injury in endocarditis. Four disease mechanisms are directly attributable to valvular vegetations. Valve destruction is a direct consequence of the damage produced by replicating bacteria present in high numbers, particularly if they are invasive pathogens (*eg*, *Staphylococcus aureus* or the pneumococcus). This damage can result in valvular insufficiency and heart failure, which are major complications of infective endocarditis. Large vegetations also may produce valvular dysfunction by obstructing the valve orifice. The vegetation also is a source of infection that directly seeds the bloodstream, allowing wide dissemination of infection to extracardiac sites (*eg*, bone, joints, lungs, brain). Fragmentation of friable vegetation leads to systemic or pulmonary embolization. Microemboli are responsible for many of the peripheral and cutaneous stigmata of endocarditis. Larger emboli can produce vasoocclusive phenomena, leading to stroke, peripheral vascular insufficiency syndromes, or pulmonary embolism. Immune-complex disease results from the presence of a large and persistent antigen load. Circulating antigen–antibody complexes can produce peripheral manifestations, most notably glomerulonephritis.

Clinical Manifestations

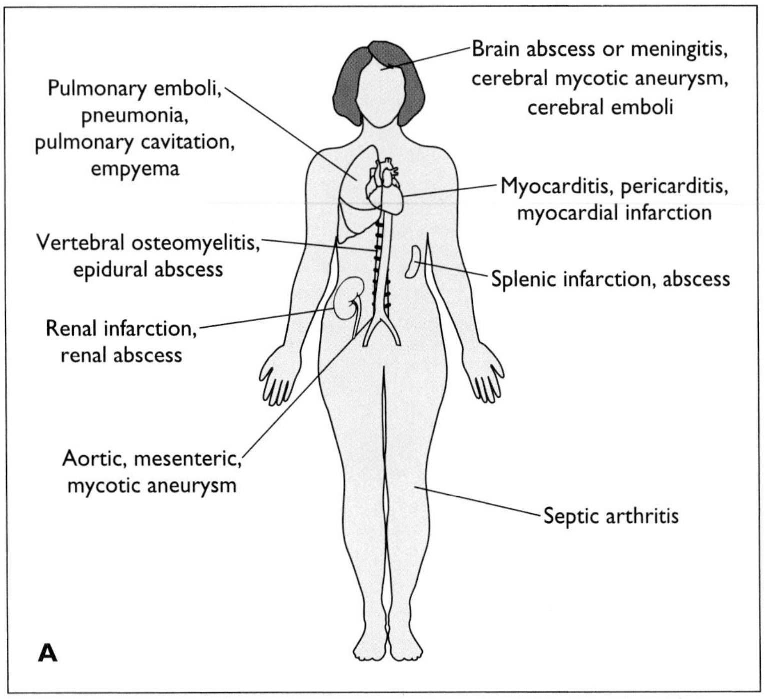

Brain abscess or meningitis, cerebral mycotic aneurysm, cerebral emboli
Pulmonary emboli, pneumonia, pulmonary cavitation, empyema
Myocarditis, pericarditis, myocardial infarction
Vertebral osteomyelitis, epidural abscess
Splenic infarction, abscess
Renal infarction, renal abscess
Aortic, mesenteric, mycotic aneurysm
Septic arthritis
A

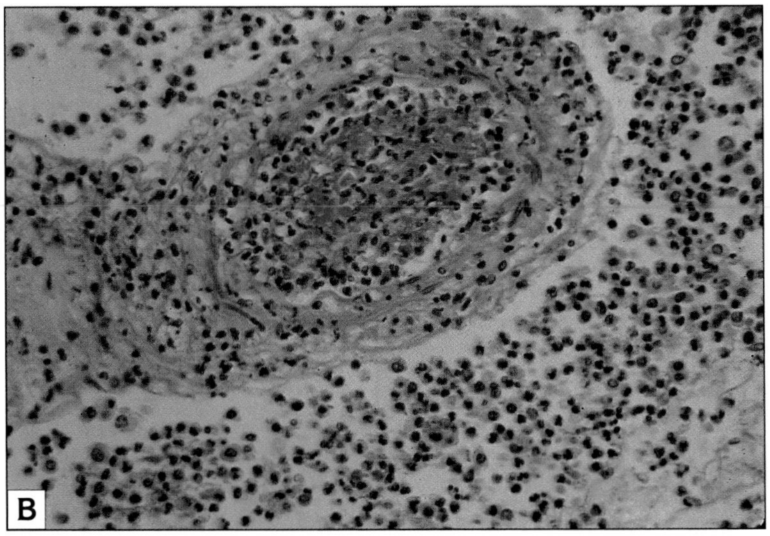

B

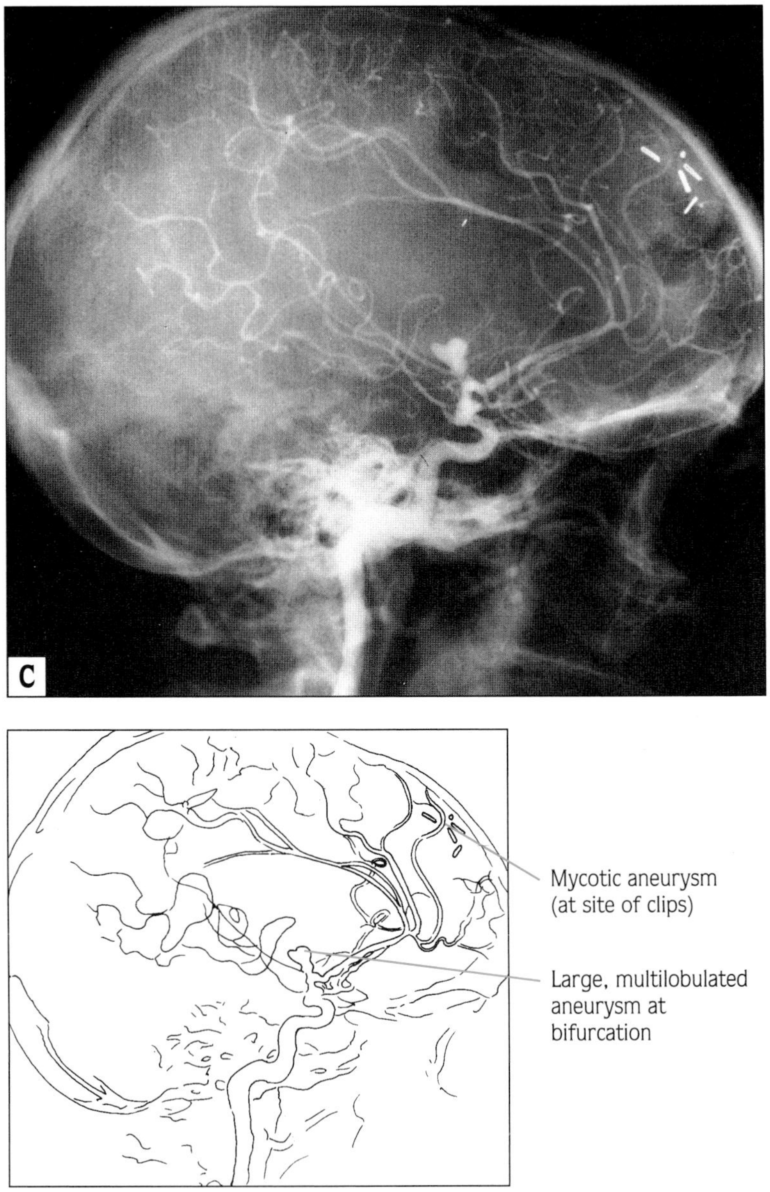

C
Mycotic aneurysm (at site of clips)
Large, multilobulated aneurysm at bifurcation

Figure 6-4 **A**, Sites of embolization and metastatic infection in infective endocarditis. Embolization and/or bacterial seeding may affect virtually any organ; the more common sites are indicated in the figure. Infection at extracardiac sites may be the predominant manifestation, thus obscuring the underlying diagnosis. Infection of extracardiac sites, particularly if blood cultures are positive for organisms that are known to be associated with endocarditis (*eg*, *Staphylococcus aureus*, enterococcus, or viridans streptococci), should prompt further evaluation for the possibility of valvular infection. Metastatic infections may provide an early clue to the bacterial etiology because some organisms are more likely to cause distant infection (*eg*, *S. aureus*) or abscesses (*eg*, *S. aureus* or *Streptococcus milleri*). **B**, Small artery embolus. A septic embolus may lodge in the arterial lumen and obstruct blood flow, leading to vascular insufficiency and infarction. The infarcted tissue may become secondarily infected from bacteria in the embolus. The arterial wall at the site of the embolus may become infected, resulting in a focal vasculitis, extension of infection to perivascular tissues, and weakening and disruption of the vessel wall with hemorrhage. **C**, Cerebral angiogram showing intracerebral mycotic aneurysms. Cerebral mycotic aneurysms typically occur at vessel bifurcations and branch points of small secondary arteries (the site of the clips in the frontal lobe area of this angiogram). Since clipping of the small vessel aneurysm, a larger multilobulated aneurysm has appeared at the bifurcation of the internal carotid artery. (Panel 4C *from* Scheld [1].)

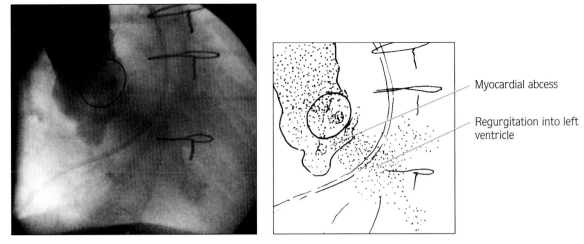

Myocardial abcess

Regurgitation into left ventricle

FIGURE 5-12 Aortic porcine bioprosthetic valve infected by *Staphylococcus epidermidis*. The radiopaque circular structure is part of the sewing ring of a porcine bioprosthetic aortic valve. A supravalvular injection of contrast material has been performed at cardiac catheterization. The contrast media outlines a myocardial abscess (thumbprint area). Furthermore, contrast flows back into the left ventricle during diastole, reflecting aortic paravalvular regurgitation.

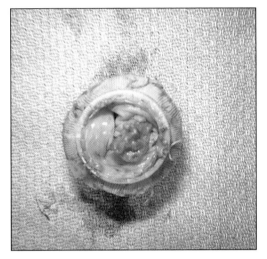

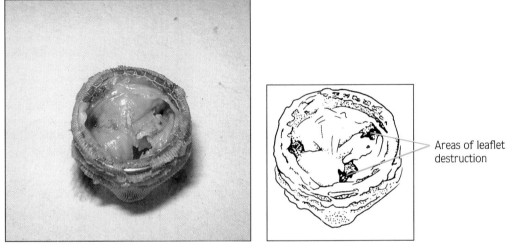

Areas of leaflet destruction

FIGURE 5-13 *Candida parapsilosis* infection of a porcine bioprosthesis. The infection has required removal of the prosthesis from the mitral position, where it had been originally placed. This large bulky vegetation resulted in hemodynamically significant obstruction of the mitral valve orifice. Valve orifice obstruction by vegetations can occur at any valve site; nevertheless, this phenomenon most commonly occurs with mitral site prosthetic valve endocarditis.

FIGURE 5-14 Bioprosthetic valve infected by enterococci. The prosthetic aortic valve endocarditis developed approximately 18 months after valve insertion. The infection only involved the valve leaflets. Although the infection was eradicated by ampicillin-gentamicin antibiotic therapy, the valve was replaced because the destruction of one porcine leaflet caused severe aortic regurgitation and congestive heart failure. The time of onset, microbiology, and pathology are typical of later-onset presentations of community-acquired porcine bioprosthetic valve endocarditis (*see* Figs. 5-3 and 5-6).

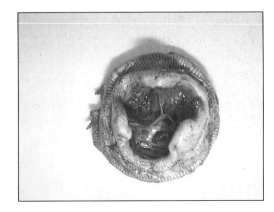

FIGURE 5-15 Porcine valve removed from the mitral position due to uncontrolled *Staphylococcus epidermidis* prosthetic valve endocarditis. A paravalvular abscess was identified at surgery. Vegetations can be seen on the ventricular side of the porcine leaflets. Although paravalvular abscesses complicate porcine valve infection (*see* Fig. 5-12), indicating infection occurring at the interface between the prosthetic valve ring and the native tissue of the valve annulus, infection at this interface is more typical for endocarditis involving mechanical valves. In contrast, infection involving bioprosthetic valves, especially infection that occurs more than 1 year after surgery, is more likely to be engrafted on the porcine leaflets themselves (*see* Figs. 5-13 and 5-14).

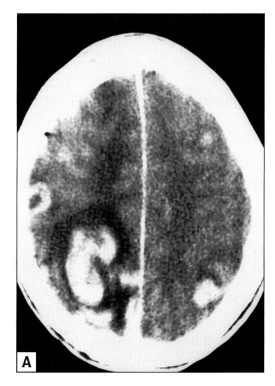

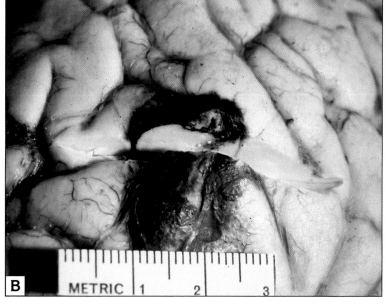

FIGURE 6-5 A, Computed tomographic brain scan showing multiple peripheral, nodular, enhancing lesions due to mycotic aneurysms. The scan also shows a large right posterior parietal intraparenchymal hemorrhage and surrounding edema from aneurysmal rupture. **B,** Brain specimen with a ruptured cerebral mycotic aneurysm. Mycotic aneurysms of cerebral vessels probably are the result of septic embolization leading to endothelial necrosis and vasculitis at the site of occlusion. An aneurysm may be asymptomatic or may manifest as headache and stiff neck, focal neurologic deficit, or intracranial hemorrhage. The diagnosis should be suspected if blood is detected by computed tomographic scan or if cerebrospinal fluid is xanthochromic or contains red blood cells. A hemorrhagic stroke due to septic embolization can produce a similar picture, and angiography is often required to make a definitive diagnosis. Aneurysms that have bled are at high risk for rebleeding and should be surgically removed if possible. Cerebral mycotic aneurysms may regress with appropriate antimicrobial therapy for endocarditis. Medical therapy is appropriate if the aneurysm is small and asymptomatic, if the aneurysm is surgically inaccessible, or if extensive neurologic damage is likely to result from its removal. (Panel 5A *courtesy of* V. McCormack, MD.)

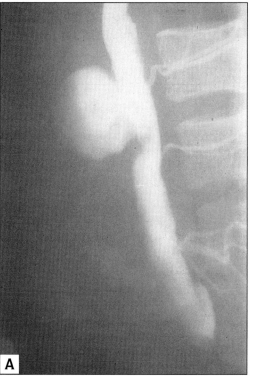

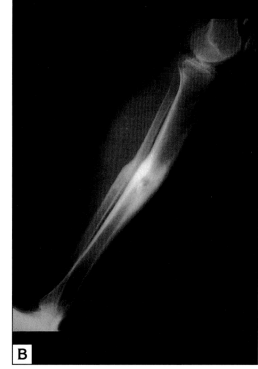

FIGURE 6-6 A, Arteriogram demonstrating an abdominal aortic mycotic aneurysm in a patient with *Staphylococcus aureus* endocarditis. Mycotic aneurysms also may occur at other sites outside the central nervous system. These aneurysms probably result from septic embolization of vasa vasorum, leading to a focal vasculitis and subsequent extension of infection to the large vessel wall. Alternatively, sites of endothelial injury and disruption (*eg,* an arteriosclerotic plaque) may become colonized and infected. Abdominal pain, occult blood loss, hypotension, gastrointestinal hemorrhage, and embolization of the vascular bed supplied by the infected artery are signs and symptoms suggestive of mycotic arterial aneurysms. Mycotic aneurysm of the aorta or other noncerebral arteries should be surgically excised to achieve a cure and to prevent catastrophic hemorrhage. **B,** Plain radiograph of the lower extremity shows soft-tissue swelling in the popliteal region. The patient had staphylococcal endocarditis and developed a mycotic aneurysm of the peroneal artery. (*continued*)

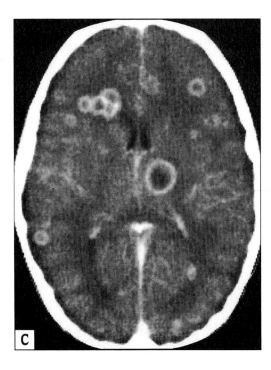

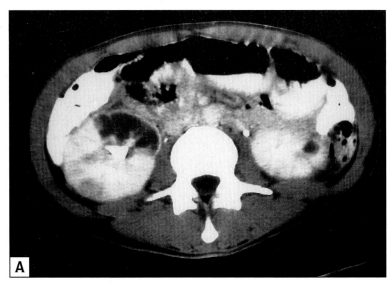

FIGURE 6-6 (*continued*) **C**, Contrast-enhanced computed tomographic scan of brain showing multiple brain abscesses. Brain abscess is among the least-common complications of infective endocarditis and is estimated to occur in less than 5% of cases. Likewise, underlying endocarditis is present in less than 5% of cases of brain abscess. Although the cause of the brain abscesses in this case was not identified, these ring-enhancing lesions are typical of those complicating endocarditis, in that they tend to be multiple, reflecting a vascular route of dissemination. *Staphylococcus aureus* and streptococci are usually isolated from brain abscesses associated with endocarditis. Signs and symptoms suggestive of brain abscess reflect both the focal nature of the disease and the increased intracranial pressure and include fever, headaches, nausea, vomiting, altered mental status, seizures, papilledema, and focal neurologic deficits. (Panel 6B *courtesy of* O.M. Korzeniowski, MD; panel 6C *from* Iagarashi [2]; with permission.)

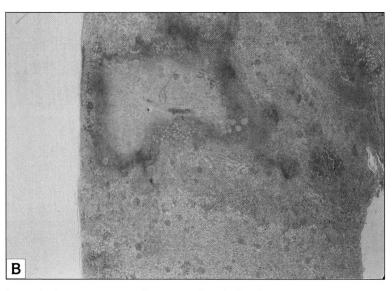

FIGURE 6-7 A, Abdominal computed tomographic scan demonstrating large peripheral wedge-shaped area of low attenuation of the right kidney extending to the renal cortex. These findings indicate renal infarction due to septic embolization of the kidney. Embolization of renal arteries is very common due to the large volume of renal blood flow, but it is asymptomatic unless emboli are large and renal infarction is present. Flank pain, hematuria, pyuria, and bacteriuria are common features of embolization to renal arteries. Renal insufficiency as a result of embolization alone, however, is uncommon. **B**, Microscopic section through a renal infarction with early abscess formation (hematoxylin-eosin stain). The central clearing is indicative of avascular necrosis. Early abscess formation is evidenced by the dense, polymorphonuclear infiltration surrounding the infarct. (Panel 7A *courtesy of* V. McCormack, MD.)

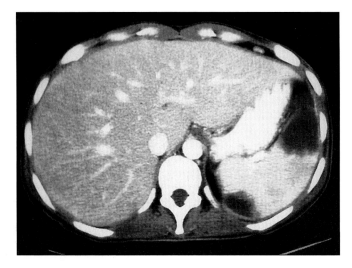

FIGURE 6-8 Abdominal computed tomographic scan demonstrating splenic infarction and abscess in a patient with tricuspid valve *Staphylococcus aureus* endocarditis and a patent foramen ovale. Multiple peripheral wedge-shaped low-attenuation defects of the spleen are present. Although systemic embolization is usually a complication of endocarditis involving aortic or mitral valves, it is occasionally seen in patients with so-called right-sided endocarditis, who typically have infection limited to the tricuspid valve (the pulmonic valve is rarely involved in endocarditis). Emboli originating from the tricuspid valve may enter the systemic arterial circulation via a right-to-left shunt. The shunt may be a permanent congenital defect, or it may be a transiently patent foramen ovale that has opened due to elevated right-sided pressures with right ventricular failure from tricuspid valve dysfunction. Differentiation of splenic infarct from abscess can be difficult radiographically, but an abscess should be suspected when there is unexplained persistent fever, particularly with accompanying bacteremia. Splenic abscess is best managed by drainage, either surgically or percutaneously using computed tomography or sonographic guidance. (*Courtesy of* V. McCormack, MD.)

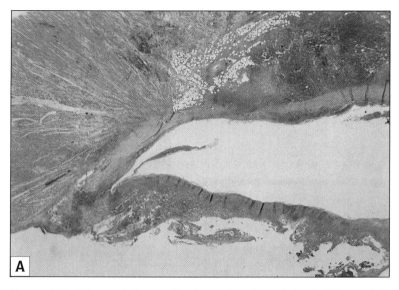

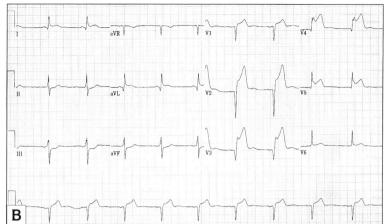

FIGURE 6-9 Myocardial complications of endocarditis. **A,** Myocarditis may result from direct extension of infection from the valve (usually aortic) and perivalvular structures (*eg,* perivalvular abscess or sinus of Valsalva aneurysm) to adjacent myocardial tissues. Extension to the intraventricular septum may lead to conduction abnormalities or formation of a left-to-right shunt. Septic microembolization of the coronary bed also may produce myocarditis. Infection may extend to involve the pericardium. **B,** Electrocardiogram of acute myocardial infarction secondary to occlusion of the left anterior descending coronary artery. Embolization of the coronary circulation, often in association with aortic valve endocarditis, may cause occlusion of a major coronary artery producing signs and symptoms of myocardial infarction. (Panel 9B *courtesy of* T. Evans, MD.)

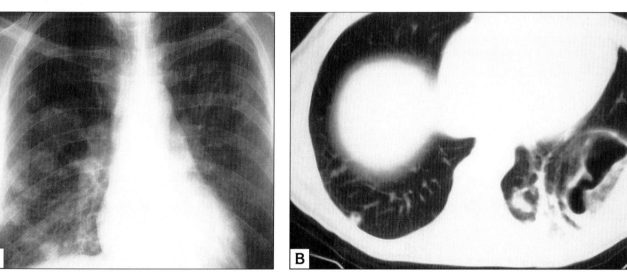

FIGURE 6-10 **A** and **B,** Septic pulmonary embolization in a patient with *Staphylococcus aureus* tricuspid valve endocarditis. Findings are demonstrated by chest radiograph (*panel 10A*) and computed tomographic scan (*panel 10B*). Approximately three quarters of patients with tricuspid valve endocarditis will present with clinical signs and symptoms of pulmonary embolism or pneumonia. Radiographically, septic pulmonary emboli appear as multiple nodular, peripheral, and often cavitary lesions (*panel 10B*). The appearance may also be that of a bacterial pneumonia with consolidation of one or more lobes. Signs of pleural effusions, such as loss of the costophrenic angle and layering in decubitus film, also may be present. These effusions usually are sterile and sympathetic. However, in patients with recurrent or persistent fevers and large pleural effusions, thoracentesis is recommended to exclude the possibility of pleural infection. Radiographic findings may continue to evolve early during the clinical course even with appropriate therapy. (*Courtesy of* V. McCormack, MD.)

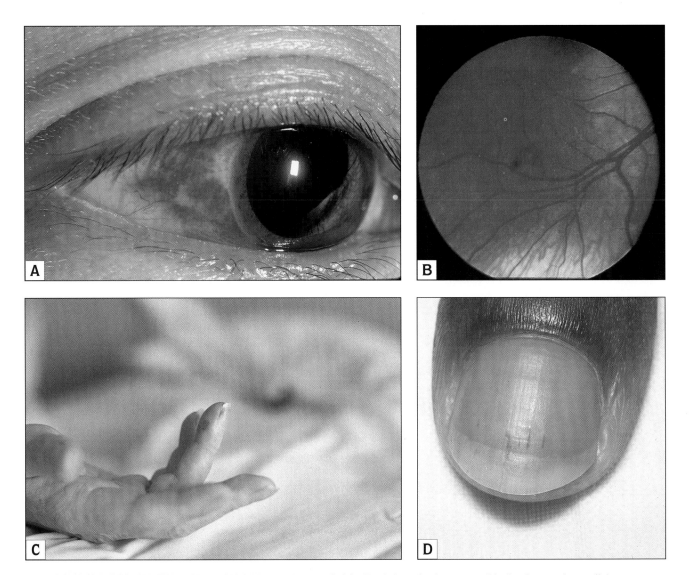

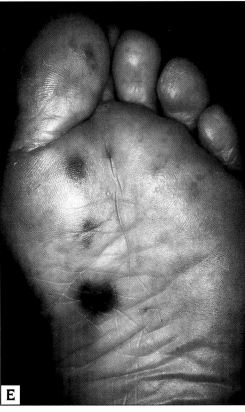

FIGURE 6-11 Peripheral stigmata of infective endocarditis.
A, Conjunctival petechiae and hemorrhage. **B**, Roth spot.
C, Osler node and a splinter hemorrhage. **D**, Splinter hemorrhages. **E**, Janeway lesions. Originally attributed to immune-
complex mediated vasculitis, these phenomena probably are
initiated by microembolization. Their presence is indicative of
infection of the aortic or mitral valve or the tricuspid valve with a
right-to-left shunt. None are pathognomonic of endocarditis. The
Roth spot (*panel 11B*), which is a small hemorrhagic lesion with
central pallor, may be seen in conditions associated with vasculitis
(*eg*, systemic lupus erythematosus) and has been reported in
patients with leukemia. Osler nodes (*panel 11C*), which are
painful, peripheral, nodular hemorrhagic or erythematous lesions
of the distal phalanges, may also be seen in systemic vasculitides.
Janeway lesions (*panel 11E*) are similar in appearance and pathogenesis to Osler nodes, but Janeway lesions are located on the
palms and soles, tend not to be painful, and can be transient. They
also may ulcerate or become hemorrhagic. Splinter hemorrhages
(*panel 11D*) are linear hemorrhages, which are similar to peripheral petechiae but occur in the distal nail bed. These hemorrhages
are nonspecific and may be seen with trauma. (Panels 11A and
11B *courtesy of* D. Char, MD; panel 11E *from* Sande and Strausbaugh [3]; with permission.)

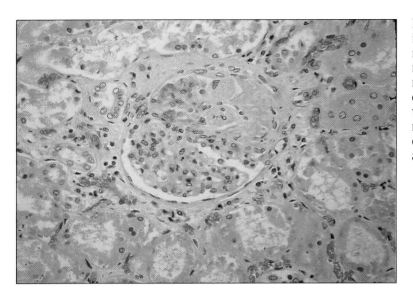

FIGURE 6-12 Focal glomerulonephritis. This lesion is due to immune complex deposition. Nephritis with renal failure, which may be rapidly progressive, may be a presenting feature. Hallmarks are red cell casts in the urinary sediment and hypocomplementemia. Other potentially reversible causes of azotemia with endocarditis that should be considered are hypovolemia, acute tubular necrosis from sepsis, drug toxicity, and heart failure with renal hypoperfusion from low cardiac output. Renal insufficiency due to glomerulonephritis usually resolves with appropriate antimicrobial therapy of the endocarditis.

REFERENCES

1. Scheld WM: Infective endocarditis. In *Atlas of Infectious Diseases*, vol 8: External Manifestations of Systemic Diseases. Edited by Mandell GL, Fekety R. Philadelphia: Current Medicine; 1996.

2. Igarashi M: Multiple brain abscesses. *N Engl J Med* 1993, 329:1083.

3. Sande MA, Strausbaugh LJ: Infective endocarditis. In *Current Concepts of Infectious Diseases*. Edited by Hook EW, Mandell GL, Gwaltney JM Jr, *et al.* New York: Wiley; 1977:60.

SELECTED BIBLIOGRAPHY

Chambers HF, Korzeniowski OM, Sande MA, and the National Collaborative Endocarditis Study Group: *Staphylococcus aureus* endocarditis: Clinical manifestations in addicts and nonaddicts. *Medicine* 1983, 62:170–177.

Mansur AJ, Grinberg M, DaLuz PL, Bellotti G: The complications of infective endocarditis: A reappraisal in the 1980s. *Arch Intern Med* 1992, 152:2428–2432.

Pruit AA, Rubin RHJ, Karchmer AW, *et al.*: Neurologic complications of infective endocarditis. *Medicine* 1978, 57:329–343.

Scheld WM, Sande MA: Endocarditis and intravascular infections. In *Principles and Practice of Infectious Diseases*, 4th ed. Edited by Mandell GL, Bennett JE, Dolin R. New York: Churchill Livingstone; 1995:740–783.

Steckelberg JM, Murphy JG, Ballard D, *et al.*: Emboli in infective endocarditis: The prognostic value of echocardiography. *Ann Intern Med* 1991, 114:635–640.

Tunkel AR, Kaye D: Neurologic complications of infective endocarditis. *Neurol Clin* 1993, 11:419–440.

CHAPTER 7

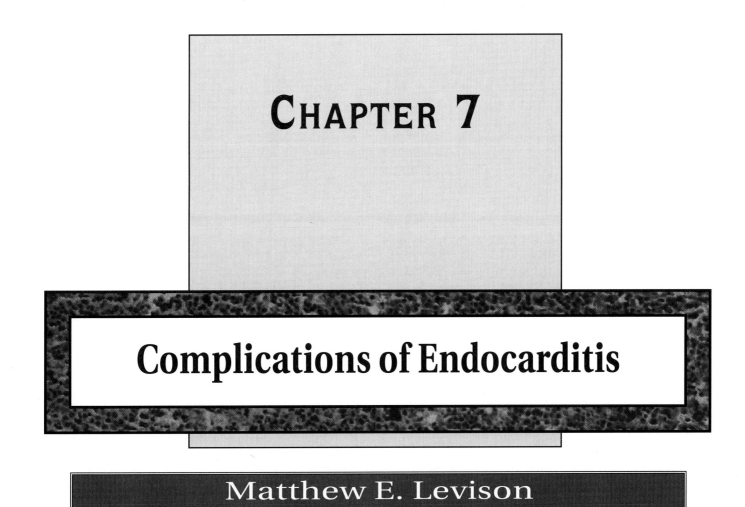

Complications of Endocarditis

Matthew E. Levison

COMPLICATIONS OF INFECTIVE ENDOCARDITIS include those complications that involve the cardiac valves themselves and those that affect extravalvular sites. These complications are the result of either 1) the valvular infection itself, 2) embolization of fragments of the infected vegetation that results in bland or suppurative infarcts of distal organs, 3) suppurative foci on the basis of hematogenous spread of infection, or 4) immunologic response to the infection in the form of immune complex vasculitis.

Valvular complications include 1) valvular insufficiency due to destruction or distortion of the valve and its supporting structures; 2) valvular stenosis due to large, bulky vegetations; and 3) persistent or relapsing infection with the same organism or recurrent infection with a new organism. Myocardial complications include valve ring abscess that extends from the valve ring into the myocardium. Periannular extension occurs more frequently with aortic than mitral or tricuspid native valve infection and more frequently with prosthetic than native valve infection. Valve ring abscess can lead to 1) persistent fever, despite appropriate antimicrobial therapy; 2) heart block as a result of destruction of conduction pathways in the area of the atrioventricular node and bundle of His in the upper interventricular septum; 3) pericarditis or hemopericardium as a result of burrowing abscesses into the pericardium; or 4) shunts between cardiac chambers or between the heart and aorta as a result of burrowing abscesses into other cardiac chambers or aorta.

Additional myocardial complications include congestive heart failure (CHF) as a result of valvular dysfunction, myocardial infarction from coronary artery embolization, myocardial abscess as a consequence of bacteremia, or diffuse myocarditis possibly as a consequence of immune-complex vasculitis. CHF is the most common complication of endocarditis, developing in approximately 60% of patients as a consequence of valvular or myocardial involvement or possibly preceding the onset of endocarditis as a consequence of the underlying cardiac lesion. CHF may progress gradually either during the course of antimicrobial therapy or in the months after its completion, or it may develop dramatically, *eg*, in patients with acute *Staphylococcus aureus* endocarditis with the sudden development of an aortic diastolic murmur, the rupture of mitral valve chordae, or sudden shunts created from fistulous tracts. CHF occurs more frequently with left-sided than right-sided endocarditis and more frequently with aortic than mitral involvement.

Extracardiac complications include embolic events that result in infarction of numerous organs, such as the lung in right-sided endocarditis or the brain, spleen, kidneys, bowel, or extremities in left-sided endocarditis; suppurative complications such as abscesses, septic infarcts, and infected mycotic aneurysms; and immunologic reactions to valvular infection such as glomerulonephritis, sterile meningitis or polyarthritis, and a variety of vascular phenomena (*eg*, mucocutaneous petechiae, splinter hemorrhages, Roth spots, and Osler nodes). Systemic embolization, often a devastating complication when it involves the cerebral circulation, occurs in approximately 20% to 40% of patients with left-sided endocarditis. Embolization occurs more frequently with mitral than aortic valve vegetations and more frequently with anterior than posterior mitral leaflet vegetations. Frank cerebral abscess is rare, except in cases of *S. aureus* endocarditis, when it occurs in 1% to 5% of patients. Septic pulmonary emboli commonly occur in patients with right-sided endocarditis. On chest radiographs, these emboli appear as multiple round infiltrates, which may undergo cavitation or be complicated by empyema. Emboli can occur at any time during the course of illness, even after completion of an otherwise successful course of antibiotic therapy—although the frequency of embolization decreases as the vegetation heals. Failure of the vegetation to stabilize or diminish in size during appropriate antimicrobial therapy by transesophageal echocardiography may predict subsequent embolization.

Mycotic aneurysms are an unusual, but important, complication of endocarditis. Mycotic aneurysms are commonly asymptomatic but can become clinically evident in 3% to 5% of patients, even months or years after completion of successful therapy. These aneurysms characteristically develop at arterial bifurcations, *eg*, in the middle cerebral, splenic, superior mesenteric, pulmonary, coronary, and extremity arteries; the abdominal aorta; and sinus of Valsalva. In a patient with endocarditis, unremitting headache, visual disturbance, or cranial nerve palsy is suggestive of an impending rupture of a cerebral mycotic aneurysm. Signs of blood loss at any site in a patient with endocarditis should suggest rupture of a mycotic aneurysm once the aneurysm has enlarged beyond a critical size, probably about 1 cm in diameter. The development of clinically apparent splenomegaly and many of the various nonsuppurative peripheral vascular phenomena is related to the duration of illness prior to presentation. The frequency of these clinical manifestations (<50%) is currently less than that in the past as a result of shorter durations of illness prior to initiation of antimicrobial therapy.

Complications of endocarditis

Valvular	Myocardial	Extracardiac
Valvular regurgitation	Valve ring abscess	Emboli
Valvular stenosis	Heart failure	Mycotic aneurysms (aorta, renal, intracranial,
Relapsing valvular infection	Myocardial abscesses and rupture	visceral, peripheral arteries)
(same organism)	Myocardial conduction defects	Metastatic infection (abscesses, septic infarcts)
Persistent valvular infection	Myocardial infarction	Central nervous system abnormalities
(same organism)	Myocarditis	Mucocutaneous abnormalities
Increased risk of recurrent infection	Pericarditis	Renal failure, hematuria
(new organism)		

FIGURE 7-1 Complications of endocarditis. (*Adapted from* Steckelberg *et al.* [1].)

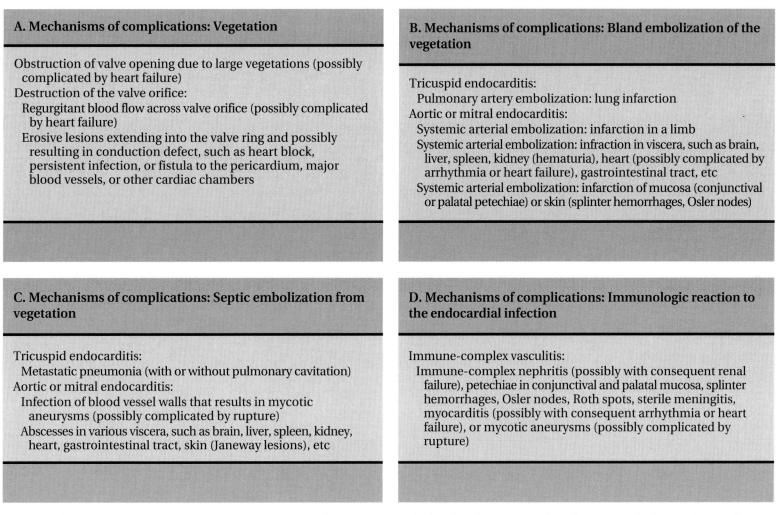

A. Mechanisms of complications: Vegetation

Obstruction of valve opening due to large vegetations (possibly complicated by heart failure)
Destruction of the valve orifice:
Regurgitant blood flow across valve orifice (possibly complicated by heart failure)
Erosive lesions extending into the valve ring and possibly resulting in conduction defect, such as heart block, persistent infection, or fistula to the pericardium, major blood vessels, or other cardiac chambers

B. Mechanisms of complications: Bland embolization of the vegetation

Tricuspid endocarditis:
Pulmonary artery embolization: lung infarction
Aortic or mitral endocarditis:
Systemic arterial embolization: infarction in a limb
Systemic arterial embolization: infraction in viscera, such as brain, liver, spleen, kidney (hematuria), heart (possibly complicated by arrhythmia or heart failure), gastrointestinal tract, etc
Systemic arterial embolization: infarction of mucosa (conjunctival or palatal petechiae) or skin (splinter hemorrhages, Osler nodes)

C. Mechanisms of complications: Septic embolization from vegetation

Tricuspid endocarditis:
Metastatic pneumonia (with or without pulmonary cavitation)
Aortic or mitral endocarditis:
Infection of blood vessel walls that results in mycotic aneurysms (possibly complicated by rupture)
Abscesses in various viscera, such as brain, liver, spleen, kidney, heart, gastrointestinal tract, skin (Janeway lesions), etc

D. Mechanisms of complications: Immunologic reaction to the endocardial infection

Immune-complex vasculitis:
Immune-complex nephritis (possibly with consequent renal failure), petechiae in conjunctival and palatal mucosa, splinter hemorrhages, Osler nodes, Roth spots, sterile meningitis, myocarditis (possibly with consequent arrhythmia or heart failure), or mycotic aneurysms (possibly complicated by rupture)

FIGURE 7-2 Mechanisms of complications in infective endocarditis. **A**, Vegetation. **B**, Bland embolization of the vegetation. **C**, Septic embolization from vegetation. **D**, Immunologic reaction to the endocardial infection.

Indications for surgery (cardiac and noncardiac) in infective endocarditis

Heart failure secondary to severe valvular incompetence

Multiple systemic embolic events despite antibiotic therapy for at least 2 wk
  Prophylactic valve replacement to prevent embolization of vegetations that are
  detected by echocardiography is generally not indicated.

Valve ring abscesses
  These intracardiac sites of suppuration, which may be complicated by conduction
  defects, persistent bacteremia, and fistulae to major vessel, cardiac chamber, or
  pericardium, are generally refractory to medical therapy alone.

Persistent bacteremia despite at least 2 wk of appropriate antibiotic therapy
  Staphylococcus aureus endocarditis, especially if treated with vancomycin, may be
  associated with persistent bacteremia for 1–2 wk, or longer, that eventually responds
  to appropriate antimicrobial therapy. Extracardiac sites of infection, such as visceral
  abscesses, should be excluded as potential sources of persistent bacteremia.

Endocarditis due to microorganisms resistant to bactericidal agents, *eg*, multidrug-
  resistant gram-negative bacilli, multidrug-resistant enterococci, *Brucella* spp,
  Coxiella burnetii

Fungal endocarditis
  Fungal endocarditis is generally refractory to medical therapy alone.

Mycotic aneurysms
  Intracranial mycotic aneurysms that are enlarging or bleeding
    Complaints of severe, unremitting, localized headache; focal neurologic events;
    "sterile" meningitis; or visual field defects may result from an enlarging or bleeding
    mycotic aneurysm and should be evaluated by cerebral angiography. Computed
    tomography, with or without contrast, likely will detect the intracerebral hemor-
    rhage but is inadequate to confirm a diagnosis of intracranial aneurysm itself.
    Conventional four-vessel angiography also has been reported to be more sensitive
    than magnetic resonance angiography to detect intracranial aneurysms [2].
  All extracranial mycotic aneurysms
    Appearance of a pulsatile mass in an extremity or bleeding at any site, which may be
    associated with pain at the site or shock, in a patient with endocarditis should
    suggest a possible mycotic aneurysm and the diagnosis confirmed by angiography.

FIGURE 7-3 Indications for surgery (cardiac and noncardiac) in infective endocarditis. Although some complications respond to antimicrobial therapy alone, others require surgical intervention as well.

Cure rates by type of valve and organism

Native valve endocarditis	
Viridans streptococci	>90%
Nonviridans streptococci	36%–50%
Enterococci	75%–90%
Staphylococcus aureus	60%–75%
Tricuspid valve	>95%
Gram-negative enteric bacilli	75%–83%
Fungi	50%
Prosthetic valve endocarditis	50%
Coagulase-negative staphylococci	80%
S. aureus	15%

FIGURE 7-4 Overall cure rates for infective endocarditis by type of valve and organism. (*Adapted from* Gold [3].)

VASCULAR COMPLICATIONS

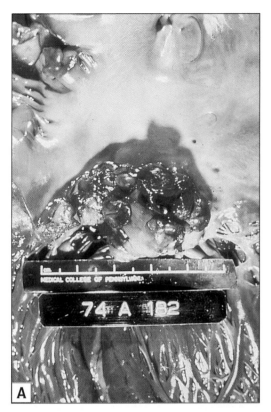

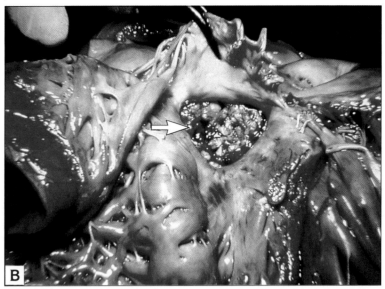

FIGURE 7-5 A, Bulky valvular vegetations on a native valve in a patient with *Staphylococcus epidermidis* endocarditis. **B**, Large valvular vegetations on a prosthetic valve in a patient with candidal endocarditis. The large vegetations (*arrow*) in endocarditis due to fungal or *Haemophilus* species tend to be friable and lead to frequent embolic occlusions of relatively large blood vessels and bland or septic infarcts of numerous organs. (Panel 5B *courtesy of* O.M. Korzeniowski, MD.)

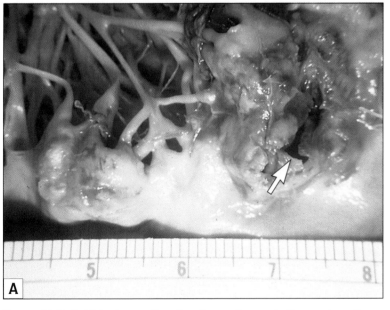

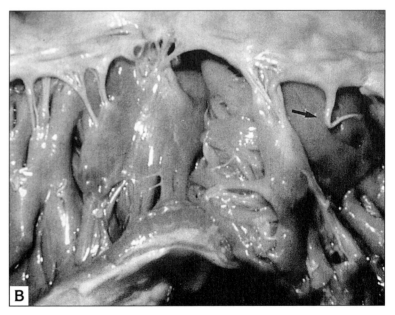

FIGURE 7-6 A, Valvular perforation (*arrow*) seen in the center of one of two granular vegetations. **B**, Mitral valve with ruptured chordae (*arrow*) in a patient with infective endocarditis. Destructive vegetative lesions can lead to valvular regurgitation and congestive heart failure. These mitral valves, which are retracted, have thickened edges, and are rolled with fused, shortened chordae, are characteristic of rheumatic heart disease. (*From* Livornese and Korzeniowski [4]; with permission.)

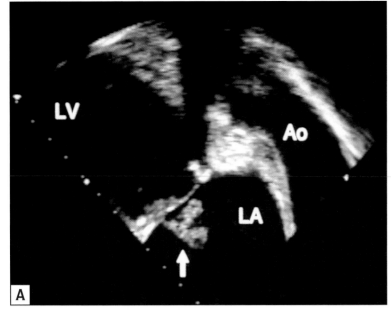

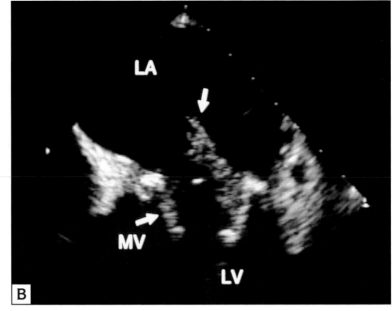

FIGURE 7-7 Lesions of infective endocarditis. The enhanced image resolution afforded by high-frequency transesophageal echocardiographic (TEE) transducers allows for better identification of vegetations in patients with infective endocarditis as compared with transthoracic echocardiography [5]. **A**, TEE long-axis view of a large vegetation (*arrow*) on a Carpentier-Edwards bioprosthesis. **B**, TEE horizontal image of the same vegetation (*arrows*). Vegetation size, extent, mobility, and texture have all been shown to be univariate predictors of complications in endocarditis. Ao—aorta; LA—left atrium; LV—left ventricle; MV—mitral valve. (*From* Nishan *et al.* [6].)

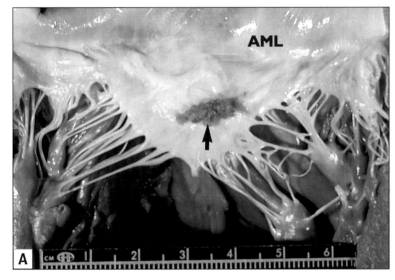

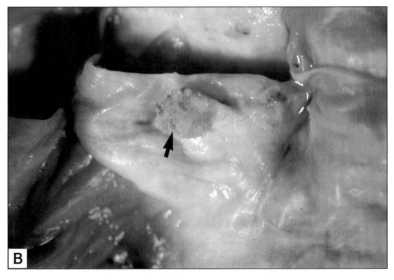

FIGURE 7-8 Endocarditis. **A**, Marantic endocarditis (nonbacterial thrombotic endocarditis). Marantic endocarditis usually occurs in patients with an underlying chronic inflammatory condition or malignancy. This mitral valve shows nonbacterial thrombotic endocarditis (*arrow*) on the anterior mitral leaflet (AML) in a patient who initially survived injuries incurred in a motor vehicle accident but died 7 days after injury. **B**, Aortic valve shows a 0.5-cm papillary fibroelastoma (*arrow*) that echocardiographically can be mistaken for bacterial endocarditis. (*From* Virmani *et al.* [7].)

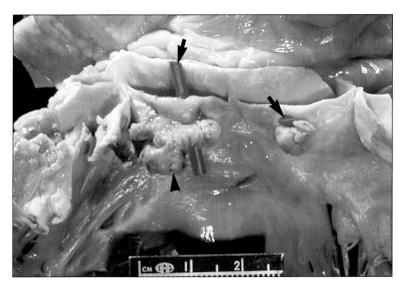

FIGURE 7-9 Infective endocarditis. This infection usually occurs on congenitally malformed valves, on valves with acquired disease, or on normal valves in intravenous drug abusers or immunocompromised patients. However, the incidence of infective endocarditis on anatomically normal heart valves is increasing. This aortic valve shows large friable vegetations of infective endocarditis (*arrowhead*) caused by *Staphylococcus aureus* in a man aged 62 years with a normal tricuspid aortic valve. The *left arrow* denotes a probe through the perforation. The *right arrow* denotes another perforation. (*From* Johnson [8]; with permission.)

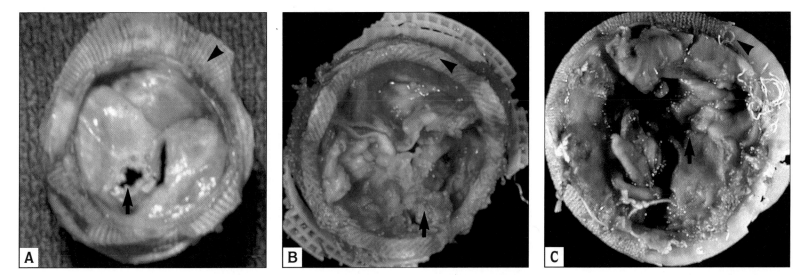

FIGURE 7-10 Bioprosthetic valve, endocarditis. **A,** Type III tear (*arrow*) in a Hancock valve with infective endocarditis. Endocarditis is a potentially disastrous complication of valve replacement. In bioprosthetic valves, it takes one of two forms: infection of valve leaflet and sewing ring abscess; in this example, the infection is localized to the leaflet. *Arrowhead* denotes stent. **B,** Porcine valve viewed from aortic aspect. Note destruction of valve leaflets by infectious vegetation (*arrow*). The infectious agent was *Staphylococcus epidermidis*; the valve was moved 1 month after insertion. Endocarditis occurs at a rate of about 5% at 5 years, and up to five times this rate in patients originally operated for endocarditis. Early infections are usually secondary to perioperative contaminants, whereas infections after 60 days result from bacteremic seeding. *Arrowhead* denotes cloth-covered stent. **C,** A woman aged 45 years had severe mitral valve prolapse treated with mitral valve replacement. Clinical symptoms of endocarditis and congestive failure occurred 2.5 years later. The figure demonstrates a Carpentier-Edwards valve infected by *Staphylococcus aureus*, with cuspal tissue destroyed by vegetation (*arrow*). Staphylococci are extremely destructive to bioprosthetic tissues and are the most common cause of infections involving either mechanical or bioprosthetic valves. *Arrowhead* denotes stent. (*From* Virmani *et al.* [7].)

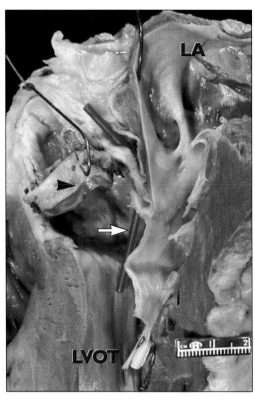

FIGURE 7-11
Healed endocarditis. A drug addict aged 34 years with recurrent bacterial endocarditis and aortic valve replacement died of narcotic intoxication. A long-axis cut through the heart demonstrates the aortic outflow, porcine valve in aortic position. A healed ring abscess (a colored probe [*arrow*]) is present, demonstrating the perivalvular leak. No active endocarditis was present on histologic examination. Perivalvular leaks can be a result in noninfectious tissue retraction, incomplete surgical seating, or endocarditis. *Arrowhead* denotes prosthetic valve. LA—left atrium; LVOT—left ventricular outflow tract. (*From* Virmani *et al.* [7].)

FIGURE 7-12 A male intravenous drug abuser aged 28 years with a history of recurrent fever and multiple admissions for *Staphylococcus aureus* sepsis. The edge of the tricuspid valve has been eroded (*arrow*) and a portion of the leaflet is absent. The adjacent tricuspid valve shows bulky and friable bacterial vegetations (*arrowhead*). (*From* Virmani *et al.* [7].)

MYOCARDIAL COMPLICATIONS

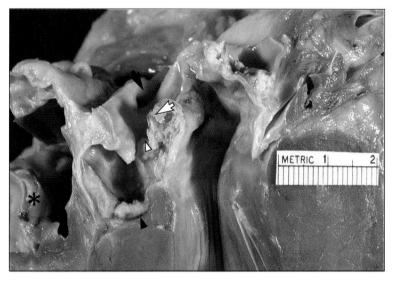

FIGURE 7-13 A bicuspid stenotic valve shows a ring abscess (*black arrowhead*) located in the sinus of Valsalva (*white arrowhead*) with extension into the myocardium in a man aged 58 years with recurrent fever. The organism was *Streptococcus bovis*. Thickened and calcified anterior and posterior aortic valve leaflets are denoted by the *black* and *white arrows*, respectively. The *asterisk* denotes anterior mitral valve. (*From* Virmani *et al.* [7].)

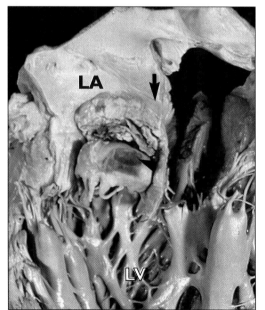

FIGURE 7-14 Infective endocarditis. A woman aged 53 years was admitted with acute myocardial infarction and died 3 days after admission. At autopsy, there was mitral valve prolapse (*arrowhead*) with superimposed friable infectious endocarditis (*arrow*) and embolic obstruction of the left anterior descending coronary artery. LA—left atrium; LV—left ventricle. (*From* Virmani *et al.* [7].)

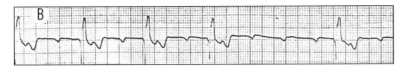

FIGURE 7-15 Electrocardiogram of a patient with viridans-type streptococcal endocarditis. The electrocardiogram illustrates heart block that may be a consequence of either invasion of the conduction system by direct extension of an aortic valve ring abscess or bland or septic emboli to the myocardium. Patients who develop conduction abnormalities should be placed in a hospital bed equipped for continuous monitoring of the cardiac electrical activity. Because development of first-degree heart block or left bundle branch block may herald sudden death, a transvenous pacemaker should be inserted if early conduction abnormalities are progressive. (*Adapted from* Levison [9]; with permission.)

EXTRACARDIAC COMPLICATIONS

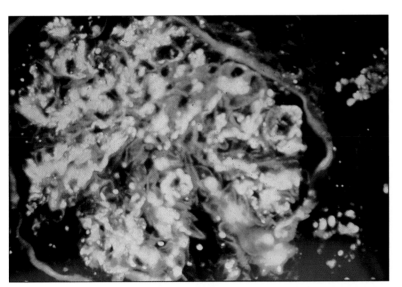

FIGURE 7-16 Microscopic section of renal glomerulus, prepared with fluorescein-tagged antihuman globulin. This section illustrates immune complexes (*yellow-green areas*) composed of immunoglobulin, particularly IgG, and complement. Immune complexes are deposited in the glomerular basement membrane and mesangium. Focal and diffuse varieties of immune complex glomerulonephritis usually occur in long-standing endocarditis and rarely can cause renal failure. Renal failure is more commonly the consequence of congestive heart failure or drug (*eg,* aminoglycoside) toxicity. Immune complex disease may be manifest by other phenomena, such as splinter hemorrhages, Osler nodes, Roth spots, sterile meningitis, myocarditis, or mycotic aneurysm, in these patients. (*From* Krause and Levison [10]; with permission.)

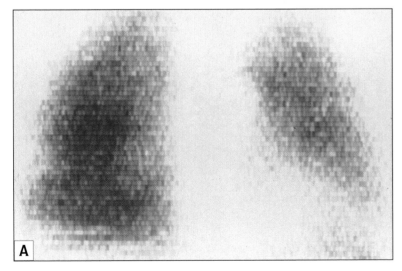

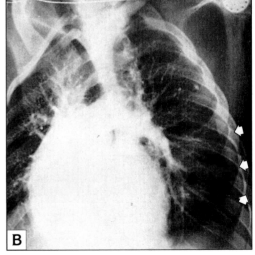

FIGURE 7-17 A, Radionuclide scan of the lungs with technetium-tagged albumen identifying a nonperfused area in the left lower lobe of a patient with tricuspid valve endocarditis who developed fever and left-sided pleuritic chest pain. Right-sided vegetations may embolize to the lungs, and the chest radiograph may or may not show a corresponding parenchymal infiltrate. **B,** Pulmonary angiogram with right atrial injection of the patient whose lung scan is shown in *panel 7A* confirms an obstruction (*black arrow*) of the pulmonary artery to the left lower lobe. The *white arrows* outline the nonperfused area. (*From* Cannon and Cobbs [11]; with permission.)

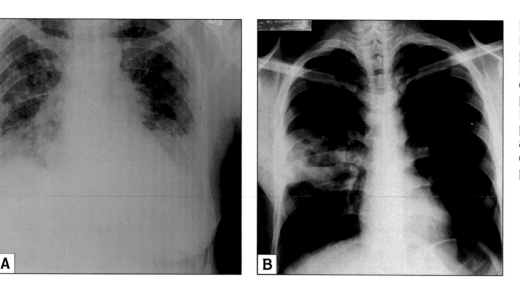

FIGURE 7-18 Radiographs of the chest showing multiple, diffusely scattered infiltrates in patients with tricuspid valve endocarditis. Embolization from right-sided vegetations due to *Staphylococcus aureus* may produce pulmonary alveolar infiltrates and abscesses. Microorganisms such as *S. aureus* tend to produce pulmonary necrosis, which eventually results in a cavity in the lung that may contain an air–fluid level. **A**, Metastatic pneumonia. **B**, Pulmonary abscess.

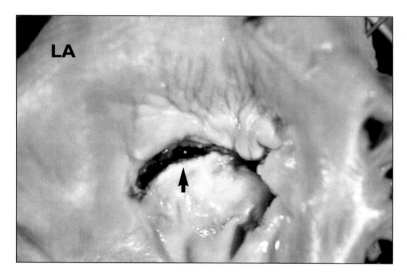

FIGURE 7-19 Infective endocarditis. Atrial view of the mitral valve in a woman aged 56 years with rheumatic mitral stenosis who had sudden onset of transient ischemic attacks. Note the vegetation on the valve margins of a stenotic valve secondary to rheumatic heart disease (*arrow*). LA—left atrium. (*From* Virmani *et al.* [7].)

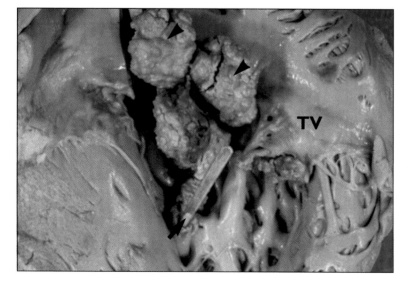

FIGURE 7-20 Foreign body endocarditis. A woman aged 58 years had abdominal pain for 1 year and recurrent pulmonary infarcts beginning 6 months prior to death. At autopsy, a toothpick (*arrow*) protruded through the tricuspid valve (TV) into the right ventricle, and the TV was surrounded by large polypoid vegetations (*arrowheads*). Microscopic examination showed the large vegetations were formed by budding yeast consistent with *Candida*. (*From* Atkinson and Virmani [12]; with permission.)

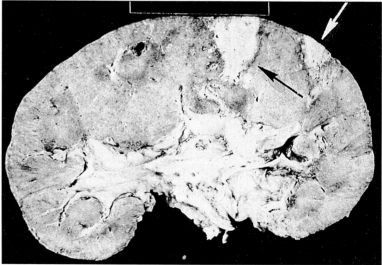

FIGURE 7-21 Hemisected kidney with two pale, wedge-shaped subcapsular infarcts (*arrows*). The infarcts developed as a consequence of embolization to the systemic circulation from left-sided vegetations. (*From* Krause and Levison [10]; with permission.)

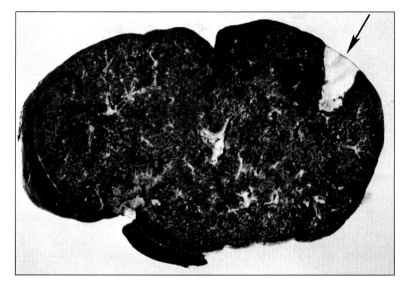

FIGURE 7-22 White, wedge-shaped, subcapsular splenic infarct (*arrow*). This infarct, like the ones shown in Fig. 7-21, also develops as a consequence of embolization to the systemic circulation from left-sided vegetations. (*From* Krause and Levison [10]; with permission.)

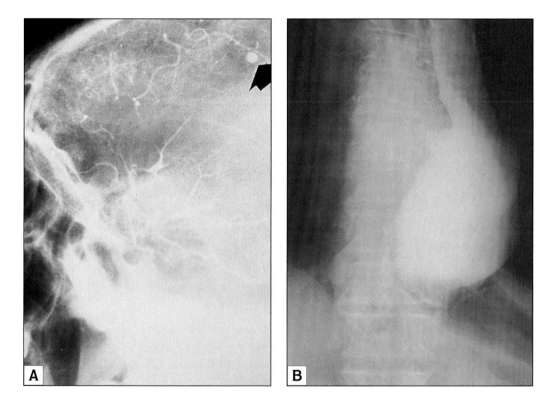

A

B

FIGURE 7-23 A and **B**, Arteriograms showing mycotic aneurysm of a cerebral artery (*arrow; panel 23A*) and of the descending aorta (*panel 23B*). Aneurysms, often called "mycotic" aneurysms, whether associated with bacterial or fungal endocarditis, can develop on an immunologic or septic basis and cause death by rupture, particularly when the cerebral arteries are involved. Mycotic aneurysms may become clinically evident (usually when rupture occurs) at anytime during the course of the infection or even years after otherwise successful antimicrobial therapy. They characteristically develop at points of arterial bifurcation. (*From* Johnson [8]; with permission.)

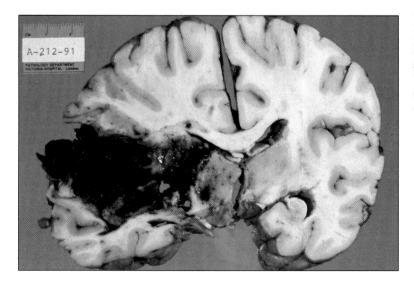

FIGURE 7-24 Gross specimen showing endocarditic intracerebral hemorrhage. Intracerebral hemorrhage occurs in approximately 5% of patients with native-valve bacterial endocarditis, and in some cases it can be predicted by radiologic identification of "mycotic" aneurysms. Most of the cerebrovascular complications of bacterial endocarditis occur early, and the risk of these complications diminishes rapidly as the infection is controlled. (*Courtesy of* D.A. Ramsay, MB, and G.B. Young, MD.)

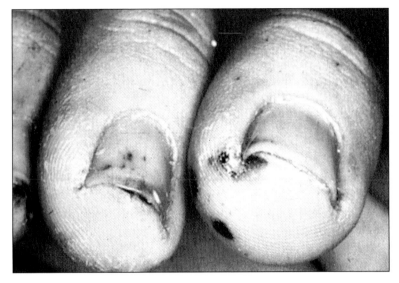

FIGURE 7-25 Splinter and cutaneous hemorrhages in a patient with infective endocarditis. Splinter hemorrhages are observed in 10% to 28% of patients with untreated infective endocarditis. Their origin is probably similar to that of other mucocutaneous hemorrhagic lesions seen in patients with infective endocarditis. Splinter hemorrhages appear as linear reddish streaks under the fingernails or toenails, but they are difficult to distinguish from lesions due to trauma. Splinter hemorrhages that are located more proximally in the nailbed are more likely due to endocarditis. (*From* Korzeniowski and Kaye [13]; with permission.)

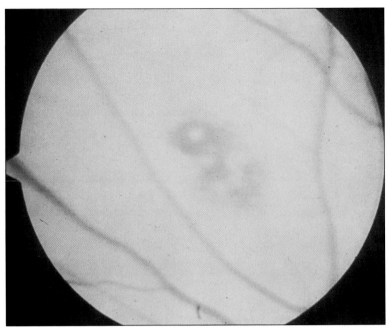

FIGURE 7-26 Roth spots. Roth spots, which are pale-centered, oval hemorrhages in the retina, are observed in less than 5% of patients with endocarditis. They typically are seen in those patients with more long-standing courses, but may also be seen in patients with collagen-vascular and hematologic disorders.

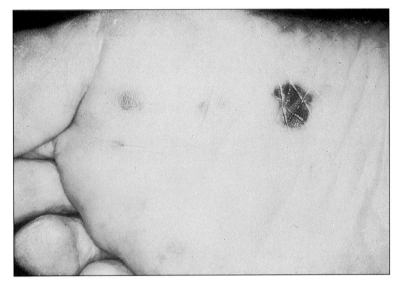

FIGURE 7-27 Janeway lesions. Janeway lesions are uncommon, painless, hemorrhagic, macular lesions on the soles or palms. They typically are seen in patients with acute endocarditis due to *Staphylococcus aureus*. (*From* Bush and Johnson [14]; with permission.)

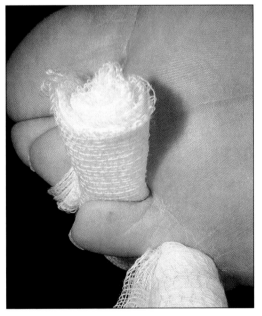

FIGURE 7-28 Osler nodes. Osler nodes are tender, small, subcutaneous nodules that develop in the pulp of the balls of digits of the hands and feet. The overlying skin may be barely discolored or reddened.

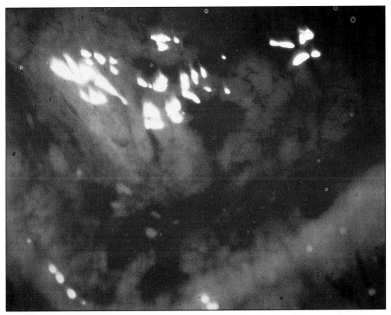

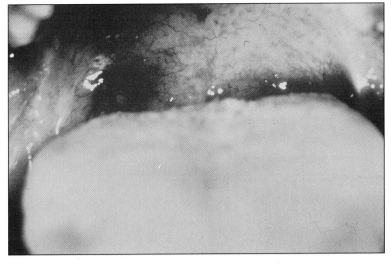

FIGURE 7-30 Palatal petechiae in a patient with infective endocarditis.

FIGURE 7-29 Subconjunctival petechiae in a patient with infective endocarditis. Mucocutaneous lesions of various types occur in about 30% of patients with untreated infective endocarditis, especially if the treatment course has been long-standing, and may continue to appear for weeks following initiation of appropriate antimicrobial therapy without indicating a poor prognosis. Petechiae are the most frequent lesions and may be found in the mouth, pharynx, conjunctivae, or anywhere on the skin. They are small, red, hemorrhagic lesions, which fail to blanch on pressure, are not painful or tender to palpation, and turn brown and fade within several days. They probably develop as a result of vasculitis or microemboli. Mucocutaneous petechiae are not specific for endocarditis, but they may be found in patients with other conditions such as trichinosis, rickettsial infections, sepsis without endocarditis, severe anemia, or thrombocytopenia.

PERSISTENT OR RECURRENT FEVER IN INFECTIVE ENDOCARDITIS

FIGURE 7-31 Causes of persistent or recurrent fever in patients with infective endocarditis.

Causes of persistent or recurrent fever in infective endocarditis

Drug fever
Persistent infection (bacteriologic failure of antimicrobial therapy)
Metastatic abscesses (*eg*, pulmonary, splenic, renal, cerebral, vertebral, etc)
Bland or septic infarcts
Phlebitis at site of intravenous drug administration
Sterile or septic abscesses at sites of intramuscular drug administration
Superinfection of the cardiac valve

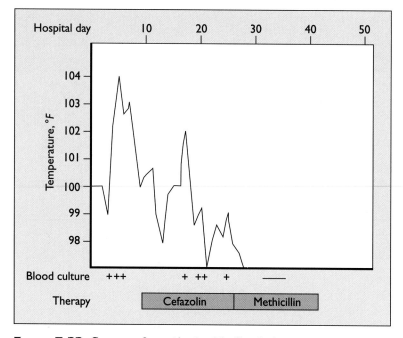

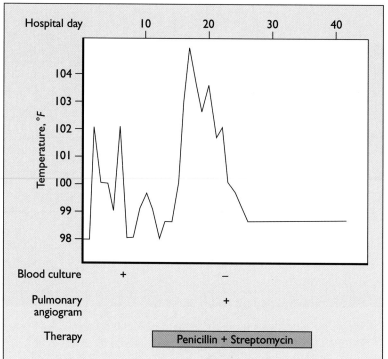

FIGURE 7-32 Course of a patient with *Staphylococcus aureus* endocarditis who had persistent fever for 4 weeks due to persistent bacteremia as a consequence of possible delayed response to or bacteriologic failure of antimicrobial therapy. The average duration of *S. aureus* bacteremia after initiation of nafcillin therapy is 3.4 days. However, prolonged bacteremia and concomitant fever, even of several weeks' duration, may occur in some patients following initiation of therapy with any antimicrobial agents to which the pathogen is susceptible on in vitro testing—but apparently occurs more commonly with vancomycin. The average duration of bacteremia following initiation of vancomycin has been reported to be 9 days. In this case, bacteremia abated within days of switching from cefazolin to methicillin, which suggests that cefazolin may have been at fault, perhaps as a result of cefazolin's greater susceptibility to inactivation by *S. aureus* β-lactamase. On the other hand, cessation of bacteremia once methicillin therapy was started may have been an adventitious event. (*From* Levison [9]; with permission.)

FIGURE 7-33 Course of a patient with tricuspid endocarditis who had recurrent fever due to a pulmonary infarct. Persistent fever is commonly associated with bland or especially septic infarctions that result from embolization of the vegetation. (*From* Levison [9]; with permission.)

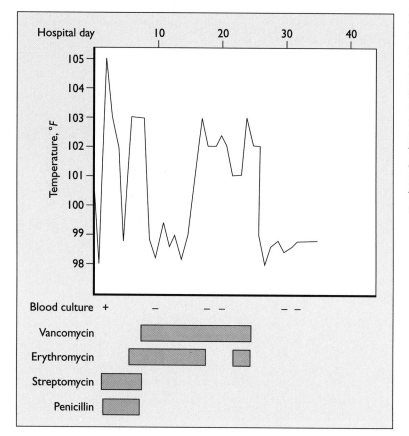

FIGURE 7-34 Course of a patient with *Staphylococcus aureus* endocarditis and persistent fever that abated within days of discontinuation of antimicrobial therapy. Prolonged exposure to the antimicrobial agent itself or certain other drugs such as quinidine or procainamide that the patient with endocarditis may be receiving are common causes of fever complicating the course of treated endocarditis. Fever usually abates within several days of discontinuing the offending drug. Drug fever is not indicative of a poor prognosis, and if unaccompanied by serious adverse drug reactions and tolerable to the patient, it is not in itself a reason to discontinue therapy with the offending drug, as long as the drug has reliable antimicrobial activity and is convenient to use, relatively inexpensive, and otherwise a relatively innocuous agent. (*From* Levison [9]; with permission.)

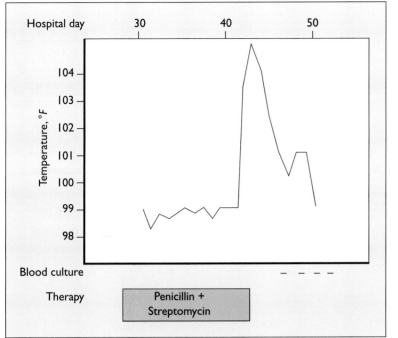

FIGURE 7-35 Course of a patient with enterococcal endocarditis and recurrent fever that abated within days of discontinuation of antimicrobial therapy. (*From* Levison [9]; with permission.)

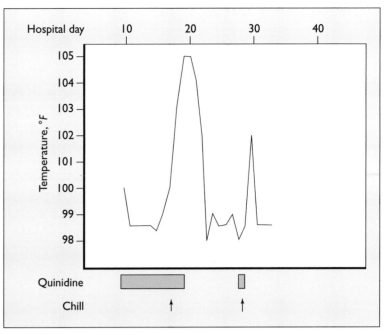

FIGURE 7-36 Course of a patient with recurrent fever associated with quinidine administration. The fever recurred when the patient was subsequently challenged with quinidine. (*From* Levison [9]; with permission.)

REFERENCES

1. Steckelberg JM, Murphy JG, Wilson WR: Management of complications in infective endocarditis. In *Infective Endocarditis*, 2nd ed. Edited by Kaye D. Philadelphia: Raven Press; 1992:435–454.

2. Huston JH III, Nichols DA, Luetmer PH, *et al.*: Blinded prospective evaluation of sensitivity of MR angiography to known intracranial aneurysms: Importance of aneurysm size. *Am J Neuroradiol* 1994, 15:1607–1614.

3. Gold MJ: Cure rates and long-term prognosis. In *Infective Endocarditis*, 2nd ed. Edited by Kaye D. Philadelphia: Raven Press; 1992:455–464.

4. Livornese LL, Korzeniowski OM: Pathogenesis of infective endocarditis. In *Infective Endocarditis*, 2nd ed. Edited by Kaye D. New York: Raven Press; 1992:19–35.

5. Erbel R, Rohmann M, Drexler S, *et al.*: Improved diagnostic value of echocardiography in patients with infective endocarditis by transesophageal approach: A prospective study. *Eur Heart J* 1988, 9:43–53.

6. Nishan PC, Nishimura RA: Role of two-dimensional echocardiography and Doppler ultrasound. In *Atlas of Heart Diseases*, vol II. Edited by Braunwald E, Rahimtoola SH. Philadelphia: Current Medicine; 1997.

7. Virmani R, Burke AP, Farb A: Pathology of valvular heart disease. In *Atlas of Heart Diseases*, vol II. Edited by Braunwald E, Rahimtoola SH. Philadelphia: Current Medicine; 1997.

8. Johnson WD: The clinical syndrome. In *Infective Endocarditis*. Edited by Kaye D. Baltimore: University Park Press; 1976:87–100.

9. Levison ME: Response to therapy. In *Infective Endocarditis*. Edited by Kaye D. Baltimore: University Park Press; 1976:185–200.

10. Krause JR, Levison SP: Pathology of infective endocarditis. In *Infective Endocarditis*. Edited by Kaye D. Baltimore: University Park Press; 1976:55–86.

11. Cannon NJ, Cobbs CG: Infective endocarditis in drug addicts. In *Infective Endocarditis*. Edited by Kaye D. Baltimore: University Park Press; 1976:111–128.

12. Atkinson JB, Virmani R: Infective endocarditis: Changing trends and general approach for examination. In *Cardiovascular Pathology. Major Problems in Pathology Series*, vol 23. Edited by Virmani R, Atkinson JB, Fenoglio J. Philadelphia: WB Saunders; 1991:435–450.

13. Korzeniowski OM, Kaye D: Infective endocarditis. In *Heart Disease*, 4th ed. Edited by Braunwald E. Philadelphia: WB Saunders; 1992.

14. Bush LM, Johnson CC: Clinical syndrome and diagnosis. In *Infective Endocarditis*, 2nd ed. Edited by Kaye D. Philadelphia: Raven Press; 1992:99–115.

SELECTED BIBLIOGRAPHY

Francioli P: Central nervous system complications of infective endocarditis. In *Infections of the Central Nervous System.* Edited by Scheld WM, Whiteley RJ, Durack DT. New York: Raven Press; 1991:515–599.

Karchmer AW, Gibbons GW: Infections of prosthetic heart valves and vascular grafts. In *Infections Associated With Indwelling Devices*, 2nd ed. Edited by Bisno AL, Waldvogel FA. Washington DC: American Society for Microbiology; 1994:213–249.

Kaye D (ed): *Infective Endocarditis*, 2nd ed. Philadelphia: Raven Press; 1992.

Wilson WR, Steckelberg JM (eds): Infective endocarditis. *Infect Dis Clin North Am* 1993, 7:1–170.

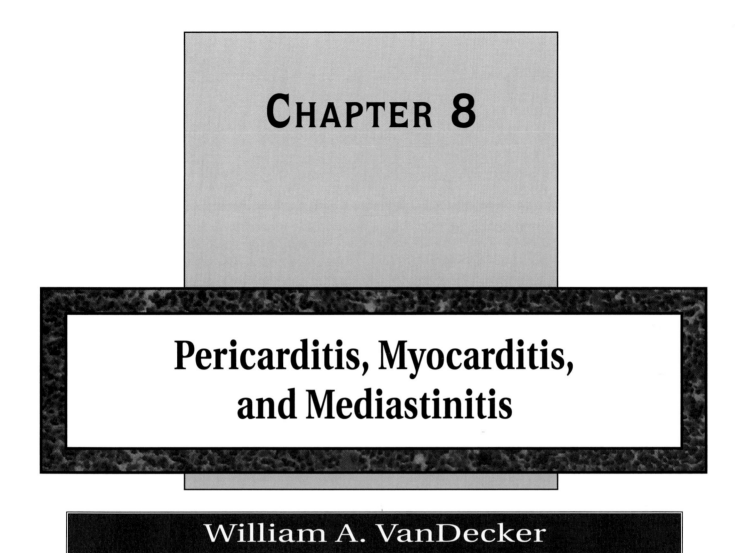

CHAPTER 8

Pericarditis, Myocarditis, and Mediastinitis

William A. VanDecker

AMONG A BROAD SPECTRUM OF POTENTIAL CARDIOVASCULAR DISEASE PROCESSES, cardiovascular infections pose one of the most difficult diagnostic challenges, and the possible underlying immunology and cellular pathophysiology are fascinating topics. This chapter deals with pericarditis, myocarditis, and mediastinitis and integrates the clinical, histologic, and pathophysiologic data of these disease states.

Pericarditis, inflammation of the protective pericardial sac surrounding the heart, is frequently infectious in nature. Viruses are the most common agent, but other etiologies are possible. Symptom relief with anti-inflammatory drugs is usually necessary, and the syndrome usually passes, but recurrences are common. Mechanical complications of cardiac tamponade from pericardial effusion and constrictive pericarditis from calcification or fibrosis need to be watched for and treated appropriately.

Myocarditis, or nonischemic inflammation of the myocardium, remains an intellectual diagnostic challenge. The symptoms are nonspecific. No noninvasive imaging technique can add specifically to the diagnosis, and patchy histologic abnormalities make endocardial biopsy interpretation difficult. Viruses are probably a leading infectious agent, but many interesting bacteria and parasites may be involved, especially in the immunocompromised host. The molecular and immunopathologic mechanisms of myocarditis are subjects of debate and investigation.

Mediastinitis is a serious infection that most often occurs after cardiothoracic surgery. It is frequently bacterial in nature, although fungus can play a role in the correct setting. Aggressive long-term antibiotics and surgical débridement are necessary.

PERICARDITIS

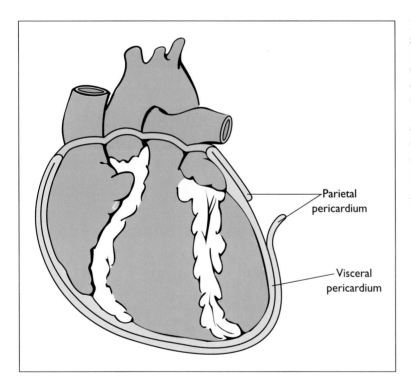

FIGURE 8-1 Pericardium. A protective, double-layered, "reflected" sac with a fibrous outer layer (parietal pericardium) attaching the pericardium to the great vessels, sternum, spinal column, and diaphragm and an inner single cell layer of serous membrane attached to the heart perform two functions vital to cardiac physiology. First, they provide structural support stability to the heart in the thoracic cavity. Second, with interposed pericardial fluid as a lubricant, they allow the pericardial membranes to slide over each other, permitting cardiac contraction. This elastic potential space also allows changes in cardiac volume and shape during contraction. The normal pericardium may contain up to 50 mL of pericardial effusion. Inflammation of this tissue defines pericarditis and may have many etiologies (frequently infectious) and many pathophysiologic presentations. The inflammation may or may not be associated with pericardial fluid.

Clinical signs and symptoms of acute pericarditis

Chest pain
Precordial but not necessarily retrosternal
May radiate to left shoulder
Usually sharp
May be pleuritic or aggravated by cough or body motion
No exertional relation
Prolonged duration
Worsened in supine position, improved by leaning forward

Dyspnea
Variable finding

Fever
May be low-grade or lacking
May include upper respiratory infection symptoms, arthralgias, malaise

Pericardial friction rub
Pathognomonic physical examination auscultatory finding
Absence does not exclude diagnosis
Superficial, leathery, scratchy, in character
Classically has three components: atrial systole, ventricular systole, and early diastolic ventricular filling
May exhibit only one or two components

FIGURE 8-2 Clinical signs and symptoms of acute pericarditis. The cardinal sign of acute pericarditis is chest pain, which a careful history in the correct clinical context differentiates from ischemic heart pain. A three-component, scratchy friction rub confirms the diagnosis but need not be present. A myriad of other findings may be present, with low-grade fever and dyspnea being most common.

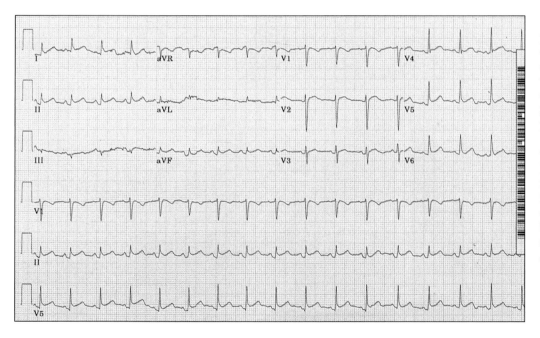

FIGURE 8-3 Electrocardiogram of acute pericarditis. Pericarditis inflammation can cause a classic diffuse pattern of myocardial injury on the resting echocardiogram thought to be secondary to contiguous epicardial irritation. It is marked by diffuse ST-segment elevation in a concave upward pattern with upright T waves in leads II, III, AVF, AVL, and V_{3-6}. In its most specific form, PR depression is seen in the inferior leads (II, III, AVF). Care in interpretation is necessary to avoid confusion with acute myocardial infarction or normal-variant early repolarization. Atrial fibrillation may be a complicating arrhythmia. The initial electrocardiogram may undergo evolutionary ST changes over time.

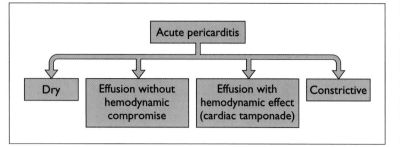

FIGURE 8-4 Acute pericarditis. The inflammation of pericarditis may take several pathophysiologic forms. Dry "bread-and-butter" fibrinous pericarditis and small effusions without compressions frequently resolve with conservative treatment, but clinical symptoms may recur in up to 20% of patients. Hemodynamically compressive effusion needs therapeutic drainage. Chronic scarring of the pericardium with fibrosis, thickening, and calcification after acute pericarditis usually restricts cardiac diastolic relaxation and filling, causing dyspnea and edema, and frequently requires surgical intervention (a possible finding with tuberculosis pericarditis).

Clinical and hemodynamic features of compressive pericardial disease

Features	Cardiac tamponade	Constrictive pericarditis
Duration of symptoms	Hours to days	Months to years
Chest pain, friction rub	Usual	Remote (none active)
Pulsus paradoxus (exaggerated increase in RV filling during inspiration at expense of LV filling)	Prominent	Slight to absent
Kussmaul's sign (systemic venous pressure as visualized in neck veins paradoxically increases with inspiration)	Absent	Often present
Early diastolic knock	Absent	Often present
Heart size on chest radiograph	Usually enlarged	Usually normal, may be enlarged
Pericardial calcification	Absent	Often present
Equal RV and LV diastolic pressures	Yes	Yes
Pericardial effusion	Yes	No
Third heart sound	Absent	Absent

LV—left ventricle; RV—right ventricle.

FIGURE 8-5 Clinical and hemodynamic features of compressive pericardial disease. Cardiac tamponade and constrictive pericarditis are two severe mechanical complications of pericarditis that frequently require procedural or surgical intervention. They can be differentiated based on a number of descriptors. In addition, constrictive pericarditis occasionally needs to be differentiated from restrictive cardiomyopathy. LV—left ventricular; RV—right ventricular. (*Adapted from* Hancock [1]; with permission.)

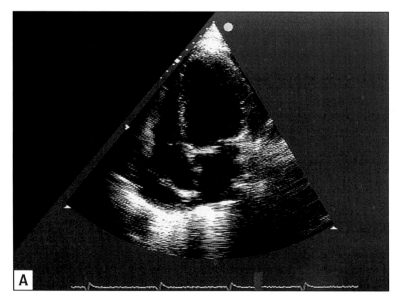
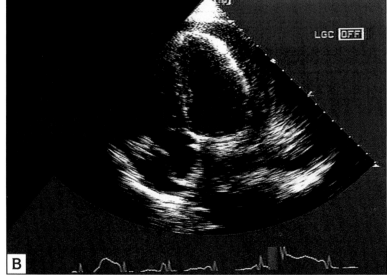

FIGURE 8-6 Echocardiographic evaluation of pericardial effusion. **A,** Small pericardial echo-free space of effusion without evidence of cardiac compression in patient with recent upper respiratory viral infection that was treated conservatively. Serial studies are occasionally helpful in tracking disease processes and resolution. **B,** Small pericardial effusion with right atrial invagination, suggesting that pericardial pressure is greater than right atrial pressure. In the advancing state, right ventricular diastolic collapse would also be seen, suggesting that pericardial pressure is higher than right ventricular end-diastolic pressure. Cardiac tamponade is a clinical diagnosis based on physical examination and pressure recordings, but echocardiography can provide highly useful information in making this diagnosis.

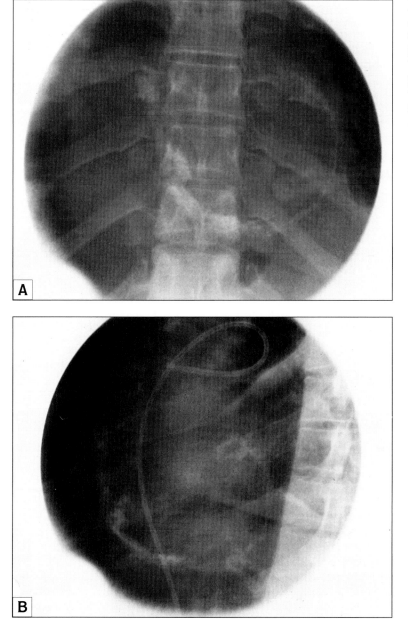

A

B

FIGURE 8-7 Radiographic evaluation of pericardial calcification. **A** and **B**, Cinefluoro images (*panel 7A*, anterior; *panel 7B*, lateral) of patient with significant dyspnea on exertion and marked pericardial calcifications on chest radiograph. Cardiac catheterization confirmed constrictive physiology with elevated and superimposable (equalized) left ventricular and right ventricular diastolic filling patterns. The patient was treated for tuberculosis, a diagnosis fully confirmed at operative pericardial stripping. (*Courtesy of* R. Mintz, MD.)

Noninfectious causes of pericarditis
Idiopathic
Uremia
Metastatic, infiltrating neoplasms
Acute myocardial infarction
Radiation therapy (to mediastinal area)
Autoimmune diseases (classically, lupus erythematosus)
Drugs (classically, procainamide and hydralazine)
Sarcoid
Trauma
Dressler's post–myocardial infarction syndrome
Postpericardiotomy syndrome
Myxedema

FIGURE 8-8 Noninfectious causes of pericarditis. Although infectious processes represent a large portion of pericarditic inflammation, a number of other disease processes may cause pericarditis. It is possible that a large portion of the idiopathic category is also infectious but that the diagnosis is unable to be made owing to inadequate tissue and serologic testing.

Infectious pericarditis

	Virus	Bacteria	Tuberculosis	Fungi	Parasites
Frequency	Common	Occasional	<5% of all pericarditis (decreasing frequency)	Rare	Rare
Risk population	Viral infection, otherwise healthy patient	1) Recent chest surgery 2) Contiguous or hematologic spread of bacterial infection	Systemic or pulmonary	Immunocompromised patients (including youth) and endemic areas	Immunocompromised patients and endemic areas
Time course	1–4 wk	Fulminant, with high temperatures over several days	Usually slow	Usually slow (histoplasmosis may be 2–6 wk)	Slow
Most common etiologic agent	Coxsackie B	Staphylococci	Tuberculosis	Histoplasmosis	*Toxoplasma gondii*
Chest pain	Extremely common	Occasional	Rare	Common	Rare
Morbidity and mortality	Overall low, but 20% symptomatic recurrence	High (50%–70%)	High (30%)	High overall (histoplasmosis may be more benign in endemic areas)	Presumably high
Diagnosis	1) Frequently presumptive on clinical presentation 2) Viral titers (acute and convalescent) 3) Culture of virus from other source (*eg*, stool)	Gram stain of pericardial effusion	1) Acid-fast bacillus stain and culture of pericardial effusion 2) Pericardial biopsy	Pericardial fluid stain	Pericardial fluid stain or pericardial biopsy

FIGURE 8-9 Infectious pericarditis. Many infectious classes of agents may cause pericarditis. The largest class is viral, which usually occurs in late summer or early fall and has a relatively rapid time course. Bacterial pericarditis usually presents as a severe toxic state that requires immediate pericardial fluid drainage and antibiotics. In addition to recent chest surgery, contiguous spread from pneumonia or endocarditis can cause bacterial pericarditis, as can hematologic spread. Tuberculosis is rapidly decreasing as a cause of pericarditis because of early antituberculous therapy in patients with pulmonary tuberculosis. Tuberculosis, however, still carries a high mortality rate and can lead to constriction physiology. Histoplasmosis as the leading cause of fungal pericarditis may have a clinical course similar to viral pericarditis; without systemic involvement, however, it usually has a benign course. Nonhistoplasmosis fungal pericarditis frequently is a progressive illness with high mortality; it is treated with intravenous amphotericin B. Parasitic infections are rare but may occur in endemic areas.

Infectious causes of pericarditis

Viruses

Coxsackie A	Varicella zoster
Coxsackie B	Cytomegalovirus
Echoviruses	Herpes simplex
Mumps	Hepatitis B
Influenza	HIV
Epstein-Barr	

Bacteria

Streptococcus pneumoniae	*Actinomyces* spp
Staphylococcus aureus	*Mycoplasma pneumoniae*
Neisseria meningitidis	*Legionella pneumophila*
Haemophilus influenzae	*Mycobacterium tuberculosis*
Enteric gram-negative rods	*Borrelia burgdorferi*
Salmonella spp	

Fungi

Histoplasma capsulatum	*Cryptococcus neoformans*
Coccidioides immitis	*Candida* spp
Blastomyces dermatitidis	*Aspergillus* spp

Parasites

Toxoplasma gondii
Entamoeba histolytica
Schistosoma spp

FIGURE 8-10 Infectious causes of pericarditis. The causes of infectious pericarditis in the literature are myriad. Most cases of viral pericarditis are probably caused by coxsackievirus or echoviruses. Viruses such as Epstein-Barr, varicella, cytomegalovirus, herpes, and hepatitis are more likely to be associated with subclinical infection or with major clinical presentations in other noncardiac organ systems. Early antibiotic therapy for bacterial pneumonias has led to less infectious pericarditis from contiguous spread from the lungs and a decreasing incidence of pneumococcus as a causative agent. Fungal infections can occur by contiguous spread from the lungs or mediastinal lymph nodes or from hematogenous inoculation in fungal sepsis. Parasitic infection must be considered in endemic areas. (*Adapted from* Savoia and Oxman [2].)

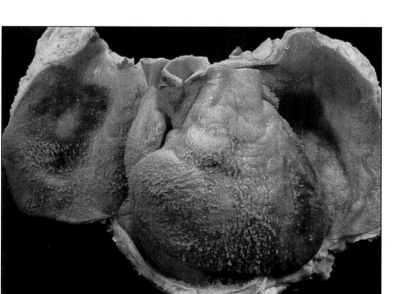

FIGURE 8-11 Gross anatomy picture of fibrinous ("dry") pericarditis, probably viral in nature, showing inflammatory changes in both the visceral and parietal pericardium. (*From* Shabetai [3]; with permission.)

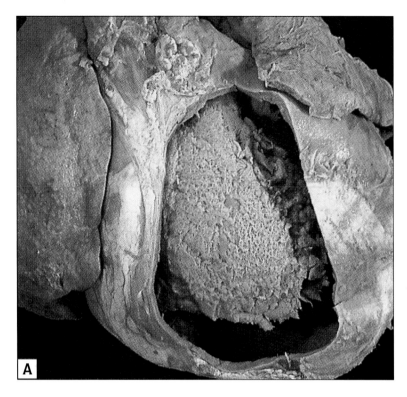

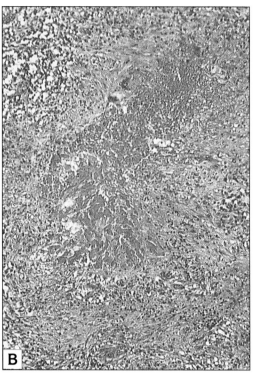

FIGURE 8-12
A, Window cut into pericardium showing tuberculosis fibrinous pericarditis.
B, Histology of the pericardium showing caseous necrosis. (*From* Becker and Anderson [4]; with permission.)

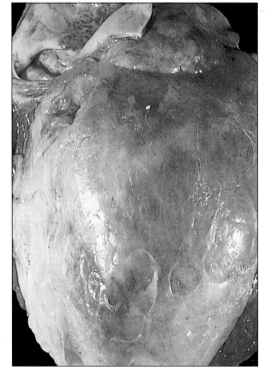

FIGURE 8-13 Acute pneumococcal pericarditis found at autopsy in a woman who died with severe pneumococcal lobar pneumonia shortly after being admitted to the hospital. Delicate, gray deposits of fibrin are apparent on the pericardium. Early and appropriate antimicrobial therapy decreases contiguous bacterial seeding of the pericardium. (*From* Belmonte *et al.* [5]; with permission.)

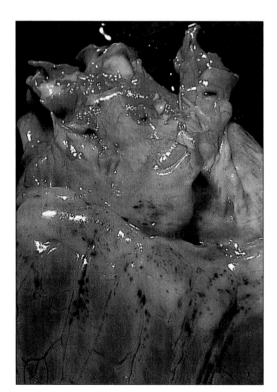

FIGURE 8-14 Petechiae seen on pericardium of elderly man with *Staphylococcus aureus* sepsis from pyelonephritis. Hematogenous spread from infectious focus or associated serologic abnormalities such as endotoxin or autoimmune reactions may cause pericarditis. (*From* Belmonte *et al.* [5]; with permission.)

Treatment of infectious pericarditis

Bed rest
Anti-inflammatory drugs (aspirin, nonsteroidal agents, steroids)
Appropriate chemotherapy based on etiologic agent
Treatment of mechanical complications

FIGURE 8-15 Treatment of infectious pericarditis. Treatment of infectious pericarditis is most frequently supportive and conservative given the high preponderance of presumed viral causes. Recurrent symptoms are common (up to 20% of cases). Purulent pericarditis that results from bacterial or fungal infection requires drainage of the effusion and may also require pericardial stripping.

MYOCARDITIS

Definition of myocarditis

A histopathologic process characterized by an inflammatory infiltrate of the myocardium with necrosis and/or degeneration of adjacent myocytes not typical of the ischemic damage associated with coronary artery disease

FIGURE 8-16 Definition of myocarditis. Inflammation of the heart, a disease state with frequent fulminant clinical findings and sequelae, is a difficult histopathologic diagnosis, perhaps related to the frequent patchiness of the disease process, the likelihood of mild cellular infiltration in simple chronic interstitial fibrotic disease states, and the difficulty in establishing an etiology [6].

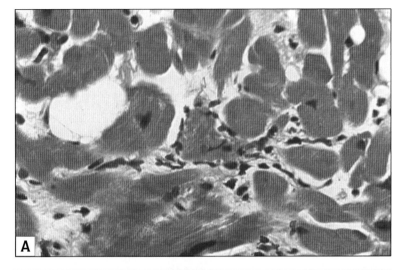

A

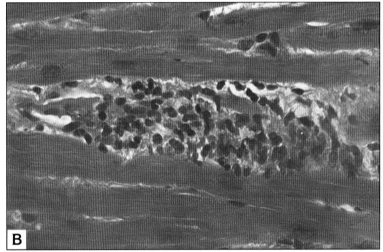

B

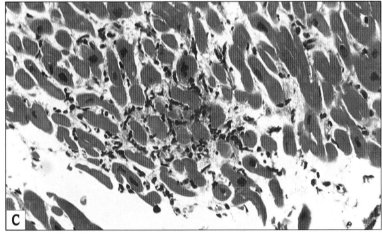

C

FIGURE 8-17 Histopathology of endomyocardial biopsy samples from patients with myocarditis. **A**, Hematoxylin-eosin high-power micrograph showing one necrotic myocyte surrounded by a mixed inflammatory infiltrate. **B**, Small cluster of myocytes with focal area of dense mononuclear inflammatory cell infiltrate. Note that the surrounding myocardium is well preserved and appears not to be involved. **C**, Cross-section of myocytes undergoing necrosis. Interstitial inflammatory cells surround the myocytes, which no longer have distinct cell outlines. The interstitial space in the affected zone contains fibrin and fibrinogen, probably from microvascular injury. Although the Dallas criteria were defined to assess idiopathic myocarditis rather than specific infectious (or noninfectious) causes, etiologic agents are rarely found on biopsy (especially viral evidence), confounding therapy even further because idiopathic myocarditis may be the best slide diagnosis possible. (*From* Herskowitz and Ansari [7]; with permission.)

Noninfectious causes of myocarditis

Sarcoidosis	Drug induced	Drug induced (hypersensitivity)
Collagen vascular disease	(direct toxin)	Isoniazid
Systemic lupus erythe-	Cocaine	Methyldopa
matosus	Alcohol	Antibiotics (amphotericin B,
Rheumatic arthritis	Catecholamines	ampicillin, tetracycline,
Thyrotoxicosis	Arsenic	sulfisoxazole, chloram-
Pheochromocytoma	Cyclophosphamide	phenicol, streptomycin)
Radiation induced	Daunorubicin	Diuretics (hydrochloro-
	Doxorubicin	thiazide, acetazolamide,
		chlorthalidone)
		Giant cell myocarditis
		Kawasaki disease

FIGURE 8-18 Noninfectious causes of myocarditis. As with pericarditis, many disease processes can cause myocarditis that are not infectious and need to be systemically excluded from the differential diagnosis. (*Adapted from* Savoia and Oxman [2].)

Infectious causes of myocarditis

Viruses

Coxsackie A	Yellow fever
Coxsackie B	Argentinian hemorrhagic fever
Echoviruses	Bolivian hemorrhagic fever
Poliomyelitis	Lymphocytic choriomeningitis
Mumps	Adenovirus
Rubeola	Varicella zoster
Influenza A and B	Cytomegalovirus
Rabies	Epstein-Barr
Rubella	Vaccinia
Dengue	Variola
Chikungunya	Hepatitis B
Herpes simplex	HIV

Rickettsiae

Rickettsia rickettsii (Rocky Mountain spotted fever)	*Rickettsia tsutsugamushi* (scrub typhus)

Bacteria

Corynebacterium diphtheriae	*Staphylococcus aureus*
Clostridium perfringens	*Mycoplasma pneumoniae*
Streptococcus pyogenes	*Chlamydia psittaci*
Neisseria meningitidis	*Tropheryma whippelii*
Salmonella spp	*Borrelia burgdorferi*
Brucella spp	

Fungi

Aspergillus spp
Candida spp
Cryptococcus spp

Parasites

Trypanosoma cruzi	*Trypanosoma rhodesiense*
Trypanosoma gambiense	*Trichinella spiralis*
Toxoplasma gondii	

FIGURE 8-19 Infectious causes of myocarditis. Although viruses are the most important infectious cause of myocarditis in the United States and Western Europe, other infectious agents can be implicated worldwide. The mechanism of the inflammatory injury differs from agent to agent. The clinical diagnosis is most often made by serology, agent isolation elsewhere, and/or classic cardiovascular complaints rather than by myocardial tissue biopsy. A careful cardiovascular history, physical examination, and screening echocardiogram are necessary when these systemic infections are suspected causes of underlying myocarditis. (*Adapted from* Savoia and Oxman [2].)

A. Mechanism of injury in infectious myocarditis

Direct cellular damage by infectious agent
Direct cellular damage by circulating toxin
Cellular damage by immune reactions or immune complexes
Cellular damage by adjacent interstitial inflammatory process

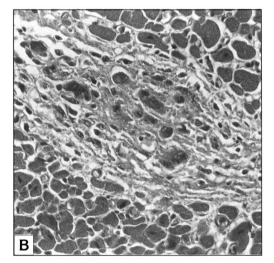

B

FIGURE 8-20 A, Mechanism of injury in infectious myocarditis. The inflammatory response may begin in a number of ways. Some viruses, like coxsackie B, infect the myocytes directly, as can parasites such as *Trypanosoma cruzi* (*see* Chapter 9, "Chagas' Disease"). Classically, diphtheria, which has cardiac involvement in more than 20% of its presentations, releases a circulating toxin that inhibits protein synthesis, causing extensive myocardial damage. Rickettsial infections frequently cause a small artery inflammation and occlusion, eventually causing an inflammatory process of the adjacent myocytes. Rheumatic fever results from the cross-reactivity of antibodies produced in response to *Streptococcus pyogenes* infections with monocytes in heart muscle. **B,** The pathognomonic lesion of acute rheumatic fever is the Aschoff body, an interstitial collection of Aschoff cells and monocytes found in the myocardium, endocardium, or valves. (*continued*)

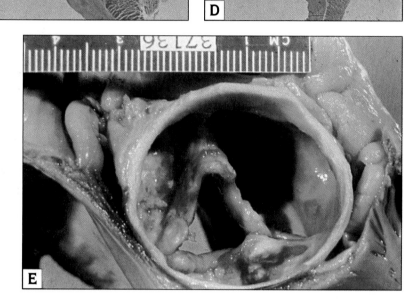

Figure 8-20 (*continued*) **C–E,** Inflammatory responses produce small, noninfected vegetations (*arrow*) on the line of closure of valves (*panel 20C*, rheumatic fever; *panel 20D*, normal) and fusion of commissures and thickening of cusps with subsequent stenosis and insufficiency (*panel 20E*). The mitral valve is most frequently affected, followed by the aortic and tricuspid valves. (Panels 20B–20E *from* Hutchins [8]; with permission.)

Nonspecific clinical manifestations of myocarditis

History
Preceding symptoms
  Fever and chills
  Influenza-like symptoms (cough, sore throat, malaise, arthralgia)
  Gastrointestinal symptoms (nausea, vomiting)
  Chest pain
Recent cardiovascular symptoms
  Shortness of breath
  Heart failure
  Palpitations
  Syncope or presyncope

Signs
S3 gallop
Pericardial friction rub
Left- or right-sided congestive heart failure (*eg*, rales, edema)
Cardiogenic shock

Laboratory findings
Increase in
  Creatine phosphokinase
  Liver enzymes
  Erythrocyte sedimentation rate
  Leukocyte count
Serologic evidence of active viral infection
Electrocardiographic abnormalities
  Atrioventricular block
  Atrial fibrillation, supraventricular tachycardia
  Low voltage
  Persistent sinus tachycardia
  Intraventricular conduction block or left bundle-branch block
  ST changes
  Ventricular tachycardia
Echocardiographic abnormalities
  Global left ventricular dysfunction
  Pericardial effusion
  Ventricular thrombi

Figure 8-21 Nonspecific clinical manifestations of myocarditis. The findings in myocarditis are frequently symptoms of heart failure or arrhythmia (bradycardic or tachycardic) and are mostly nonspecific. Serologic evidence of viral infections requires a greater than fourfold rise in specific antibody in paired acute (<1 week) and convalescent (>2 weeks) serum specimens. Initially, IgM antibody is present, peaking at 2 to 3 weeks. IgG antibody predominates after the first month of infection. (*Adapted from* Herskowitz and Ansari [7].)

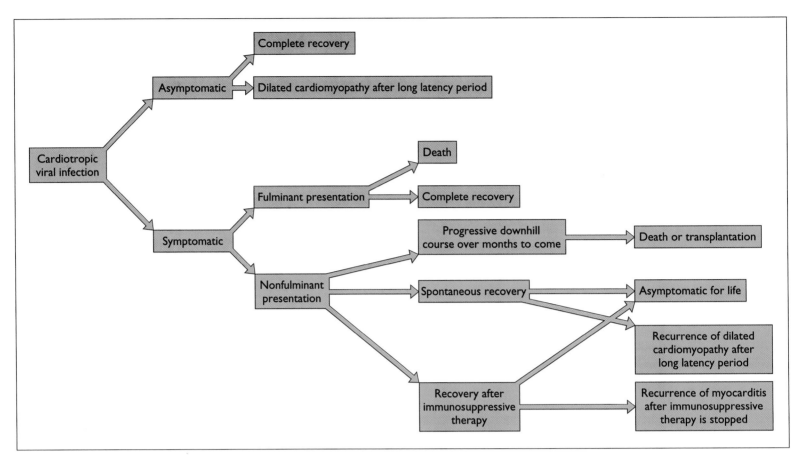

FIGURE 8-22 The natural history of human myocarditis. Most patients with mild symptoms of acute myocarditis are not seen by cardiologists, and most of these patients appear to recover fully. Of the patients with symptomatic heart disease typically seen by cardiologists, a small number have fulminant presentations and either die in the acute stage or appear to recover fully. Of the remaining patients with myocarditis, a few are characterized by a progressive downhill course over a period of months to years that ends in death from heart failure or intractable arrhythmias [9,10]. Some spontaneously recover and remain asymptomatic for life, and others have an asymptomatic period followed by development of dilated cardiomyopathy. The heterogeneity of clinical presentations and natural history in human myocarditis probably reflect the genetic predisposition of the individual, the virulence of the cardiotropic virus, and environmental factors. With the advent of molecular viral probes, it will be critical to relate the presence of persistent enterovirus RNA with the patterns of the natural history of myocarditis. (*From* Herskowitz and Ansari [7].)

FIGURE 8-23 Inflammatory infiltrates and differential diagnosis in myocarditis. Clues to the myocarditic etiologic agent can be sought in the histopathologic cellular milieu of the biopsy. (*Adapted from* Aretz [11].)

Inflammatory infiltrates and differential diagnosis in myocarditis

Lymphocytic	Neutrophils present	Eosinophils present	Giant cells present
Idiopathic	Idiopathic (early)	Hypersensitivity	Idiopathic
Viral	Viral (early)	Parasitic infection	Sarcoidosis
Toxic	Pressor effect	Hypereosinophilic	Hypersensitivity
Collagen vascular	Ischemia	syndrome	Rheumatic fever
Sarcoidosis	Bacterial infections	Idiopathic	Rheumatoid diseases
Kawasaki disease			Granulomatous infections (*eg*, tuberculosis)

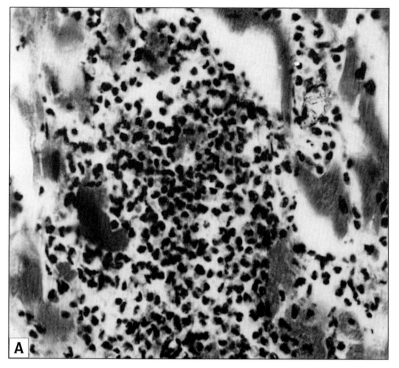

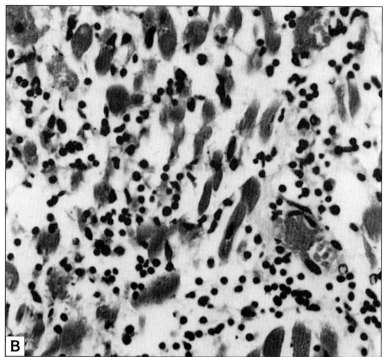

FIGURE 8-24 Two types of extensive myocarditic cellular infiltration and damage. **A,** Cellular response almost exclusively of polymorphonuclear leukocytes, suggesting bacterial infection.

B, Predominance of lymphocytes, suggesting viral infection. (Hematoxylin-eosin stain, ×230.) (*From* Becker [12]; with permission.)

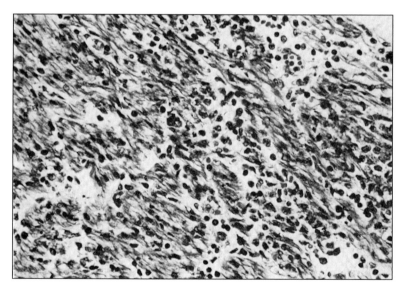

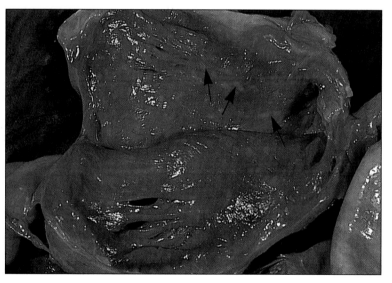

FIGURE 8-25 Coxsackievirus myocarditis with extensive infiltration of mononuclear cells, plasma cells, lymphocytes, and some eosinophils in the interstitial tissue (×250). These small, nonenveloped, single-stranded RNA viruses of the picornavirus family appear to have a high affinity for specific receptors on myocardial cells and are the leading cause of viral myocarditis. Mouse models of coxsackie B3 have shown that susceptibility is age dependent and genetically determined and that exercise and corticosteroids worsen mortality in the model. (*From* Bloor [13]; with permission.)

FIGURE 8-26 Macroscopic view of acute myocarditis. This acute myocarditis is the result of bacterial embolization from a necrotic mass of adenocarcinoma and gram-negative bacilli. The myocardium has multiple small yellow spots (*arrows*), which are early abscesses. Hematologic spread (sepsis) would be a common mechanism for bacterial myocarditis. (*From* Belmonte *et al.* [5]; with permission.)

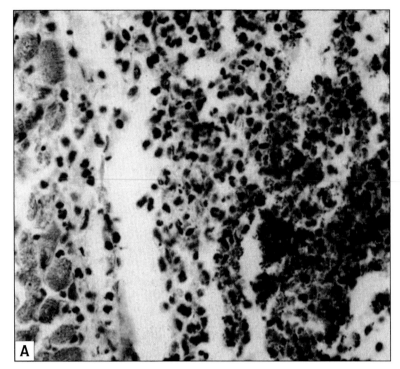

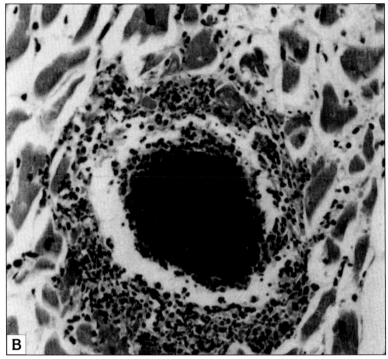

FIGURE 8-27 **A** and **B**, Bacterial myocarditis. The most common bacterial organisms in myocarditis are staphylococci, streptococci, pneumococci, and meningococci. They cause an inflammatory response of polymorphonuclear leukocytes, with visualization of microorganisms (*panel 27A*), or they can form microabscesses, as in the patient with staphylococcal sepsis seen in *panel 27B*. (Hematoxylin-eosin stain, *panel 27A*, ×350; *panel 27B*, ×230.) (*From* Becker [12]; with permission.)

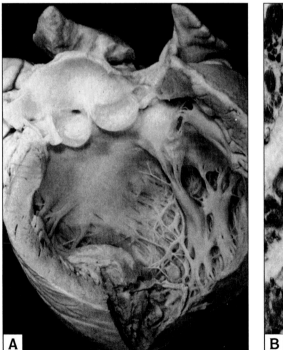

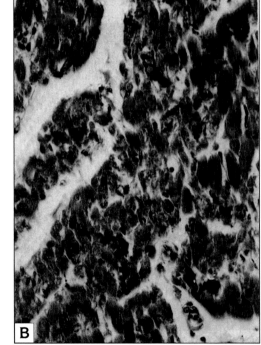

FIGURE 8-28 Diphtheria myocarditis in a child. **A**, Dilated left ventricle with apical thrombosis. **B**, Histology showing extensive patchy hyaline and granular degeneration of myocytes. *Cornebacterium diphtheriae* produces a potent endotoxin that has direct action on myocytes and leads to their granular degeneration. As is also true with Lyme disease (*Borrelia burgdorferi*), frequent atrioventricular node block and even complete heart block may occur. Heart block can occur years after active infection from presumed conduction tissue fibrosis. (Hematoxylin-eosin stain, ×350.) (*From* Becker [12]; with permission.)

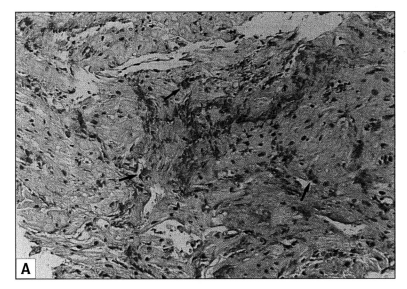

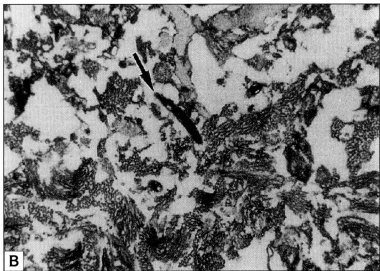

FIGURE 8-29 A, Periodic acid–Schiff staining of right ventricle myocardial biopsy showing macrophages and bacilli, suggesting *Tropheryma whippelii* infection. **B**, Electron microscopy of myocardial biopsy showing Whipple's bacillus (*arrow*). Cardiac involvement in abdominal Whipple's disease can manifest as pancarditis (valve, myocardium, pericardium), congestive heart failure, and atrioventricular block. (*From* Silvestry *et al.* [14]; with permission.)

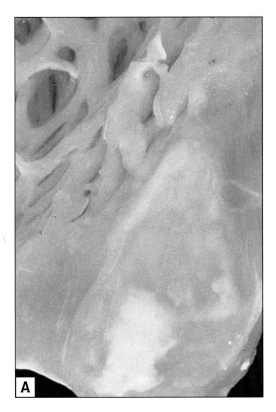

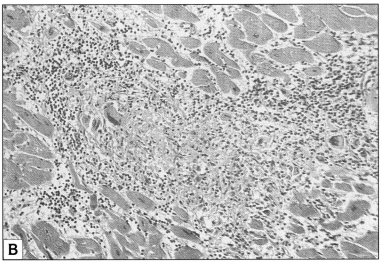

FIGURE 8-30 A, Macroscopic tuberculoma in left ventricle myocardium. **B**, Histology of tuberculosis: caseating granuloma with necrosis and giant cells. Tuberculous involvement of myocardium is extremely rare; it may occur more often in children. The most common cause may be direct extension from hilar lymph nodes. Tuberculous myocarditis is usually clinically silent but may occasionally lead to arrhythmias. (*From* Becker and Anderson [4]; with permission.)

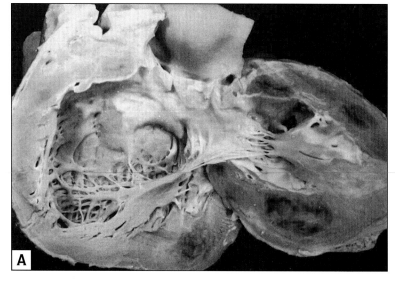

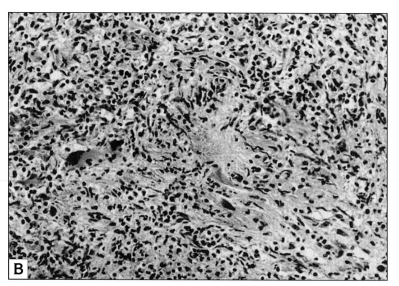

FIGURE 8-31 Syphilitic myocarditis. **A,** Partitioned left ventricle with gummata in wall. This is a rare finding that is usually unsuspected clinically. It typically involves the interventricular septum, which may result in damage to the conduction system and atrioventricular block. **B,** Histology of a gumma shows liquefaction necrosis and cellular infiltrate with predominance of lymphocytes and occasional multinucleated giant cells. The possible existence of diffuse myocarditis without gummata in adults with syphilis is controversial. (*From* Becker [12]; with permission.)

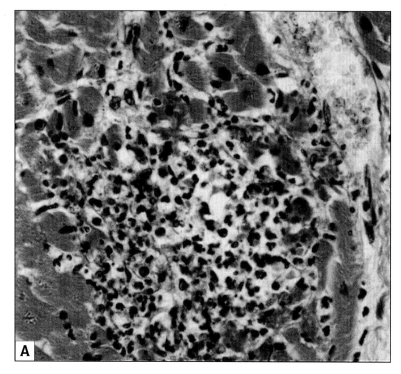

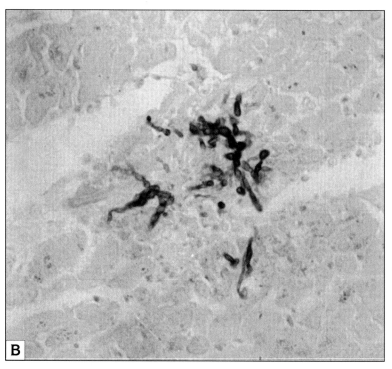

FIGURE 8-32 Fungal myocarditis. **A,** Nonspecific inflammatory focus. (Hematoxylin-eosin stain, ×350.) **B,** Special staining showing fungal elements. (Grocott's stain, ×350.) This most frequently occurs in patients with malignant disease or in immunosuppressed patients. Cardiac surgery and HIV infection may also be risk factors. Contiguous (from mediastinal lymph nodes) or hematologic spread can occur. Myocardial involvement is common in systemic aspergillosis. Actinomycosis, blastomycosis, cryptococcosis; candidiasis; coccidioidomycosis, and histoplasmosis may all have cardiac involvement with resulting arrhythmias or congestion. (*From* Becker [12]; with permission.)

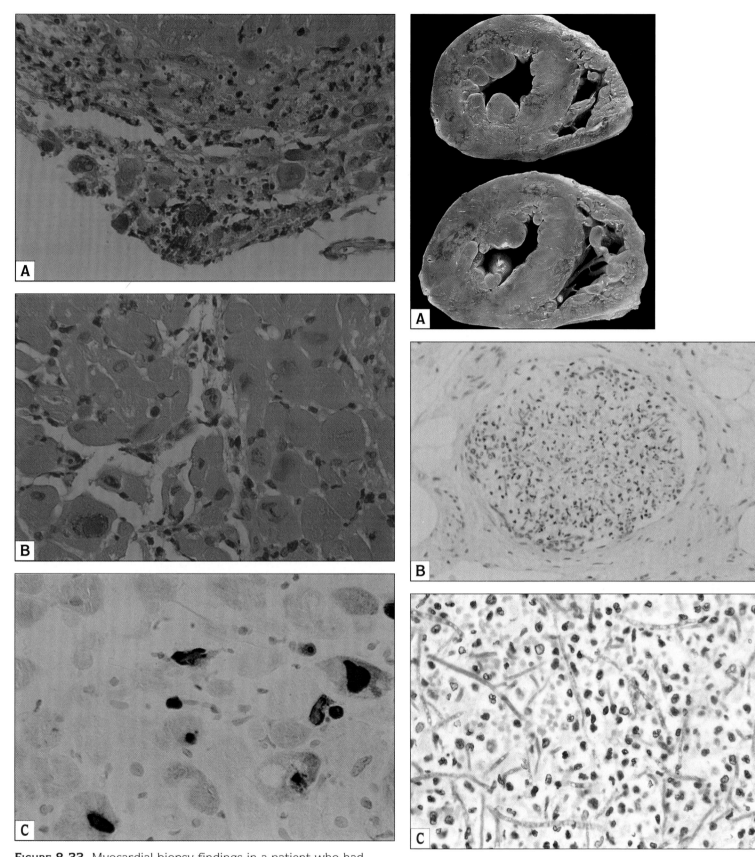

FIGURE 8-33 Myocardial biopsy findings in a patient who had undergone heart transplantation 6 weeks previously. Patients taking immunosuppressive drugs for cardiac transplantation are prone to opportunistic infections. **A**, Large abnormal nuclei in both the surface macrophages and underlying myocardial cells. **B**, Abnormally large, swollen myocardial nuclei with obvious inclusions. **C**, Immunoperoxidase-labeled anticytomegalovirus monoclonal antibody localizing to the nuclei. Interestingly, the patient and the donor both tested positive for cytomegalovirus. (*See* Chapter 12, "Infections Associated With Coronary Artery Disease.") (*Courtesy of* J. Caulfield, MD.)

FIGURE 8-34 Gross and microscopic pathology of transplanted heart from a patient with disseminated *Aspergillus fumigatus.* **A**, Areas of necrosis were palpable throughout the myocardium at autopsy. These abscesses are seen here. **B**, Low-power appearance of a small abscess. **C**, Hematoxylin-eosin stains show the hyphae. As is frequently the case in transplant patients who develop disseminated fungal disease, this patient had required aggressive antirejection therapy. Although the heart valves were not infected in this patient, aspergillus is a recognized cause of endocarditis in intravenous drug abusers and patients with prosthetic intracardiac material. (*Courtesy of* C.G. Cobbs, MD.)

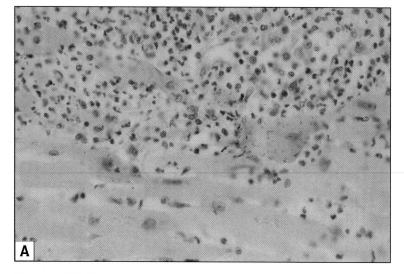

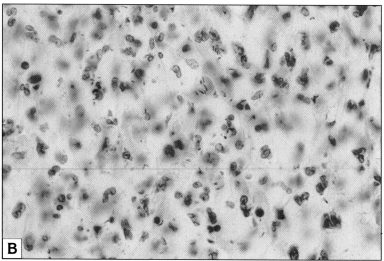

FIGURE 8-35 Listerial myocarditis. The patient previously underwent heart transplantation. **A**, Tissue Gram stain shows the intense lymphocyte response. **B**, Hematoxylin-eosin stain from the same patient. The rod-shaped bacteria, although visualized in *panel 35A*, are more clearly visible in *panel 35B*. The patient was successfully treated by repeat transplantation. (*Courtesy of* C.G. Cobbs, MD.)

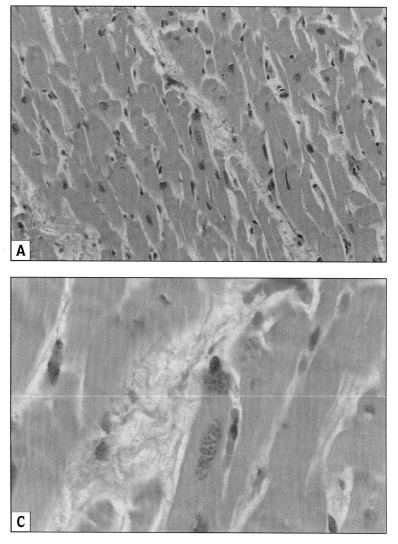

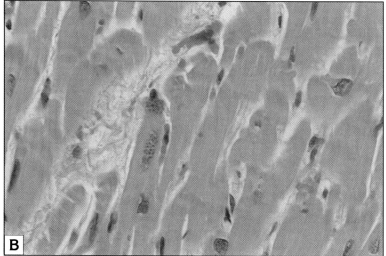

FIGURE 8-36 A–C, Acute systemic toxoplasmosis. A cystozoite is seen. This patient recently underwent heart transplantation and suffered almost immediate severe rejection. Toxoplasmosis was found to be widely disseminated at autopsy. (*Courtesy of* S.D. Reilly, MD.)

MEDIASTINITIS

Causes of acute mediastinitis

Oropharyngeal infection complication
Perforation of the esophagus
Cardiac surgery
Infection from contiguous structures

FIGURE 8-37 Causes of acute mediastinitis. Most cases of acute mediastinitis in the current era are the result of complications from cardiothoracic surgery, the incidence of which ranges from 0.4% to 5.0%. Sternal débridement and prolonged antimicrobial therapy are needed for cure.

Possible clinical signs of acute mediastinitis

Fever
Tachycardia
Brawny edema of neck or chest wall
Purulent pleural or pericardial effusions
Pneumonitis
Postoperative sternal instability
Widening mediastinum on chest radiograph

FIGURE 8-38 Possible clinical signs of acute mediastinitis. Patients are often severely ill and toxic. Aggressive care is necessary, but mortality is high. (*Adapted from* Savoia and Oxman [2].)

Potential acute mediastinitis organisms

Anaerobes (after esophageal perforation and oropharyngeal infection)
Staphylococcus aureus
Gram-negative organisms, including *Pseudomonas aeruginosa*
Staphylococcus epidermidis (postoperative)

FIGURE 8-39 Potential acute mediastinitis organisms. The origin of the infection and whether it is postoperative helps identify the infecting organism. Postoperative complications usually occur several weeks after the procedure. (*Adapted from* Savoia and Oxman [2].)

Fibrosing mediastinitis

Most common etiologic agents
 Histoplasma capsulatum
 Tuberculosis
Common presentations
 Asymptomatic mediastinal mass
 Occlusion of major mediastinal structures (superior vena cava syndrome)
Histology
 Intense inflammatory reaction, perhaps in response to rupture of caseating lymph nodes in area

FIGURE 8-40 Fibrosing mediastinitis. Granulomatous and fibrosing mediastinitis may account for 10% of all primary mediastinal masses. Surgery may help if performed early but may only be palliative if offered late. (*Adapted from* Savoia and Oxman [2].)

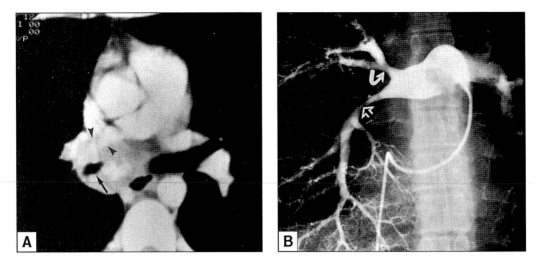

FIGURE 8-41 Fibrosing mediastinitis. Granulomatous and fibrosing mediastinitis may account for 10% of all primary mediastinal masses. The leading infectious causes are tuberculosis and histoplasmosis. Clinical compromise results from entrapment of mediastinal vascular structures. Surgery may help if performed early but may only be palliative if offered late. **A,** Contrast-enhanced chest computed tomographic scan of a man aged 55 years with mediastinal fibrosis due to histoplasmosis shows a calcified subcarinal mass encasing the bronchus intermedius (*arrow*) and compressing the right pulmonary artery (*arrowheads*). **B,** Pulmonary arteriogram shows severe stenosis (*open arrow*) of the interlobar pulmonary artery and mild stenosis (*solid arrow*) at the origin of the truncus anterior (right upper lobe pulmonary artery). (*From* McAdams *et al.* [15]; with permission.)

REFERENCES

1. Hancock EW: On the elastic and rigid forms of constructive pericarditis. *Am Heart J* 1980, 100:917.

2. Savoia M, Oxman M: Myocarditis, Pericarditis, and Mediastinitis. In *Principles and Practice of Infectious Diseases*, 3rd ed. Edited by Mandell GL, Bennett JE, Dolin R. New York: Churchill Livingstone; 1990:721–728.

3. Shabetai R: Diseases of the pericardium. In *The Heart*, 6th ed. Edited by Hurst JW. New York: McGraw Hill, 1986:1249–1275.

4. Becker AE, Anderson R: *Cardiac Pathology: An Integrated Text and Colour Atlas*. London: Raven Press; 1983.

5. Belmonte R, Bikowski J, Clements DA, *et al.*: *Color Atlas of Infectious Disease*, vol. 3. Greenwich, CT: Clinical Communications Inc.; 1995.

6. Artez HT, Billingham ME, Edwards WD, *et al.*: Myocarditis: A histopathologic definition and classification. *Am J Cardiovasc Pathol* 1987, 1:3.

7. Herskowitz A, Ansari A: Myocarditis. In *Atlas of Heart Diseases*, vol 2. Edited by Braunwald E, Abelmann WH. Philadelphia: Current Medicine; 1996.

8. Hutchins GM: Cardiovascular Pathology. Part II: Acquired Heart Disease. New York: Medcom; 1972.

9. Strain JE, Grose RM, Factor SM, *et al.*: Results of endomyocardial biopsy in patients with spontaneous ventricular tachycardia but without apparent structural heart disease. *Circulation* 1983, 68:1171–1181.

10. Smith WG: Coxsackie B myopericarditis in adults. *Am Heart J* 1980, 80:34–36.

11. Aretz HT: Myocarditis: The Dallas criteria. *Hum Pathol* 1987, 18:619.

12. Becker AE: Myocarditis. In *Cardiovascular Pathology*. Edited by Silver M. New York: Churchill Livingstone; 1991:719–741.

13. Bloor CM: Pericarditis and myocarditis. In *Cardiac Pathology*. Philadelphia: JB Lippincott; 1978:265–295.

14. Silvestry F, Kim B, Pollack B, Haimowitz J: Cardiac Whipple disease: Identification of Whipple bacillus by electron microscopy in the myocardium of a patient before death. *Ann Intern Med* 1997, 126(3):214–215.

15. McAdams HP, Rosado-de-Christenson ML, Lesar M, *et al.*: Thoracic mycoses from endemic Fungi: Radiologic-pathologic correlation. *Radiographics* 1995, 15:255–270.

SELECTED BIBLIOGRAPHY

Becker AE: Myocarditis. In *Cardiovascular Pathology*. Edited by Silver M. New York: Churchill Livingstone; 1991:719–741.

Becker AE, Anderson R: *Cardiac Pathology: An Integrated Text and Colour Atlas*. London: Raven Press; 1983.

Herskowitz A, Ansari A: Myocarditis. In *Atlas of Heart Diseases*, vol 2. Edited by Braunwald E, Abelmann WH. Philadelphia: Current Medicine; 1996.

Savoia M, Oxman M: Myocarditis, Pericarditis, and Mediastinitis. In *Principles and Practice of Infectious Diseases*, 3rd ed. Edited by Mandell GL, Bennett JE, Dolin R. New York: Churchill Livingstone; 1990:721–728.

Wynne J, Braunwald E: The Cardiomyopathies and myocarditis. In *Heart Disease*. Edited by Braunwald E. Philadelphia: WB Saunders; 1988:1410–1470.

CHAPTER 9

Chagas' Disease

Harry Acquatella

IN 1909, the Brazilian physician Carlos Chagas described a disease, which is caused by the protozoan *Trypanosoma cruzi*. Confined within ecologic units composed of infected sylvatic or peridomestic mammals and sylvatic triatomid vectors, it exists only in the Americas. Human infection occurs by penetration of these ecotopes. In Latin America it is estimated that about 16 million people are infected and another 90 million are at risk of acquiring the parasite. The initial infection occurs largely unnoticed in childhood only to become clinically manifest in adulthood. Chagas' disease mainly affects people of the lowest socioeconomic level.

In recent decades substantial migration of infected rural dwellers to urban communities has occurred. After living several decades in nonendemic areas, subjects with chronic Chagas' disease may be misdiagnosed as having ischemic heart disease or idiopathic dilated cardiomyopathy. Exposed to urban risk factors, these individuals may also present in combination with other cardiac disorders. A positive epidemiology and serology thus does not necessarily mean that cardiac symptoms are of chagasic origin in a particular patient. The diagnosis must also rely on a combination of clinical findings known as the *chagasic syndrome*. Peculiar to chagasic myocarditis is the frequently focal nature of the scarring lesions at the left ventricular apex.

Transmission of Chagas' disease via blood transfusion is a real threat even in nonendemic countries. Because at present neither a cure nor eradication is possible, prophylactic measures are of the utmost importance. Programs to control Chagas' disease are based on good epidemiologic data, housing improvement, elimination of the vectors, and community education. Only a few countries have implemented these preventive measures on a large scale.

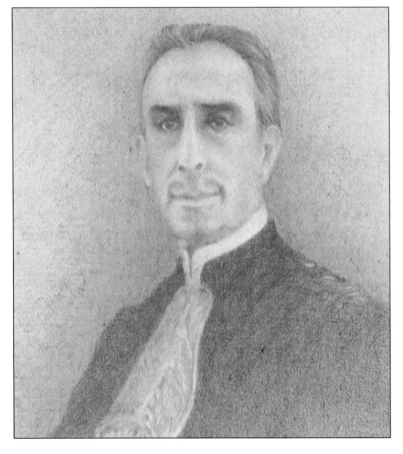

FIGURE 9-1 Carlos Chagas (1879–1934). The discovery of American trypanosomiasis (the parasite, transmitting vectors, and human clinical manifestations) is "an extraordinary chapter in the history of modern epidemiology and a tribute to the powers of observation and deduction of one man" [1,2]. Carlos Chagas, while on a mission to control malaria in Lassance (a shantytown in Minas Gerais), noticed the abundance of blood-sucking insects (*Panstrongylus megistus*), containing innumerable flagellate forms of an unknown parasite in the insect gut. Exposure of these insects to a monkey and other laboratory mammals was followed by the appearance of trypanosome forms in peripheral blood. Finally in 1909, Chagas examined a 9-month-old girl, Berenice, suffering from fever, increased glands, and hepatosplenomegaly, and he detected the same flagellate in peripheral blood smears. He proposed the name *Trypanosoma cruzi* to honor his mentor, Dr. Oswaldo Cruz [3]. Berenice died of advanced age. (*From* Gomez [4]; with permission.)

ETIOLOGY

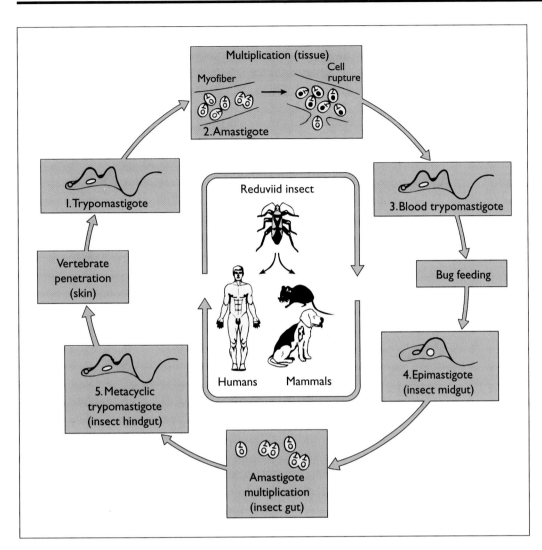

FIGURE 9-2 Parasite cycle. Chagas' disease is caused by *Trypanosoma cruzi*, a protozoan present in sylvatic mammals of the Americas such as armadillos, rodents, and opossums, as well as in domestic animals. It has vertebrate and invertebrate cycles. Transmission to humans is by reduviid bugs while feeding, by fecal contamination rather than inoculation. After initial trypomastigote (flagellate form) parasitemia (*1*), the parasites penetrate cardiac muscle and other tissue cells where they transform into amastigotes (aflagellate form) (*2*). Intracellular parasite multiplication may lead to cell rupture with passage into the circulation or parasitism of other tissues including various ganglionic plexuses and segments of the alimentary tract. The cycle is completed when feeding bugs pick up blood trypomastigotes (*3*). The trypanosomes become epimastigotes in the insect midgut (*4*), and then multiply and migrate to the hindgut where they become metacyclic trypomastigotes (*5*), the infective form in humans. Continuous transmission is independent of human infection [5].

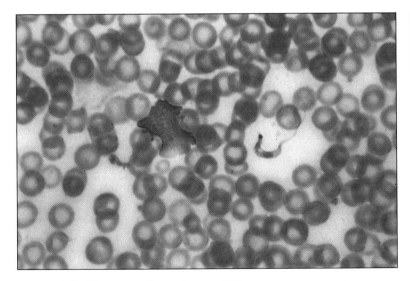

FIGURE 9-3 Trypomastigote form of *Trypanosoma cruzi* in a peripheral blood smear. Various parasite strains are recognized by different morphologic and histopathologic behavior in mice [6], of which the Y strain is particularly aggressive. Nuclear *T. cruzi* DNA fingerprinting allows characterization of distinct parasite strains. Individual clones of the Y form shows that the strain is heterogeneous [7]. (*From* The Pan American Health Organization [8]; with permission.)

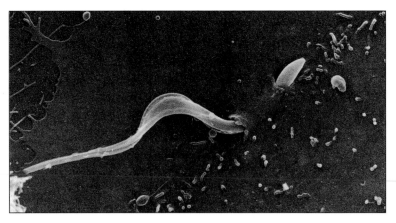

FIGURE 9-4 Scanning electron micrograph of *Trypanosoma cruzi* trypomastigotes actively entering mammalian cells. Immediately after invasion, the parasites can be found inside endocytic vacuoles in macrophages, fibroblasts, epithelial and endothelial cells, muscle, and nerve cells. Attachment of the parasite is an active process that requires energy, which can be inhibited by drugs affecting *T. cruzi* energy conservation. (*From* Schenkman *et al.* [9]; with permission.)

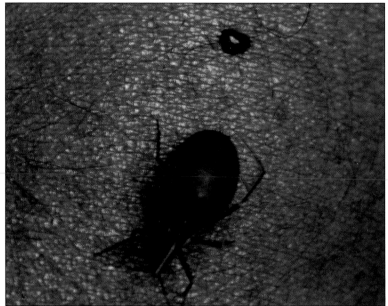

FIGURE 9-5 *Rhodnius prolixus* (nymph stage) after having a meal. The abdomen is greatly swollen from sucked blood even after defecation (dark bright spot behind the insect). The infection is acquired through the skin or mucosa by penetration of infecting forms of *Trypanosoma cruzi* present in the insect feces. (*From* The Pan American Health Organization [8]; with permission.)

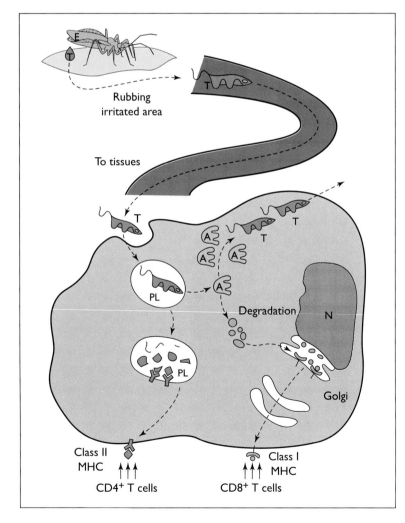

FIGURE 9-6 Aspects of the life cycle of *Trypanosoma cruzi* and the potential for antigen presentation to CD4+ and CD8+ T cells. Epimastigotes (E), which multiply in the midgut of insects vectors, and blood-borne trypomastigotes (T), which enter tissue macrophages by phagocytosis, are shown. In the phagolysosomes (PL), trypomastigotes, by a mechanism that is unclear, enter the cytoplasm and convert to replicating amastigotes (A), which eventually produce new trypomastigotes. In the phagolysosome system, there is opportunity for trypanosome antigens to be presented by class II major histocompatibility complex (MHC) molecules to CD4+ T cells; during replication in the cytoplasm, there is the possibility for trypanosome antigens to be presented by class I MHC molecules. N—nucleus. (*Adapted from* Parham [10]; with permission.)

EPIDEMIOLOGY

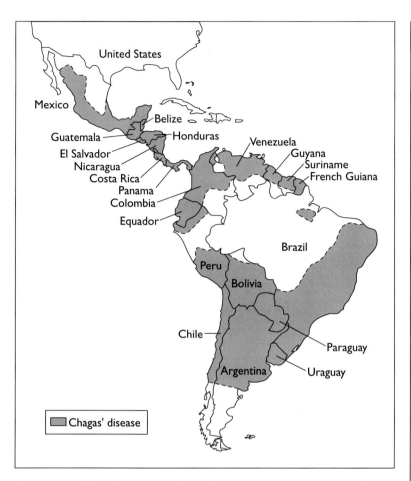

FIGURE 9-7 Distribution of Chagas' disease in the Americas. The extent of Chagas' disease depends on the geographic distribution of the triatomid vectors of *Trypanosoma cruzi* (*shaded areas*). There are significant differences among insect species of ecotope habitats: *Triatoma infestans* (southern South America) and *Rhodnius prolixus* (northern South America) are well adapted to human dwellings, whereas *T. protracta* (North America) is sylvatic. *T. dimidiata*, *T. sordida*, *T. brasiliensis*, and *Panstrongylus megistus* are in the process of adapting to the human habitat while preserving an extensive sylvatic ecotope [11]. These differences have implications for both human infection and control programs. In geographic areas where domiciliary vectors predominate, high rates of human infection exist, but insect eradication programs are more prone to be effective. Areas harboring vectors living in mixed ecotopes are the most challenging to control. Human infection is rare in areas having exclusively sylvatic (woodland) vectors. (*Adapted from Epidemiol Bull PAHO* [12].)

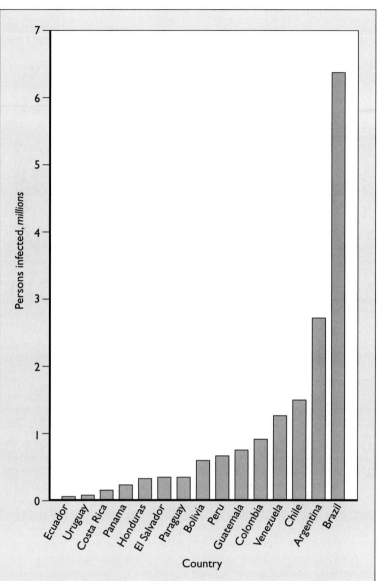

FIGURE 9-8 Prevalence of human *Trypanosoma cruzi* infection in Latin America from 1980 to 1986 [13]. The countries with the four highest rates have established prophylactic control programs. Although the prevalence in the United States is not known [14], emigration of about 5 million people from Latin America in the past three decades allows for an estimate that 50,000 to 100,000 immigrants have *T. cruzi* infection in the United States [15].

PATHOGENESIS AND PATHOPHYSIOLOGY

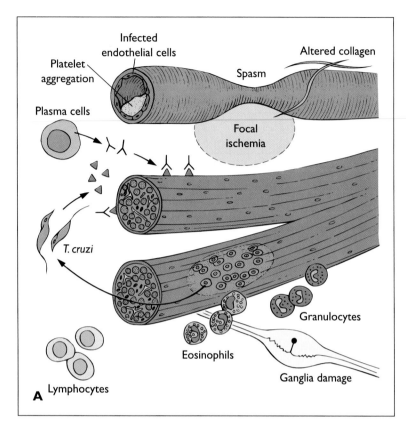

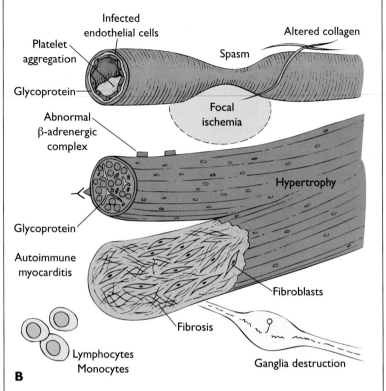

FIGURE 9-9 Pathophysiologic mechanisms proposed to explain the cardiac damage induced by *Trypanosoma cruzi* [16]. **A**, Acute Chagas' disease. The penetration of the parasite into the cardiocyte exerts direct mechanical damage and may lead to myofibrillar rupture. Intense inflammation of the endomysium is denoted by infiltration composed of granulocytes, eosinophils, lymphocytes, histiocytes, and macrophages. Cytotoxic T lymphocytes are sensitized by *T. cruzi* antigens (*triangles*). Antibodies (*inverted Ys*) are produced by plasma cells, which might cross-react with tissue. T lymphocytes release lymphokines attracting and activating macrophages and platelet activator factor, which may promote platelet aggregation and thromboxane A₂ release. Intense vasculitis and abnormalities in the coronary microcirculation may lead to microvascular hyperactivity (spasm). These microvascular changes may lead to focal ischemia. Infected endothelial cells have an increased platelet-binding and enhanced endothelium-platelet interaction. Intracardiac lesions of the autonomic nervous system (ganglia damage) include periganglionitis, perineuritis, neuronal cell depletion, and Schwann cell damage. **B**, Chronic Chagas' disease. Destruction of cardiocytes and fibrotic replacement are accompanied by hypertrophy of the remaining myocardial cells.

Myocyte hypertrophy and fibrosis interplay in a ventricular remodeling process that may take years. Myocyte ultrastructural abnormalities include mitochondrial atrophy, edema, and severe contractile system lysis. Deposition of a glycoprotein-like substance may appear in the tubular T system, and in the basement membrane of cardiac myocytes and of the endothelium. A mononuclear and lymphocytic infiltrate predominates. The absence of parasites has stimulated the concept of an autoimmune myocarditis, by virtue of cross-reactivity with mammalian tissue antigens. *T. cruzi* epimastigote forms may share antigenic determinants with mammalian striated and cardiac muscle sarcoplasmic reticulum. Extensive vagal aganglionosis and intracardiac autonomic damage may induce autonomic dysfunction (slow heart rate response to exercise, postural hypotension). Alteration of the β-adrenergic receptor complex in acute and chronic Chagas' disease may occur. Extracellular matrix abnormalities (altered collagen) have been observed in chronic murine chagasic myocarditis and in vitro *T. cruzi*–infected endothelial cells. This could allow cardiac muscle fiber slippage, fiber realignment, and wall thinning, leading to ventricular remodeling. (*Adapted from* Weber *et al.* [17].)

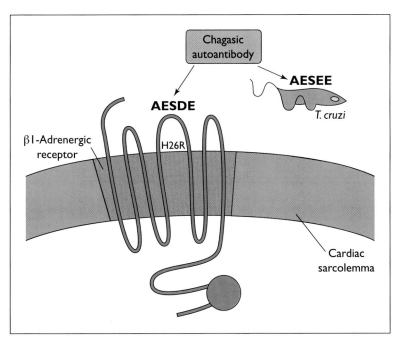

FIGURE 9-10 Schematic representation of β_1-adrenergic receptor complex. The host humoral immune response may modify the mechanical and biochemical activity of the heart in Chagas' disease. Chagasic antibodies recognize by molecular mimicry both the second extracellular loop of the human β_1-adrenergic receptor (H26R) and the carboxyl-terminal part of the ribosomal PO protein of *Trypanosoma cruzi* [18]. AESDE denotes a pentapeptide derived from human β_1-adrenoreceptor and AESEE, a pentapeptide from PO *T. cruzi* proteins (PO-β and PO-14i). In vitro experiments adding sera containing chagasic autoantibodies from rats showed that autoantibody deposited on myocardial neurotransmitter receptors may behave like an agonist that desensitizes and/or downregulates these receptors. Furthermore, a monoclonal antibody (MAbCAK20.12, not shown) that recognizes a *T. cruzi* antigen interferes with the binding of β-adrenoreceptor and muscarinic cholinergic receptors, leading to increased intracellular levels of cyclic AMP [19]. (*Adapted from* Ferrari *et al.* [18] and Wisler *et al.* [20].)

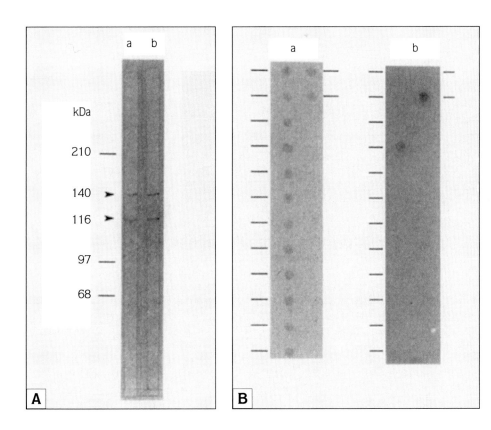

FIGURE 9-11 Molecular mimicry in Chagas' disease between the human cardiac myosin heavy chain and *Trypanosoma cruzi* B13 protein [21]. **A**, Immunoblot with *T. cruzi* trypomastigote lysate incubated with antimyosin antibody purified from sera from a patient with chronic chagasic heart disease (*strip a*) and a rabbit antiserum to B13 recombinant protein (*strip b*). A doublet of bands of 140/116-kDa (*arrowheads*) was recognized by antimyosin antibodies in 61% of patients with severe heart damage but only in 9% of Chagas' asymptomatic subjects (*P*= 0.005). **B**, Dotblots with *T. cruzi* B13 recombinant protein incubated with antimyosin antibodies were positive in all 14 chronic chagasic cardiac patients (*strip a*) but only in two of 14 asymptomatic Chagas' subjects (*strip b*) (*P*= 0.000002). Cross-reactive antibody recognition restricted to chagasic patients with heart damage defines the human cardiac myosin heavy chain and *T. cruzi* protein B13 as an antigen pair of potential relevance in the pathogenesis of chronic Chagas' heart disease. Molecular mimicry with other host components (skeletal muscle, neurons) are described [22]. (*From* Cunha-Neto *et al.* [21]; with permission)

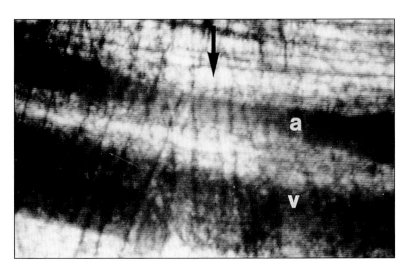

FIGURE 9-12 Videomicrograph of microvasculature changes observed in the cremaster muscle of a mouse acutely infected with *Trypanosoma cruzi* showing areas of segmental arteriolar (a) vasospasm (*arrow*). There was a significant decrease in red cell velocity in first- and third-order arterioles and venules (v) and an intense inflammatory response. These changes were reversed by verapamil. Scale bar = 20 μm. (*From* Tanowitz *et al.* [23]; with permission.)

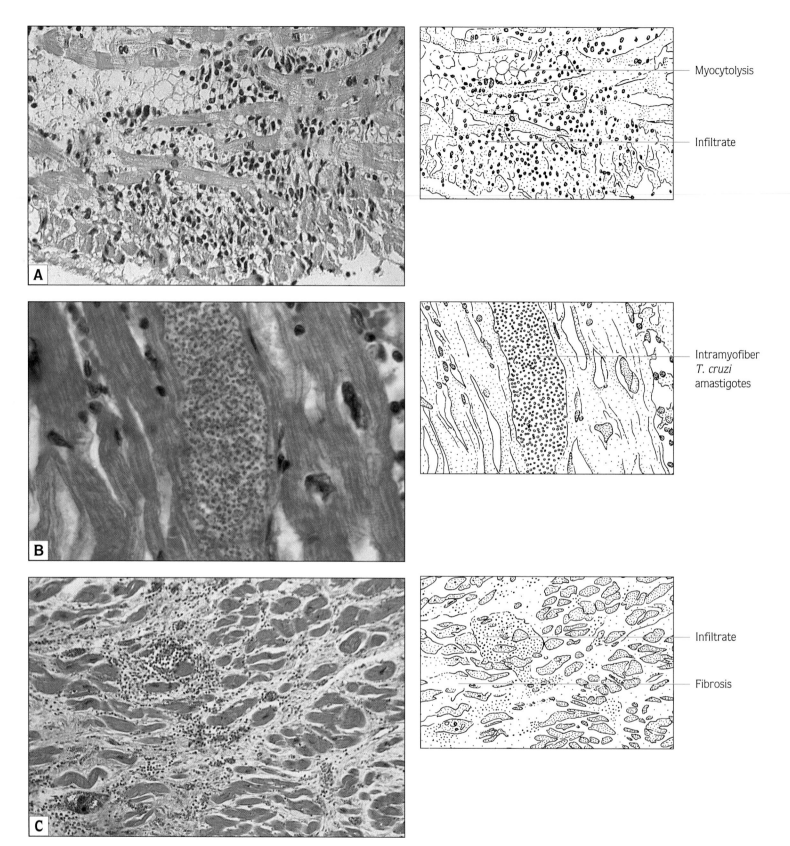

FIGURE 9-13 A, Endomyocardial biopsy section obtained from a patient with a 1-month clinical history of acute chagasic infection. Extensive myocardial fiber necrosis (myocytolysis) is accompanied by an inflammatory lymphocytic infiltrate. **B**, Autopsy section from a patient with chronic chagasic myocarditis shows an intramyofiber *Trypanosoma cruzi* amastigote nest. Parasites are rarely detected histologically in chronic cases. **C**, The chronic form may have diffuse or focal inflammatory infiltrates, predominantly of mononuclear cells (lymphocytes, monocytes, and plasma cells). Degeneration, fragmentation, and destruction of myocardial fibers are present along with interstitial fibrosis. (*Courtesy of* J.A. Suarez, MD.)

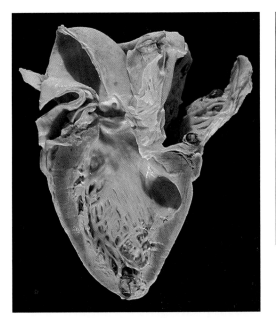

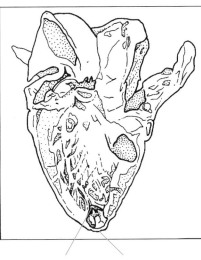

FIGURE 9-14 The heart from a patient who died suddenly shows a narrow-neck typical chagasic left ventricular apical aneurysm that is partially thrombosed. Approximately half of all patients with chronic Chagas' disease have an apical lesion. Various pathophysiologic mechanisms have been suggested to explain its origin, such as a dysautonomic imbalance with increased sympathetic drive, increased wall stress on the apex, microvascular lesions, and herniation through the apical myocardial spiral bundles. Right ventricular apical aneurysms are found at autopsy in about 10% to 20% of patients.

Thrombus   Apical aneurysm

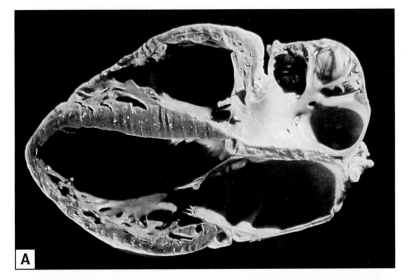

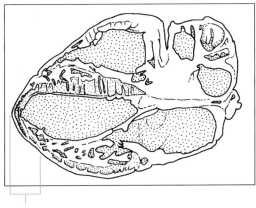

Apicoposterior scarring

A

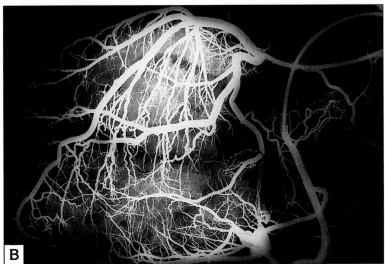

B

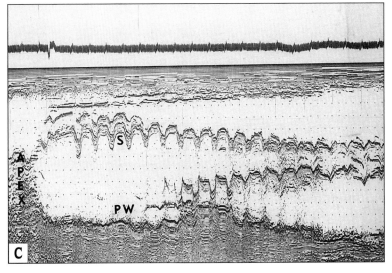

C

FIGURE 9-15 Fibrosis of the left ventricular apicoposterior wall from a patient dying in congestive heart failure. **A,** Left ventricular long-axis slice displays the apicoposterior scarring. Septal thickness is normal. **B,** Postmortem barium filling of the coronary arteries shows absence of obstruction. **C,** Slow-sweep M-mode echocardiogram scan of the long axis of the left ventricle shows preserved inward systolic thickening of the septum (S) in contrast to the noncontracting thin fibrotic posterior wall (PW). Approximately 20% of chagasic patients in heart failure may have free wall left or right ventricular localized areas of fibrosis. (Panels 15A and 15C *from* Acquatella *et al.* [24]; with permission.)

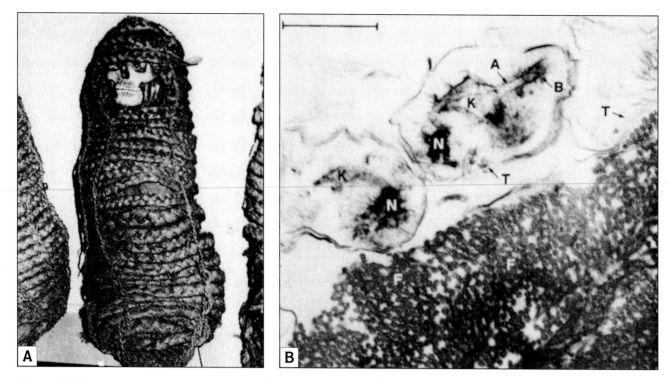

FIGURE 9-16 Chagas' disease in a Peruvian Inca mummy. **A**, Woman aged approximately 20 years, probably from 15th to 16th century AD. Megavisceral syndrome was found (cardiomegaly, megaesophagus, gastric ectasia, and megacolon with enormous amounts of feces). **B**, Ultrastructural study of the esophagus wall showed a large deposit of collagen fibers (F) and a group of *Trypanosoma cruzi* amastigote forms showing double peripheral membrane, microtubules (T), electrodense material identifiable as nucleus (N), a semilunar body identified as kinetoplast (K), and a cylindric structure identifiable as axoneme (A) with a basal body (B). Scale bar= 0.5 μm. (*From* Fornaciari *et al.* [25]; with permission.)

NATURAL HISTORY AND DIAGNOSIS

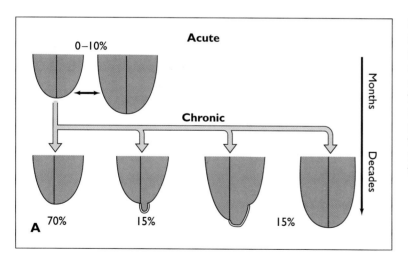

FIGURE 9-17 A, Scheme of the natural history of Chagas' heart disease represented by relative ventricular size. Primary infection occurs mostly unrecognized. Clinically apparent acute chagasic myocarditis may appear in up to 10% of persons (usually children) living in endemic areas. Chronic Chagas' disease takes years to develop into three clinical groups. A latent asymptomatic phase (indifferentiate form) develops in about 70% of seropositive persons. The rest become symptomatic with mild to moderate to severe heart damage. The main symptoms arise from arrhythmias, embolism, or heart failure. The *yellow border* represents the left ventricular apical aneurysm. (*continued*)

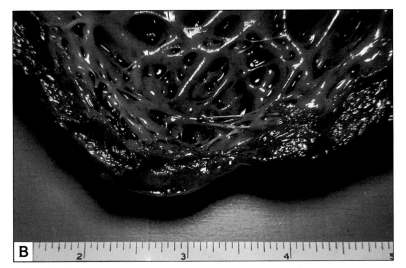

FIGURE 9-17 (*continued*) **B**, Thinning and hemorrhage of the apical ventricular muscle in a patient with Chagas myocarditis. Weakening in this area usually progresses to aneurysm formation (Panel 17B *courtesy of* O.M. Korzeniowski, MD.)

Diagnosis of acute and chronic Chagas' disease

	Acute	Chronic
Epidemiology		
Infection acquisition		
Natural	Endemic area	Endemic area
Through blood transfusion, pregnancy, or accident	Yes	Yes
Parasite		
Blood (Giemsa stain)	Possible	Extremely rare
Culture	Possible	Extremely rare
Xenodiagnosis	>50%	About 20%–30%
Polymerase chain reaction	Under investigation	About 90%
Serology		
Immunoglobulins	IgM-IgG after 2–3 wk	IgG
Serology		Highly sensitive and specific in 97%, titers 1:32
Complement fixation		or more, false-positive found in leishmaniasis,
Immunofluorescence		schistosomiasis, and immunologic disorders
Hemagglutination		
Clinical findings		
Acute symptoms	Fever, malaise, nodes, generalized swelling, Romaña's sign (highly suspicious)	None
Heart size	Normal or enlarged	Normal or enlarged
Presentation	Acute myocarditis or chronic changing due to acute immune depression by AIDS, transplantation, or cancer chemotherapy	Asymptomatic, arrhythmias, embolism, heart failure
Apical lesion	Possible	Aneurysm in about 50%
Electrocardiogram	Tachycardia, nonspecific ST-T changes	Right bundle branch block, left anterior hemiblock, ventricular extrasystoles, abnormal Q, AV block

FIGURE 9-18 Diagnosis of acute and chronic Chagas' disease. The clinical diagnosis of Chagas' disease is based on the triad of positive epidemiology, positive serology, and a combination of clinical findings (*eg*, suggestive electrocardiographic abnormalities, apical aneurysm). Xenodiagnosis involves noninfested reduviid bugs that are fed with blood from presumed infected humans (or animals). After several weeks *Trypanosoma cruzi* may be demonstrated in the bugs. Polymerase chain reaction laboratory technique allows amplification of a specific DNA genome sequence of the parasite present in tissue or other material [26].

CLINICAL MANIFESTATIONS

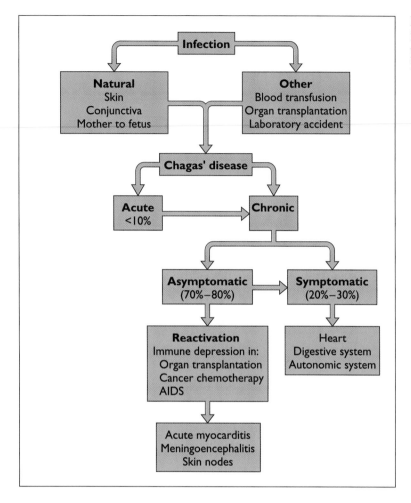

FIGURE 9-19 Mechanisms of infection and clinical manifestations in Chagas' disease. Numbers in parentheses denote approximate percentages. Disease reactivation leading to acute disease by immune depression was relatively unknown until a few decades ago.

Acute Disease

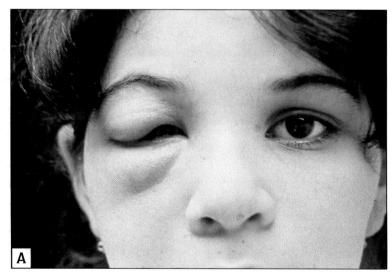

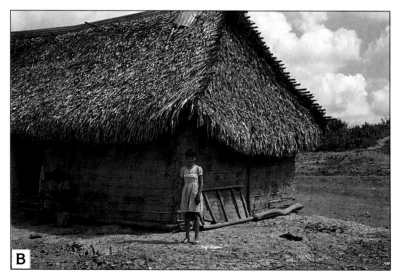

FIGURE 9-20 A, Romaña's sign. Romaña's sign is indicative of *Trypanosoma cruzi* conjunctival penetration seen during acute Chagas' disease. It consists of unilateral bipalpebral edema of abrupt onset, pink-violescent color, conjunctival congestion, and swelling of satellite nodes. It is a most useful clinical sign. Auto-inoculation by eye scratching with contaminated hands is possible. It has been reproduced experimentally in monkeys. B, Primitive housing made of mud-plastered walls and a ceiling of dried palm tree leaves. This type of housing is ideal for harboring reduviid insects. Infective bug droppings that fall from the ceiling may also contaminate the eye. Natural acute Chagas' infection almost always occurs in persons living in these ranchos or favelas. (Panel 20A *from* The Pan American Health Organization [8]; with permission.)

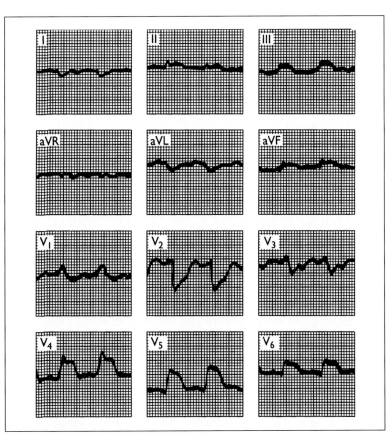

FIGURE 9-21 Electrocardiogram from a physician aged 25 years accidentally infected in the laboratory with *Trypanosoma cruzi* cultures who died after 5 weeks of heart failure from acute chagasic myocarditis. Right bundle branch block and monophasic extreme ST segment shift suggestive of a recent acute myocardial infarction are present. At autopsy, acute necrotizing panmyocarditis was more intense in the anterolateral and posterior walls of the left ventricle. Intramyocardial *T. cruzi* amastigote nests were seen. The majority of patients with acute disease do not present with this extremely aggressive form. (*Adapted from* Rosenbaum [27]; with permission.)

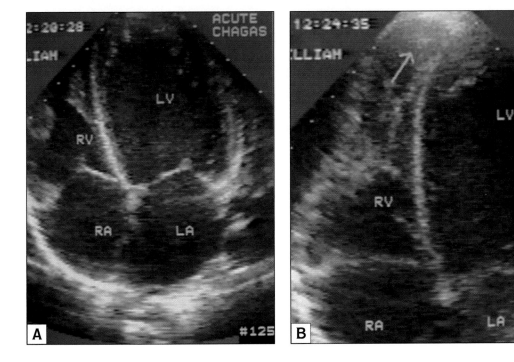

FIGURE 9-22 Two-dimensional echocardiographic four-chamber apical view from an boy aged 11 years with a 1-month history of acute chagasic myocarditis. **A**, The left ventricle (LV) was moderately dilated and diffusely hypokinetic, with intracavitary echoes. Moderate mitral regurgitation was present on Doppler studies. **B**, The right ventricular (RV) apex had a systolic bulge (*arrow*), suggesting that apical abnormalities may appear early in the disease. Both atria were dilated. The echocardiographic examination has also proved to be of great diagnostic help in chronic cases. LA—left atrium; RA—right atrium.

Chronic Disease

Clinical classification and findings in chronic Chagas' disease

	Asymptomatic	Symptomatic	
Group	A or I	B or I	C or III
Clinical history	Unremarkable, referral by positive serology	Palpitations, dizziness, syncope, fatigue, asthenia, shortness of breath, embolism	
NYHA classification	—	I–II	III–IV
Physical examination	Unremarkable	Regurgitant murmurs, S_3, venous and liver congestion, edema, pulmonary rales	
Electrocardiogram	N-A	N-A	A
Heart size (by radiography)	N	N/increased	Increased
Echocardiography and ventricular angiography			
Apical lesion	Akinesis/dyskinesis	Akinesis or aneurysm in approximately 50%	
Other focal scarring	No	Posterior wall in approximately 10%–20%	
Chamber size	N	N/increased	Increased
Ejection fraction	N	N/decreased	Decreased
Apical thrombus	Rare	10%–30%	
Diastolic function	N-A	Abnormal relaxation and filling	
Endomyocardial biopsy			
Light microscopy	N/chronic myocarditis		
Ultrastructure	N/T-tubules incipient dilatation, mitochondrial and nuclear changes	Chronic myocarditis, progression of changes, glycoprotein-like deposits, contractile system lysis	

A—abnormal; N—normal; NYHA—New York Heart Association.

FIGURE 9-23 Classification into three groups (A, B, C or I, II, III) is most useful because each group has a different clinical course (*see* Fig. 9-44). Epidemiologic surveys show that about three quarters of seropositive people are asymptomatic (indeterminate form). Approximately half of asymptomatic people have normal electrocardiograms, but cardiac damage may be demonstrated by other methods such as echocardiography, left ventriculography, or myocardial biopsy. The presence of other cardiac disorders (hypertension, ischemic heart disease) may pose clinical difficulties in ascertaining the contribution of Chagas' disease to the heart damage of a particular patient.

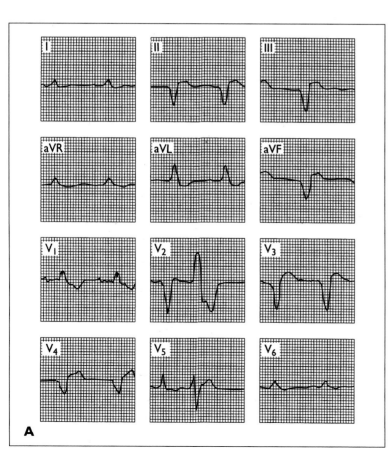

A

FIGURE 9-24 A, Electrocardiogram typical of chronic Chagas' disease shows right bundle branch block, left anterior hemiblock, poor precordial R-wave progression, ST segment elevation on precordial leads, and ventricular extrasystoles. (*continued*)

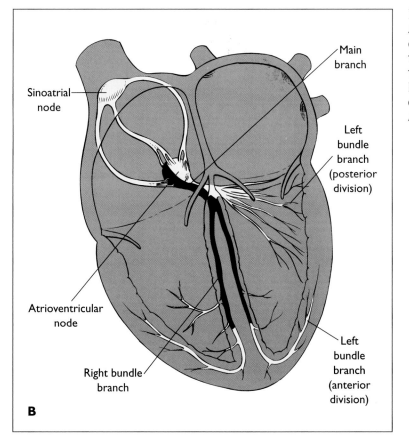

B

FIGURE 9-24 (*continued*) **B**, Diagram of the conduction system. Autopsy of the same patient revealed scattered lymphocytes, mild diffuse and distal fibrosis of the inferior portion of the atrioventricular node, and selective involvement of the right portion of the His bundle and right bundle and of the anterior portion of the left bundle were seen. A good correlation existed between the electrocardiographic and histopathologic findings. (*Adapted from* Andrade *et al.* [28]; with permission.)

Electrocardiographic findings in endemic areas

ECG abnormality		Abnormal		RBBB		LAHB		VPC	
Serology		+	-	+	-	+	-	+	-
Study	Persons studied, *n*								
Diaz *et al.* [29]	280	32.7	3.4	13.5	0.0	—	—	15.4	1.1
Rosenbaum and Cerisola [30]	1354	27.7	10.9	9.7	0.9	—	—	7.3	2.0
Pifano *et al.* [31]	7000	22.9	6.1	7.1	2.2	—	—	4.2	0.6
Maguire *et al.* [32]	644	20.2	6.0	10.7	0.3	3.2	2.7	7.5	5.4
Baruffa *et al.* [33]	1332	30.2	9.9	4.7	0.1	8.9	1.8	5.7	0.6
Acquatella *et al.* [34]	1698	30.2	2.4	16.8	1.3	16.5	3.9	18.2	4.3
Estimated risk ratio		2.8	—	13.0	—	3.3	—	4.0	—

ECG—electrocardiogram; LAHB—left anterior hemiblock; RBBB—right bundle branch block; VPC—ventricular premature contraction.

FIGURE 9-25 Electrocardiographic (ECG) surveys performed in Brazil, Argentina, and Venezuela before (1949–1985) and after (1987) the introduction of Chagas' control measures. The ECG combination of right bundle branch block, left anterior hemiblock, first- or second-degree atrioventricular block (not shown), and ventricular premature contraction is highly suggestive of chagasic origin. ECG has become the epidemiologic method of choice for screening heart damage in rural areas because it is inexpensive, transportable, and easy to read. Comparison of the age-related rates of ECG abnormalities before and after Chagas' control programs were introduced did not differ significantly [34].

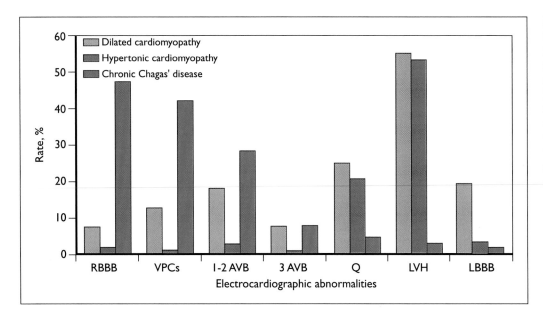

FIGURE 9-26 Differences in the rates of some electrocardiographic abnormalities found in patients with dilated cardiomyopathy, hypertrophic cardiomyopathy [35], and chronic Chagas' disease [36]. LBBB—left bundle branch block; LVH—left ventricular hypertrophy; Q—pathologic Q wave; RBBB—right bundle branch block; VPCs—ventricular premature contractions; 1-2 AVB—first- and second-degree atrioventricular block; 3 AVB—third-degree atrioventricular block.

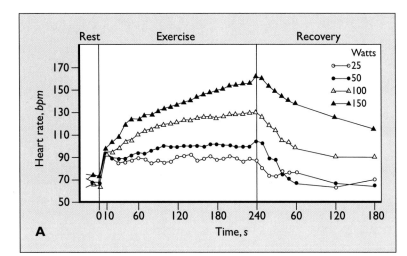

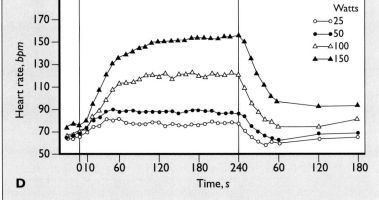

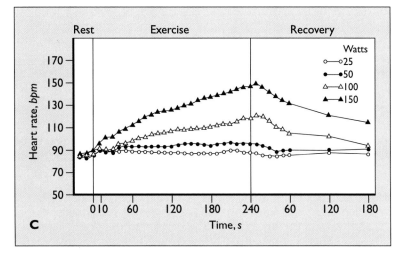

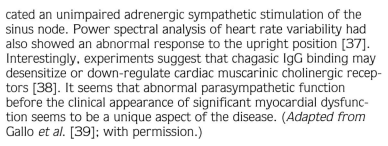

FIGURE 9-27 Changes in heart rate response during bicycle exercise. **A**, Normal control patient. **B**, Asymptomatic chagasic patient without cardiac disease. **C** and **D**, Chagasic patients with typical electrocardiograms but normal echocardiograms. Chagasic patients had a significantly abnormal lower heart rate increase in the first 10 seconds of cycle exercise at different workloads. Heart rate responses at 1 to 4 minutes of exercise were unaltered in all patients. The abnormal initial heart rate response was attributed to depression of parasympathetic efferent action on the sinus node, whereas the preserved late heart response indicated an unimpaired adrenergic sympathetic stimulation of the sinus node. Power spectral analysis of heart rate variability had also showed an abnormal response to the upright position [37]. Interestingly, experiments suggest that chagasic IgG binding may desensitize or down-regulate cardiac muscarinic cholinergic receptors [38]. It seems that abnormal parasympathetic function before the clinical appearance of significant myocardial dysfunction seems to be a unique aspect of the disease. (*Adapted from* Gallo *et al.* [39]; with permission.)

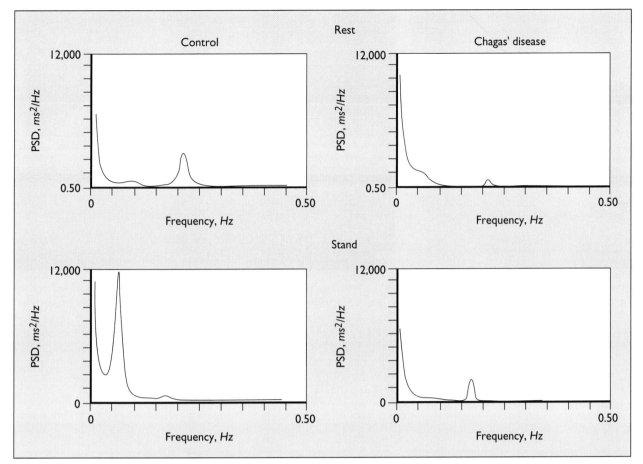

FIGURE 9-28 Power spectral density (PSD) of heart rate RR variability in a control subject (*left panels*) and in a patient with Chagas' disease (*right panels*) at rest (*top panels*) and during standing (*bottom panels*). Note that the low-frequency component does not increase in the chagasic subject during standing. (*Adapted from Guzzetti et al.* [37].)

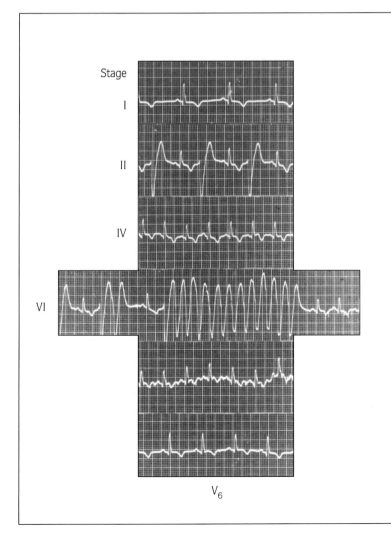

FIGURE 9-29 Electrocardiographic lead V_6 tracings obtained during a treadmill stress test (Naughton protocol) from a patient aged 37 years with chronic Chagas' disease. Upper strip shows T-wave inversion at rest. Ventricular bigeminy appears at stage II. The fourth strip, obtained at peak exercise, shows a couplet preceding a run of nonsustained rapid ventricular tachycardia, which prompted the interruption of the test. The fifth strip, taken immediately after exercise, shows an atrial flutter with a 4:1 conduction ratio. Normal sinus rhythm reappeared in the last strip. The patient hardly complained of symptoms. Contrary to coronary heart disease, Chagas' patients seldom develop ischemic ST-segment elevation or depression during electrocardiographic stress tests, which are useful for arrhythmia detection.

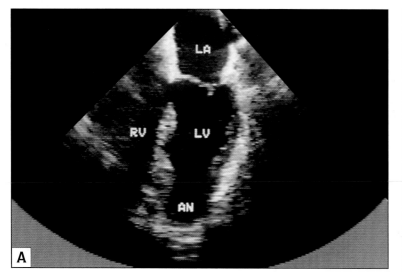

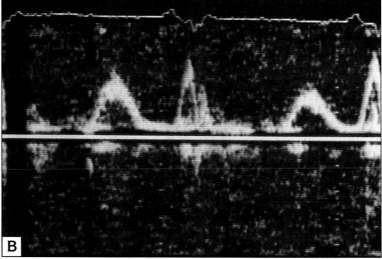

FIGURE 9-30 Two-dimensional echocardiography is helpful in characterizing ventricular function and morphology, especially of the apical lesions [24]. **A,** Transesophageal echocardiogram (transverse plane) of the long axis of the heart of a patient with a chagasic apical aneurysm (AN) of the left ventricle (LV) who had sustained multiple cerebral embolisms despite oral anticoagulation. Notice the relative shape preservation of the superior two thirds of the ventricle and the systolic bulging of the apex. No cavitary thrombus was found at the time of the examination.

B, Pulsed Doppler examination at the tip of the mitral valve is useful in analyzing the left ventricular inflow filling characteristics. This tracing obtained from a young adult shows a lower peak velocity at early diastole than at late diastole, suggesting abnormal early filling (relaxation). The reverse occurs when left atrial pressure is increased in heart failure, whereas in early diastole peak velocity inflow is high and deceleration time is short. LA—left atrium; RV—right ventricle.

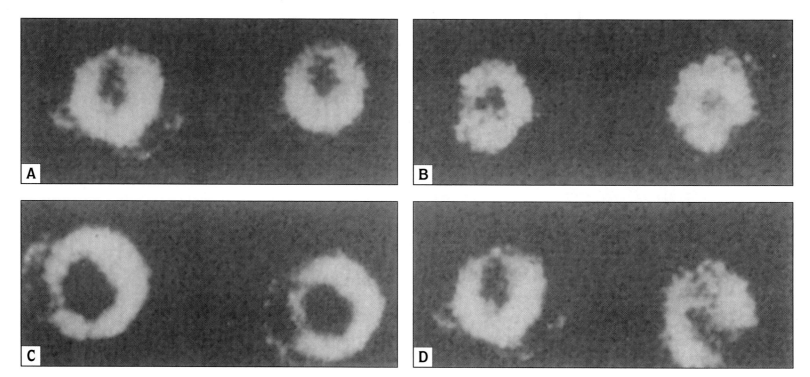

FIGURE 9-31 **A–D,** Examples of normal (*panel 31A*) thallium-201 effort-redistribution uptake and each type of perfusion defect found in a group of patients with Chagas' disease complaining of atypical chest pain: reversible (*panel 31B*) and fixed (*panel 31C*) septal defects and a paradox defect (*panel 31D*) in the posterolateral region. The *left* and *right frames* represent scintigraphic left anterior oblique views for effort and redistribution, respectively, in all panels. (*From* Marin-Neto *et al.* [40]; with permission.)

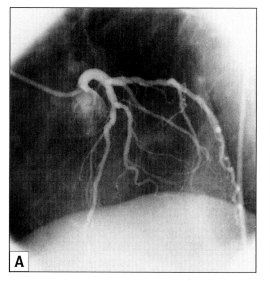
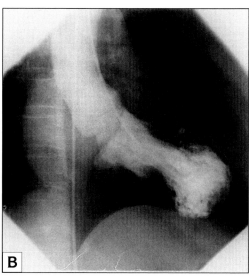

FIGURE 9-32 Chronic Chagas' disease simulating ischemic heart disease in a woman aged 55 years who complained of atypical chest pain. The electrocardiogram had QS morphology in several precordial leads suggestive of anteroseptal myocardial infarction. **A,** Angiogram of a normal left anterior coronary artery. **B,** Right anterior view angiogram of the left ventricle shows a large apical aneurysm. This and similar patients may pose difficulties in the differential diagnosis [41]. Coronary vasospasm secondary to autonomic imbalance [40,42–44], coronary embolism with recanalization, and abnormalities in the coronary microcirculation have been suggested to explain these findings [43–45].

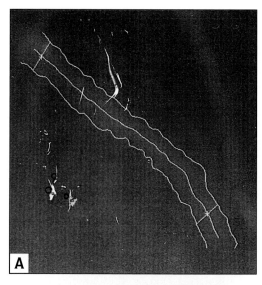
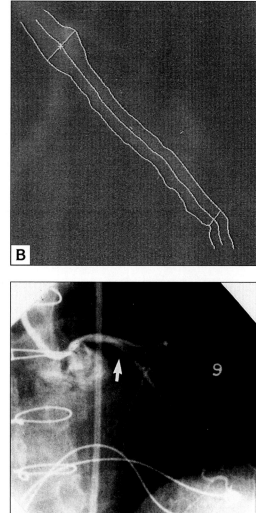
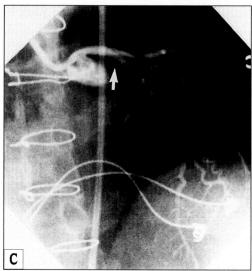

FIGURE 9-33 Abnormal endothelium-dependent coronary vascular reactivity in Chagas' disease shown by the effects of intracoronary infusion of acetylcholine. **A,** Baseline quantitative angiogram of the left anterior descending coronary artery in a patient with chronic Chagas' heart disease. **B,** A significant paradoxical decrease in diameter of the same artery occurred during the intracoronary infusion of increasing concentrations of acetylcholine up to 10^{-6} mol/L. **C** and **D,** corresponding angiograms before and at peak acetylcholine infusion. The *arrows* indicate the artery segment studied; number 6 is inverted in *panel 33D*. The reduction in coronary blood flow surpassed 40%. This abnormality in endothelium-dependent coronary vasodilation suggests that epicardial and microvascular responses are abnormal in these patients. *Trypanosoma cruzi*–induced abnormalities of endothelial cell structure and function have been demonstrated in animal models of Chagas' disease (*see* Fig. 9-12) [23,46]. These findings support a role for ischemic mechanisms in the pathophysiology of the disease. (*From* Torres *et al.* [45]; with permission.)

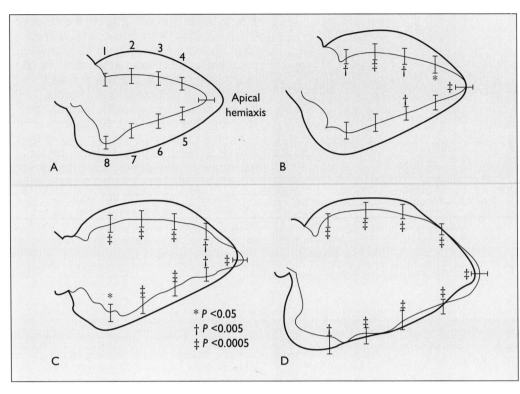

FIGURE 9-34 Cineventriculographic left ventricular outline analysis of segmental myocardial shortening of 126 chronic chagasic patients divided into groups of increasing damage. Continuous and interrupted lines denote end-diastolic and end-systolic frames, respectively. Enumeration corresponds to hemiaxes according to the Leighton method. **A** and **B**, Asymptomatic subjects with normal electrocardiograms and chest radiographs; few had atypical chest pain. In *panel 34A*, all 30 had normal segmental shortening and volumes. In *panel 34B*, among 21 subjects, 95% had asynergy at the apex, combined or not, with significant hypokinesis of the anterior and inferomedial segments. **C** and **D**, Patients with and without heart failure, respectively. Extensive asynergy, ventricular dilatation, decreased distensibility, and depressed contractility of increased severity were found. Large apical aneurysms were found in 40%, with thrombosis in 20%. *T-bars* represent the mean percent segmented shortening ±1 SD. (*Adapted from* Carrasco *et al.* [47]; with permission.)

FIGURE 9-35 Gadolinium-enhanced magnetic resonance imaging (short-axis view) showing an intense inflammatory process in the basal region of inferolateral left ventricular wall (*arrows*) in a patient with chronic Chagas' heart disease. Endomyocardial biopsy guided by transesophageal echocardiography of this wall disclosed severe myocarditis and the presence of *Trypanosoma cruzi* antigens by immunoperoxidase staining using rabbit antiserum. A significant correlation was found between the presence of *T. cruzi* antigens and moderate or severe myocarditis, supporting an active role of the parasite, even in the chronic form of the disease. (*From* Bellotti *et al.* [48]; with permission.)

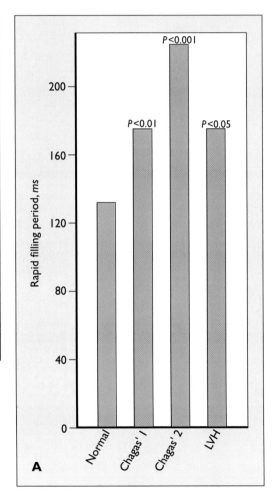

FIGURE 9-36 Abnormalities in early isovolumic relaxation assessed by left ventricular diastolic time intervals were shown by digitized simultaneous M-mode echocardiograms, phonocardiograms, and apexcardiograms in Chagas' 1 (asymptomatic) subjects, Chagas' 2 (with arrhythmias) subjects, and non-Chagas' subjects with left ventricular hypertrophy (LVH), and were compared with a normal control group. **A**, Significantly prolonged rapid filling time. (*continued*)

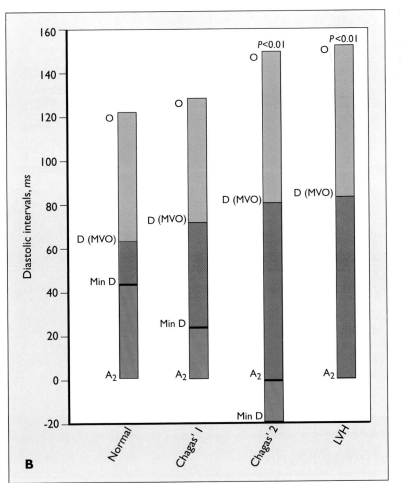

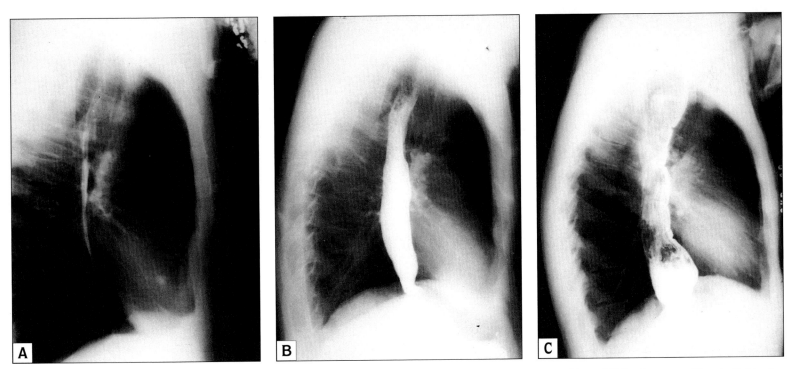

Disease Reactivation

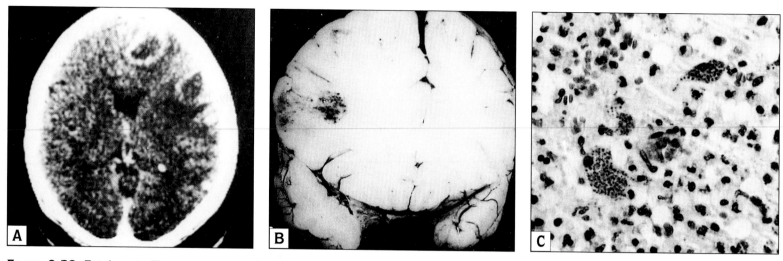

FIGURE 9-38 Fatal acute *Trypanosoma cruzi* meningoencephalitis in a man aged 37 years with hemophilia who has been positive for HIV for 21 months. The patient (known to have chronic Chagas' disease) developed headache, fever, and abnormal cerebrospinal fluid. **A,** Computed tomographic scan of the brain showed multiple hypodense nodular lesions with ring-shaped enhancement after intravenous injection of contrast material. **B,** Autopsy brain section disclosed a large lesion of the right parietal lobe and multiple small lesions scattered in subcortical areas of both hemispheres. **C,** Histopathology showed severe meningoencephalitis with numerous intracellular pseudocysts filled with amastigote forms of *T. cruzi*. (*From* Ferreira *et al.* [51]; with permission.)

THERAPY AND MANAGEMENT

Therapeutic modalities	
Parasiticide drugs	Nifurtimox (15 mg/kg for 120 d)
	Benznidazole (5 mg/kg for 60 d)
	High rate of secondary effects with both drugs [52]
	Indications: acute Chagas' disease, accidental contamination
	Uncertain benefit in chronic cases
Arrhythmias	Amiodarone: ventricular extrasystoles or tachycardia, efficacious in over 50% of treated patients [53,54]
	Mexiletine [55]
	Quinidine, disopyramide, and other class I antiarrhythmic drugs have induced a high incidence of *torsades de pointes* [53,55]
	Aneurysmectomy in selected cases [56]
	Chemical ablation in selected patients [57]
	Implantable defibrillator in evaluation [58]
Complete atrioventricular block	Survival improvement in the absence of heart failure [59]
	Atrioventricular sequential pacing in heart failure
Heart failure	Traditional treatment: low salt, diuretics, digitalis
	ACE inhibitors seem to improve survival [60]
	Oral anticoagulants
	Cardiomyoplasty [61]
	Heart transplantation [62,63]
Dysautonomic symptoms	Gangliosides appear to ameliorate dysautonomic symptoms in selected patients [64]
Disease reactivation	Immunosuppression and transplantation may require use of benznidazole or nifurtimox in cancer chemotherapy [65], AIDS immune depression [51,66–68], and organ transplant chemotherapy [14,62,63]

ACE—angiotensin converting enzyme.

FIGURE 9-39 Therapeutic modalities in Chagas' disease. Heart transplantation for chronic Chagas' heart disease is associated with a high rate of *Trypanosoma cruzi* infection of the graft despite preoperative parasiticidal treatment.

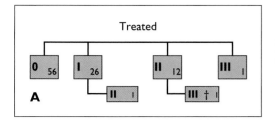

A

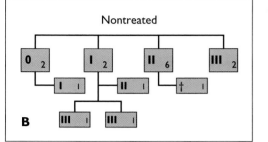

B

FIGURE 9-40 Changes in clinical group classification of Chagas' seropositive patients (age ≤50 years) whether or not they were treated with benznidazole (5 mg/kg/d for 30 days). **A**, Treated patients. **B**, Nontreated patients. Mean follow-up was nearly 8 years. Comparison of treated and nontreated subjects disclosed advancing clinical deterioration in 2.1% and in 17% ($P<0.01$), appearance of new electrocardiographic abnormalities in 4.2% and 30% ($P<0.001$), and conversion to seronegative in 19.1% and 6% ($P<0.05$), respectively. These results contrast with the inability of benznidazole treatment before cardiac transplant to prevent *Trypanosoma cruzi* reactivation in the host recipient [62]. *Dagger* denotes death. Group 0—no abnormality; I—electrocardiographic abnormality; II—plus chest radiograph cardiomegaly; III—plus heart failure. (*Adapted from* Viotti *et al.* [69]; with permission.)

Effects of antiparasite drugs on a murine model of short-term Chagas' disease

Treatment	Survival (105 days)	Negative parasitologic, serologic tests (105 days)
None (control)	0/27*	0/27
Nifurtimox (50 mg/kg/d)	6/10	0/10
Ketoconazole (30 mg/kg/d)	13/27	1/27
DO870 (10 mg/kg/d)	24/28	11/28

*Numbers indicate number of mice.

FIGURE 9-41 Experimental results of different chemotherapeutic agents in mice infected with *Trypanosoma cruzi*. It appears that the new agent DO870 is highly effective in both experimental models of short-term and long-term (not shown) murine models of Chagas' disease. In the long-term model, DO870 (≥15 mg/kg/d) provided more than 80% protection from death and parasitologic cure. Nifurtimox and benznidazole are nitrofurans commonly used in the treatment of human Chagas' disease. Ketoconazole is a sterol biosynthesis inhibitor used in the treatment of fungal disease. DO870 a *bis*-triazole derivative able to affect the metabolism of endogenous *T. cruzi* sterols. Human studies are pending.(*Adapted from* Urbina *et al.* [70].)

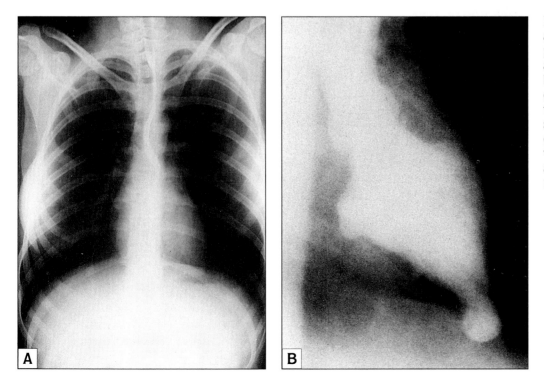

A

B

FIGURE 9-42 Seventeen-year follow-up of a woman who required various therapeutic procedures. **A**, Heart size was normal at age 25 years when she initially consulted because of palpitations. This normal radiographic aspect is misleading because two-dimensional echocardiography showed an apical aneurysm. **B**, Angiography demonstrated a narrow-neck left ventricular apical aneurysm, normal basal and midventricular wall contractility, and normal ejection fraction. (*continued*)

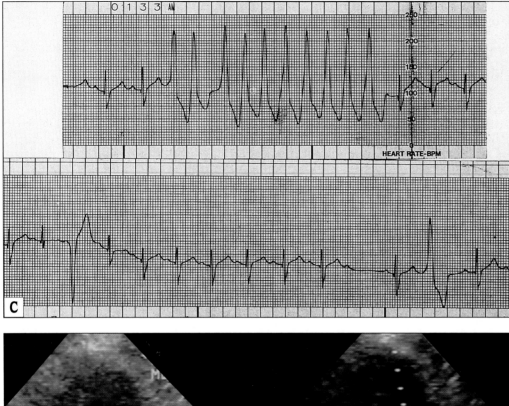

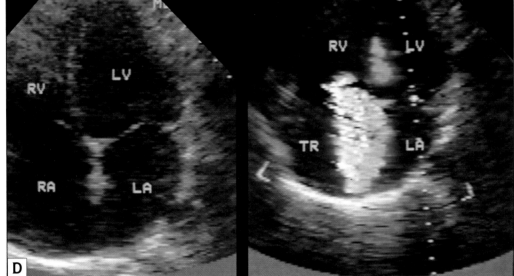

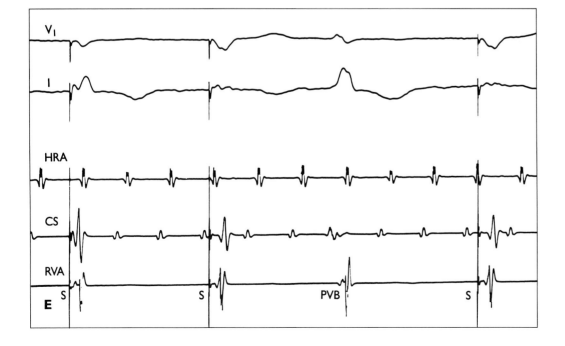

FIGURE 9-42 (*continued*) **C,** At age 27 years she developed severely symptomatic runs of sustained and nonsustained ventricular tachycardia resistant to antiarrhythmic therapy. Results of an electrophysiologic study led to an aneurysmectomy with subsequent disappearance of the malignant arrhythmias. Two years later the patient needed a pacemaker because of multiple syncopal attacks secondary to intermittent atrioventricular block. **D,** At age 37 years two-dimensional echocardiography disclosed an increase in ventricular size, moderately depressed ejection fraction, greatly enlarged atria (*left panel*), and severe tricuspid regurgitation on color Doppler (*right panel*). Notice the postaneurysmectomy rounded apex. **E,** At age 42 years the patient had drug-resistant incessant atrial tachyarrhythmias with intermittent rapid ventricular response and congestive heart failure. His bundle electrogram obtained after radiofrequency ablation of the conduction system below the atrioventricular node shows a decrease in the ventricular response. CS—coronary sinus; HRA—high right atria; I—lead I; LA—left atrium; LV—left ventricle; PVB—premature ventricular beat; RA—right atrium; RV—right ventricle; RVA—RV apex; S—pacemaker spikes; TR—tricuspid regurgitation. (Panel 42B *from* Acquatella *et al.* [24]; with permission; panel 42D *courtesy of* V. Medina, MD.)

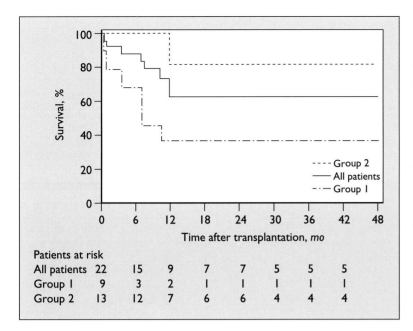

FIGURE 9-43 Kaplan-Meier survival curves of 22 patients with chronic Chagas' heart disease submitted to cardiac transplantation [62]. Group 1 underwent transplantation from 1985 to 1991 and group 2 from 1991 to 1995. Group 2 had a significantly better survival (*P*=0.008 by log-rank test). Immunosuppression was based on cyclosporine A and azathioprine. Parasitemia, reactivation of Chagas' disease with myocarditis, and neoplasias (lymphoma, Kaposi's sarcoma) were more common in group 1. The reduction of cyclosporine dose and steroids and increased experience improved survival. Chagas' disease reactivation was successfully treated with benznidazole. This agent is effective in reducing parasitemia but not in elimination of *Trypanosoma cruzi* tissue forms. In other series, survival rates were 78% at 2 years and 68% at 10 years, and rejection was less frequent in chagasic than in age- and sex-matched control patients (*P*=0.0001)[63]. (*Adapted from* Bocchi *et al.* [62]; with permission.)

MORTALITY AND PREVENTION

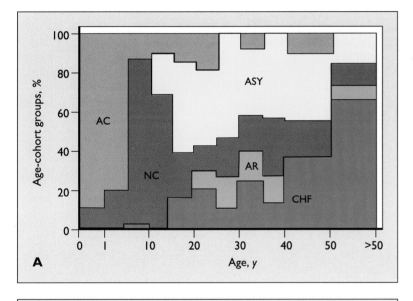

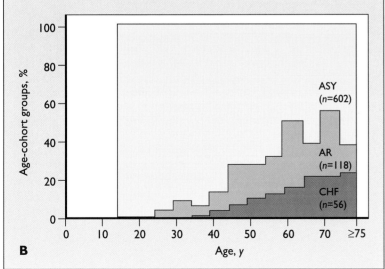

FIGURE 9-44 Changing clinical presentation of Chagas' disease observed in Roscio county (Venezuela) before and after a prophylactic control program aimed to eliminate transmitting vectors in a time span of nearly 50 years. **A,** Between 1934 and 1958, 291 subjects were collected with positive *Trypanosoma cruzi* xenodiagnosis before sanitary action. Infection with acute Chagas' disease (AC) before age 5 years was common and was associated with a high mortality of 23%. Chronic disease appearing as congestive heart failure (CHF) was observed in late adolescents, increasing in percentage in young adults. **B,** Clinical classification of 776 subjects with positive Chagas' serology studied between 1981 and 1984, living under 20 years of a prophylactic control program [34]. No acute Chagas' disease was observed. Severe cardiac compromise in young adults was "shifted" to mid–late adulthood. Moderate forms of clinical presentation as arrhythmias (AR) were more common. Although both series are not strictly comparable, these changes suggest a beneficial role of sanitary measures by diminishing transmission and reinfection of *T. cruzi.* ASY—asymptomatic; NC—not clinically classified (probably asymptomatic).

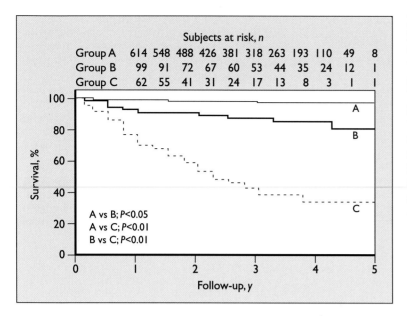

FIGURE 9-45 Survival of 775 Chagas' seropositive subjects according to clinical group classification. Group A denotes asymptomatic; Group B, moderately symptomatic; and group C, severely symptomatic patients, respectively. Survival rates among the three groups were significantly different at 3 and 5 years ($P<0.01$). The 95% confidence limits at 5-year follow-up were 97% to 98.7% for group A, 72.3% to 86.2% for group B, and 14.2% to 48.8% for group C. Mortality predictors (Cox regression model) in a series of chagasic patients with abnormal electrocardiograms [71] included systolic blood pressure of less than 120 mm Hg, atrial fibrillation, cardiothoracic index greater than 55%, and an angiographic left ventricular end-diastolic volume of greater than 110 mL/m² ($P=0.0228$). (*Adapted from* Acquatella *et al.* [34]; with permission.)

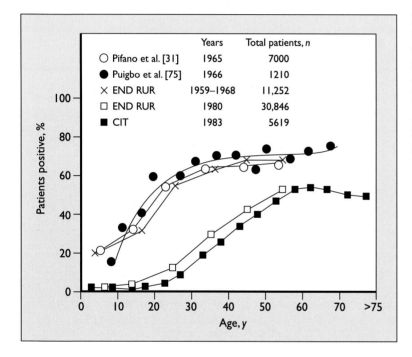

FIGURE 9-46 Decrease in the percentage of Chagas' seropositivity before and after a control program carried out in endemic communities of Venezuela between 1959 and 1983. Results of serologic surveys performed at the beginning (upper three series) and after 20 years (lower two series) show a decrease in the proportion of seropositive subjects at each age cohort, especially in subjects born during the program. Prophylactic control programs rely on housing improvement, elimination of domestic triatomid bugs, and community education [34,72–74]. CIT— Centro Investigaciones Torrealba (unpublished serology survey); END RUR—Endemias rurales (unpublished serology surveys).

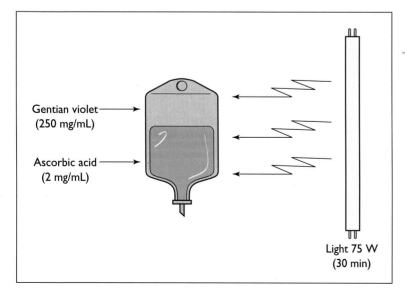

FIGURE 9-47 Sterilization of donated *Trypanosoma cruzi*–infected blood. Prevention of transfusion-associated Chagas' disease includes clinical and serologic screening of blood donors and/or inactivation of *T. cruzi* in collected blood using gentian violet [76]. In areas of high endemicity or where serologic screening is not possible, the use of gentian violet to collected blood (1:4000) for 24 to 48 hours decreases the risk of disease transmission. Further addition of ascorbic acid and blood photoradiation with a 75-W fluorescent light shortens the blood sterilization process to about 30 minutes [77]. In Brazil it has been estimated that the number of Chagas' infection acquired through blood transfusion may be as high as 20,000 new cases per year, or 10% of the yearly total [78].

REFERENCES

1. Hagar JM, Rahimtoola SH: Chagas' heart disease. *Curr Prob Cardiol* 1995, 20:825–928.

2. Iglesias JS, Storino R, Rigou D: Antecedentes históricos. In *Enfermedad de Chagas.* Edited by Storino R, Milei J. Buenos Aires: Doyma Argentina; 1994:9–30.

3. Chagas C: Nova espécie mórbida do homen produzida por um trypasonoma (*Trypanosoma cruzi*). Nóta previa. *Brasil Med* 1909, 23:161.

4. Gomez A: Carlos Chagas. In *Miocardiopatias.* Edited by Acquatella H, Pulido P. Barcelona: Salvat Editores SA; 1982.

5. Brener Z: O parasito: Relacoes hospedeiro-parasito. In *Trypanosoma cruzi e Doenca de Chagas.* Edited by Brener Z, Andrade A: Rio de Janeiro (Brazil): Editora Guanabara Koogan SA; 1979:1–41.

6. Andrade SG: Influence of *Trypanosoma cruzi* strain on the pathogenesis of chronic myocardiopathy in mice. *Mem Inst Oswaldo Cruz* 1990, 85:17–27.

7. Macedo AM, Martins MS, Chiari E, Pena SD: DNA fingerprinting of *Trypanosoma cruzi*: A new tool for characterization of strains and clones. *Mol Biochem Parasitol* 1992, 55:147–153.

8. Pan American Health Organization: La Historia Natural, la Epidemiologia y el Control de la Enfermedad de Chagas (curso de niveles multiples) [slides series 92]. Washington, DC: Pan American Health Organization.

9. Schenkman S, Robbins ES, Nussenzweig Y: Attachment of *Trypanosoma cruzi* to mammalian cells requires parasite energy, and invasion can be independent of the target cell cytoskeleton. *Infect Immun* 1991, 59:645–654.

10. Parham P: Defense cuts begin to bite. *Nature* 1992, 356:291–292.

11. Sherlock IA: Vetores. In *Trypanosoma cruzi e Doenca de Chagas.* Edited by Brener Z, Andrade Z. Rio de Janeiro: Editora Guanabara Kogan SA; 1979:42–88.

12. Status of Chagas' disease in the region of the Americas. *Epidemiol Bull PAHO* 1984, 5:5–9.

13. Moncayo A: Chagas' disease: Epidemiology and prospects for interruption of transmission in the Americas. *World Health Stat Q* 1992, 45:276–279.

14. Kirchhoff LV: American trypanosomiasis (Chagas' disease): A tropical disease now in the United States. *N Engl J Med* 1993, 329:639–644.

15. Milei J, Mautner B, Storino R, *et al.*: Does Chagas' disease exist as an undiagnosed form of cardiomyopathy in the United States? *Am Heart J* 1992, 123:1732–1735.

16. Acquatella H, Piras R: Chagas' disease. *Curr Opin Cardiol* 1993, 8:463–472.

17. Weber KT, Brilla CG, Janicki JS: Myocardial remodeling and pathologic hypertrophy. *Hosp Pract* 1991, 26: 73–80.

18. Ferrari I, Levin MJ, Wallukat G, *et al.*: Molecular mimicry between the immunodominant ribosomal protein P0 of *Trypanosoma cruzi* and a functional epitope on the human beta1-adrenergic receptor. *J Exp Med* 1995, 182:59–65.

19. Cremaschi G, Zwirner NW, Gorelik G, *et al.*: Modulation of cardiac physiology by an anti–*Trypanosoma cruzi* monoclonal antibody after interaction with myocardium. *FASEB J* 1995, 9:1482–1488.

20. Wisler PL, Green FJ, Watanabe AM: Cardiovascular adrenergic and muscarinic cholinergic receptors. In *Cardiology, An Illustrative Text/Reference.* Edited by Chatterjee K, *et al.* Philadelphia: JB Lippincott; New York: London Gower Medical Publishing; 1991.

21. Cunha-Neto E, Duranti M, Gruber A, *et al.*: Autoimmunity in Chagas' disease cardiopathy: Biological relevance of a cardiac myosin-specific epitope crossreactive to an immunodominant *Trypanosoma cruzi* antigen. *Proc Natl Acad Sci U S A* 1995, 92:3541–3545.

22. Kalil J, Cunha-Neto E: Autoimmunity in Chagas' disease cardiomyopathy: Fulfilling the criteria at last? *Parasitol Today* 1996, 12:396–399.

23. Tanowitz HB, Kaul DK, Chen B, *et al.*: Compromised microcirculation in acute murine *Trypasonoma cruzi* infection. *J Parasitol* 1996, 82:124–130.

24. Acquatella H, Schiller NB, Puigbo JJ, *et al.*: M-mode and two-dimensional echocardiography in chronic Chagas' heart disease. *Circulation* 1980, 62:787–799.

25. Fornaciari G, Castagna M, Viacava P, *et al.*: Chagas' disease in a Peruvian Inca mummy. *Lancet* 1992, 339:128–129.

26. Britto C, Cardoso MA, Monteiro-Vanni CM, *et al.*: Polymerase chain reaction detection of *Trypanosoma cruzi* in human blood samples as a tool for diagnosis and treatment evaluation. *Parasitology* 1995, 110:241–247.

27. Rosenbaum MB: Chagasic myocardiopathy. *Prog Cardiovasc Dis* 1964, 7:199–225.

28. Andrade ZA, Andrade SG, Oliveira GB, Alonso DR: Histopathology of the conducting tissue of the heart in Chagas' myocarditis. *Am Heart J* 1978, 95:316–324.

29. Diaz E, Laranja FS, Pellegrino J: Primera reunion Panamericana sobre enfermedad de Chagas, Tucuman (Argentina). Tucuman; 1949:I:33–34.

30. Rosenbaum MB, Cerisola JA: Epidemiologia de la enfermedad de Chagas en la Republica Argentina. *O Hospital* 1961, 60:55–99.

31. Pifano F, Anselmi A, Maekelt GA, *et al.*: Estudios sobre la miocardiopatia chagasica en el medio rural venezolano. *Arch Ven Med Trop Parasitol Med* 1965, 5:3–67.

32. Maguire JH, Mott KE, Lehman JS, *et al.*: Relationship of electrocardiographic abnormalities and seropositivity to *Trypanosoma cruzi* within a rural community in Northeast Brazil. *Am Heart J* 1983, 105:287–294.

33. Baruffa G, Alcantara-Filho A, de Aquino-Neto JO: Estudo pareado da cardiopatia chagasica no Rio Grande do Sul, Brasil. *Mem Inst Oswaldo Cruz* 1985, 80:457–463.

34. Acquatella H, Catalioti F, Gomez-Mancebo JR, *et al.*: Long-term control of Chagas' disease in Venezuela: Effects on serologic findings, electrocardiographic abnormalities, and clinical outcome. *Circulation* 1987, 76:556–562.

35. Flowers NC, Horan LG: Electrocardiographic and vectorcardiographic features of myocardial diseases. In *Myocardial Diseases.* Edited by Fowler NO. New York: Grune & Stratton; 1973:181–211.

36. Laranja FS, Dias E, Nobrega G, *et al.*: Chagas' disease: A clinical, epidemiologic, and pathologic study. *Circulation* 1956, 14:1035–1060.

37. Guzzetti S, Iosa D, Pecis M, *et al.*: Impaired heart rate variability in patients with chronic Chagas' disease. *Am Heart J* 1991, 121:1727–1734.

38. Sterin-Borda L, Gorelik G, Borda ES: Chagasic IgG binding with cardiac muscarinic cholinergic receptors modifies cholinergic-mediated cellular transmembrane signals. *Clin Immunol Immunopathol* 1991, 61:387–397.

39. Gallo L Jr, Morel-Filho J, Maciel BC, *et al.*: Functional evaluation of sympathetic and parasympathetic system in Chagas' disease using dynamic exercise. *Cardiovasc Res* 1987, 21:922–927.

40. Marin-Neto JA, Marzullo P, Marcassa C, *et al.*: Myocardial perfusion abnormalities in chronic Chagas' disease as detected by thallium-201 scintigraphy. *Am J Cardiol* 1992, 69:780–784.

41. Hagar JM, Rahimtoola SH: Chagas' heart disease in the United States. *N Engl J Med* 1991, 325:763–768.

42. Oliveira JSM, dos Santos M, Mucillo G, *et al.*: Increased capacity of the coronary arteries in chronic Chagas' disease: Further support for the neurogenic pathogenesis concept. *Am Heart J* 1985, 109:304–308.

43. Bestetti RB, Ariolli MT, do Carmo JL, *et al.*: Clinical characteristics of acute myocardial infarction in patients with Chagas' disease. *Int J Cardiol* 1992, 35:371–376.

44. Morris SA, Tanowitz HB, Wittner M, *et al.*: Pathophysiological insights into the cardiomyopathy of Chagas' disease. *Circulation* 1990, 82:1900–1909.

45. Torres FW, Acquatella H, Condado J, *et al.*: Coronary vascular reactivity is abnormal in patients with Chagas' heart disease. *Am Heart J* 1995, 129:995–1001.

46. Rossi MA, Ramos SG: Coronary microvascular abnormalities in Chagas' disease. *Am Heart J* 1996, 132:207–210.

47. Carrasco HA, Barboza JS, Inglessis G, *et al.*: Left ventricular cineangiography in Chagas' disease: Detection of early myocardial damage. *Am Heart J* 1982, 104:595–602.

48. Bellotti G, Bocchi EA, de Moraes AV, *et al.*: In vivo detection of *Trypanosoma cruzi* antigens in hearts of patients with chronic Chagas' heart disease. *Am Heart J* 1996, 131:301–307.

49. Combellas I, Puigbo JJ, Acquatella H, *et al.*: Echocardiographic features of impaired left ventricular diastolic function in Chagas' heart disease. *Br Heart J* 1985, 53:298–309.

50. Miles MA: The epidemiology of South American trypanosomiasis-biochemical and immunological approaches and their relevance to control. *Trans Royal Soc Trop Med Hyg* 1983;77:5–23.

51. Ferreira MS, Nishioka SDA, Rocha A, *et al.*: Acute fatal *Trypanosoma cruzi* meningoencephalitis in a human immunodeficiency virus-positive hemophiliac patient. *Am J Trop Med Hyg* 1991, 45:723–727.

52. Ferreira H de O: Treatment of the undetermined form of Chagas' disease with nifurtimox and benznidazole. *Rev Soc Bras Med Trop* 1990, 23:209–211.

53. Chiale PA, Halpern S, Nau GJ, *et al.*: Efficacy of amiodarone during long-term treatment of malignant ventricular arrhythmias in patients with chronic chagasic myocarditis. *Am Heart J* 1984, 107:656–665.

54. Giniger AG, Retyk EO, Laino RA, *et al.*: Ventricular tachycardia in Chagas' disease. *Am J Cardiol* 1992, 70:459–462.

55. Mendoza I, Camardo J, Moleiro F, *et al.*: Sustained ventricular tachycardia in chronic chagasic myocarditis: Electrophysiologic and pharmacologic characteristics. *Am J Cardiol* 1986, 57:423–427.

56. Milei J, Pesce R, Valero E, *et al.*: Electrophysiological-structural correlations in chagasic aneurysms causing malignant arrhythmias. *Int J Cardiol* 1991, 32:65–73.

57. dePaola AAV, Gomes JA, Miyamoto MH, *et al.*: Transcoronary chemical ablation of ventricular tachycardia in chronic chagasic myocarditis. *J Am Coll Cardiol* 1992, 20:480–482.

58. Valero de Pesce EM, Favaloro M, Pesce RA, Favaloro RG: Automatic implantable cardioverter-defibrillator: 4 year experience. *Rev Arg Cardiol* 1991, 59:4–11.

59. Greco OT, Ardito RV, Garzon SA, *et al.*: Follow-up of 991 patients with multiprogrammable artificial cardiac pacemaker. *Arq Bras Cardiol* 1987, 49:327–331.

60. Roberti RR, Martinez EE, Andrade JL, *et al.*: Chagas cardiomyopathy and captopril. *Eur Heart J* 1992, 13:966–970.

61. Moreira LF, Stolf NA, Braile DM, Jatene AD: Dynamic cardiomyoplasty in South America. *Ann Thorac Surg* 1996, 61:408–412.

62. Bocchi EA, Bellotti G, Mocelin AO, *et al.*: Heart transplantation for chronic Chagas' heart disease. *Ann Thorac Surg* 1996, 61:1727–1733.

63. Carvalho VB, Sousa EFL, Vila JHA, *et al.*: Heart transplantation in Chagas' disease: 10 years after the initial experience. *Circulation* 1996, 94:1815–1817.

64. Iosa D, Massari DC, Dorsey FC: Chagas' cardioneuropathy: Effect of ganglioside treatment in chronic dysautonomic patients: A randomized, double blind, parallel, placebo-controlled study. *Am Heart J* 1991, 122:775–785.

65. Villalba R, Fornées G, Alvarez MA, *et al.*: Acute Chagas' disease in a recipient of a bone marrow transplant in Spain: Case report. *Clin Infect Dis* 1992, 14:594–595.

66. Rosemberg S, Chaves CJ, Higuchi ML, *et al.*: Fatal meningoencephalitis caused by reactivation of *Trypanosoma cruzi* infection in a patient with AIDS. *Neurology* 1992, 42:640–642.

67. Gluckstein D, Ciferri F, Ruskin J: Chagas' disease: Another cause of cerebral mass in the acquired immunodeficiency syndrome. *Am J Med* 1992, 92:429–432.

68. Oddo D, Casanova M, Acuna G, *et al.*: Acute Chagas' disease (Trypanosomiasis americana) in acquired immunodeficiency syndrome: Report of two cases. *Hum Pathol* 1992, 23:41–44.

69. Viotti R, Vigliano C, Armenti H, Segura E: Treatment of chronic Chagas' disease with benznidazole: Clinical and serologic evolution of patients with long-term follow-up. *Am Heart J* 1994, 127:151–162.

70. Urbina JA, Payares G, Molina J, *et al.*: Cure of short- and long-term experimental Chagas' disease using D0870. *Science* 1996, 273:969–971.

71. Espinosa RA, Pericchi LR, Carrasco HA, *et al.*: Prognostic indicators of chronic chagasic cardiopathy. *Int J Cardiol* 1991, 30:195–202.

72. Mota EA, Guimaraes AC, Santana OO, *et al.*: A nine year prospective study of Chagas' disease in a defined rural population in northeast Brazil. *Am J Trop Med Hyg* 1990, 42:429–440.

73. Chuit R, Paulone I, Wisnivesky-Colli C, *et al.*: Result of a first step toward community-based surveillance of transmission of Chagas' disease with appropriate technology in rural areas. *Am J Trop Med Hyg* 1992, 46:444–450.

74. Control of Chagas' disease: Report of a WHO expert committee. *World Health Organ Tech Rep Ser* 1991, 811:1–95.

75. Puigbo JJ, Nava-Rhode JR, Garcia-Barrios H, *et al.*: Clinical and epidemiologic study of chronic heart involvement in Chagas' disease. *Bull WHO* 1966, 34: 655–669.

76. Nussenzweig V, Sonntag R, Biancalana A, *et al.*: Action of certain dyes on *T. cruzi* in vitro. The use of gentian violet to prevent the transmission of Chagas' disease by blood transfusion. *Hospital* (Rio J) 1953, 44:731–744.

77. Ramirez LE, Lages-Silva E, Pianetti GM, *et al.*: Prevention of transfusion-associated Chagas' disease by sterilization of *Trypanosoma cruzi*–infected blood, with gentian violet, ascorbic acid, and light. *Transfusion* 1995, 35:226–230.

78. Hayes RJ, Schofield CJ: Estimación de las tasas de incidencia de infecciones y parasitosis crónica a partir de la prevalencia: La enfermedad de Chagas' en América Latina. *Bol Oficina Sanit Panam* 1990, 108:308–316.

SELECTED BIBLIOGRAPHY

Control of Chagas' disease: Report of a WHO expert committee. *World Health Organ Tech Rep Ser* 1991, 811:1–95.

Storino R, Milei J (eds): *Enfermedad de Chagas.* Buenos Aires (Argentina): Doyma Argentina; 1994.

Hagar JM, Rahimtoola SH: Chagas' heart disease. *Curr Prob Cardiol* 1995, 20:825–928.

Kirchhoff LV: American trypanosomiasis (Chagas' disease): A tropical disease now in the United states. *N Engl J Med* 1993, 329:639–644.

Laranja FS, Dias E, Nobrega G, *et al.*: Chagas' disease: A clinical, epidemiologic, and pathologic study. *Circulation* 1956, 14:1035–1060.

CHAPTER 10

Echocardiography

Alexis B. Sokil

ECHOCARDIOGRAPHIC images are produced when high-velocity sound waves generated by a piezoelectric crystal in the transducer reflect off an acoustic target and return to the transducer. These sound waves are processed and displayed on a video monitor, then recorded on standard commercial videotape or optical disk. Although other imaging modalities, such as cineangiography, radionuclide imaging, and magnetic resonance imaging, have been used for endocarditis and have been found to be of some benefit, echocardiography with Doppler has emerged as the imaging modality of choice in patients with suspected or confirmed infective endocarditis. Its universal clinical acceptance results from its widespread availability, diagnostic accuracy, relatively low cost, and noninvasive nature as well as the presence of a solid database that has grown remarkably during the past 25 years.

Although the diagnosis of infective endocarditis is based on clinical signs and symptoms and positive blood cultures, the echocardiographic documentation of vegetations provides an enhanced degree of certainty toward making the diagnosis. The earliest descriptions of the echocardiographic appearance of vegetations were made by Dillon and colleagues [1] in 1973. Echocardiographic imaging has been shown to be increasingly useful since that time. The two-dimensional echocardiographic appearance of vegetations was first described in 1977 by Gilbert and associates [2]. Various morphologies of the infected masses known as vegetations have been described, including shaggy, irregular, linear, and globular. Although vegetations as small as 1 mm occasionally are recorded, a vegetation generally must be at least 2 to 3 mm in diameter to be detected by conventional transthoracic echocardiography.

Not only does the presence of vegetations confirm the diagnosis, but important prognostic information can also be gained from the echocardiogram. Serial studies can be performed for follow-up purposes. Clinical investigations have also shown that the echocardiographic confirmation of endocarditis implies an adverse prognosis. Patients with vegetations have a higher rate of developing embolic complications and congestive heart failure, and they require surgical intervention more often [3]. A vegetation size greater than 10 mm in its maximal dimension appears to signify a significantly increased risk of embolization [4]. Complications of the destructive process, including abscess formation, cusp perforation, dehiscence of a prosthetic valve, chordal rupture, and fistula formation, can be visualized echocardiographically. Pulsed, continuous-wave, and color-flow Doppler add tremendously to the echocardiographic examination [5]. Progressive infectious destruction results in valvular regurgitation, which is sometimes dramatically depicted by Doppler and can be a most compelling indication for surgical intervention in this disease.

Transesophageal echocardiography (TEE) has emerged as an even more sensitive procedure to enhance our ability to visualize smaller vegetations and other complications of endocarditis. Although this is an invasive procedure, it is still of low risk. It uses a higher-frequency transducer, and because there is no interposed lung tissue between the transducer and the heart, images are reliably of high quality. TEE has consistently been shown to improve the diagnostic accuracy of echocardiography for native valve and, especially, prosthetic valve endocarditis [6,7].

The TEE probe is positioned in the esophagus directly behind the left atrium and has an unobstructed view of the heart from a posterior approach, as contrasted with an anterior view with standard transthoracic echocardiography. This technique is performed in patients safely, with topical anesthesia and mild conscious sedation, and can be done on an awake outpatient or at the bedside of a critically ill patient in a brief period of time. TEE is probably more accurate early in the course of endocarditis, when vegetations are more likely to be smaller. Complications, such as satellite lesions, fistulas, valvular perforations, ring abscesses, and aneurysms, can be detected more readily. A normal TEE examination makes the diagnosis of infective endocarditis extremely unlikely.

DIAGNOSTIC UTILITY

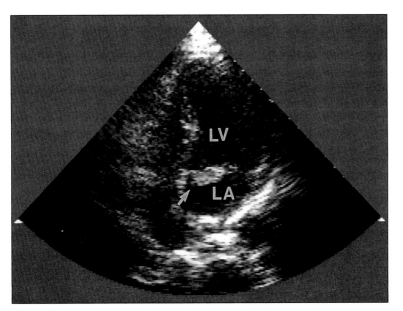

FIGURE 10-1 Transthoracic apical four-chamber echocardiogram illustrating a large vegetation (*arrow*) on the anterior mitral valve leaflet. This vegetation moved with the mitral valve in real-time. LA—left atrium; LV—left ventricle.

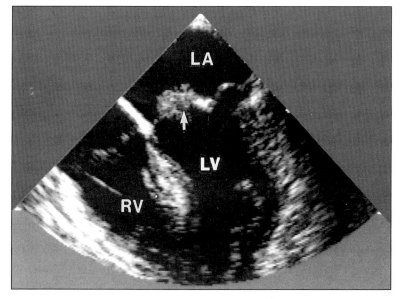

FIGURE 10-2 Transesophageal echocardiogram of same patient shown in Fig. 10-1, showing the large vegetation (*arrow*) on the left anterior mitral valve leaflet. LA—left atrium; LV—left ventricle; RV—right ventricle.

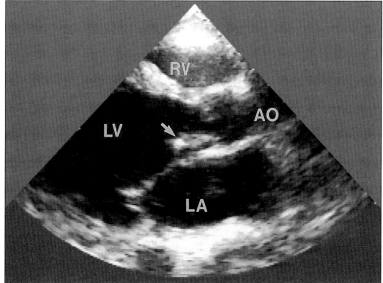

FIGURE 10-3 Transthoracic parasternal long-axis recording showing a large vegetation (*arrow*) on the left ventricular side of the aortic valve. AO—aorta; LA—left atrium; LV—left ventricle; RV—right ventricle.

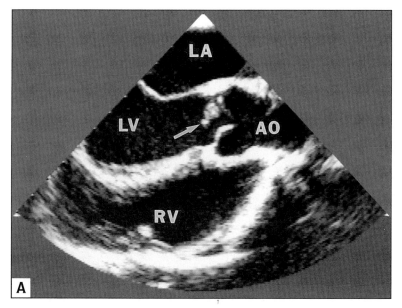

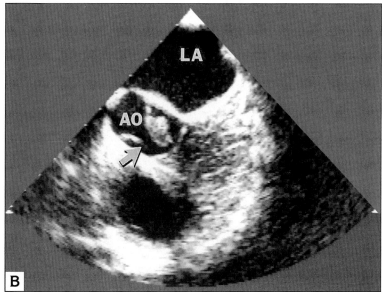

FIGURE 10-4 **A** and **B**, Long-axis (*panel 4A*) and short-axis (*panel 4B*) views from a transesophageal echocardiogram of a patient with a moderate-sized vegetation (*arrows*) on the aortic valve. AO—aorta; LA—left atrium; LV—left ventricle; RV—right ventricle.

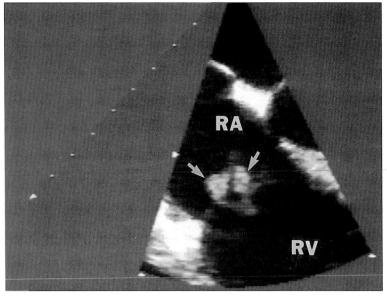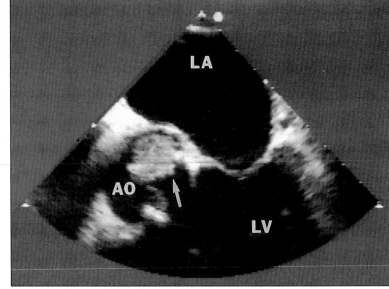

FIGURE 10-5 Transesophageal echocardiographic view showing multiple tricuspid valve vegetations (*arrows*) in a patient with intravenous drug abuse and endocarditis. RA—right atrium; RV—right ventricle.

FIGURE 10-6 Transesophageal echocardiographic appearance of a vegetation (*arrow*) attached to a leaflet of a bioprosthesis in the aortic position. AO—aorta; LA—left atrium; LV—left ventricle.

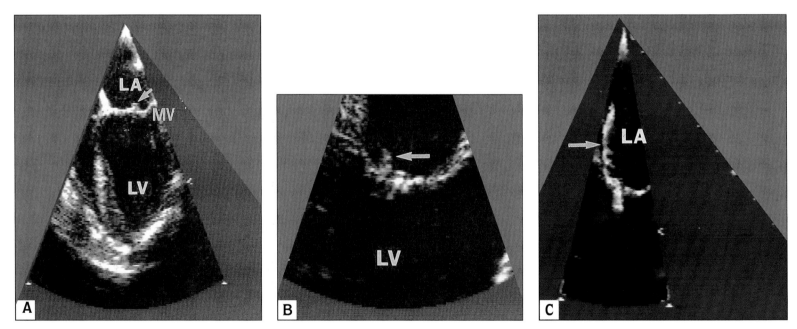

FIGURE 10-7 A, Transesophageal echocardiographic view of the left atrium (LA) and left ventricle (LV) in a patient with a transthoracic echocardiogram negative for evidence of vegetation. Mitral valve (MV) is notable for small vegetative growth (*arrow*) on left atrial side of leaflets. **B,** Close-up of mitral valve reveals attachment of this small vegetation (*arrow*) to the left atrial side of the posterior leaflet of the mitral valve. Erratic motion during the cardiac cycle was seen in real-time. **C,** Color-flow Doppler of the same patient shown in *panel 7B* showing abnormal jet of mitral regurgitation (*arrow*) in the vicinity of the abnormal leaflet with vegetation. The severity of the mitral regurgitation was judged to be mild, despite the eccentric direction of the jet along the posterior left atrial wall.

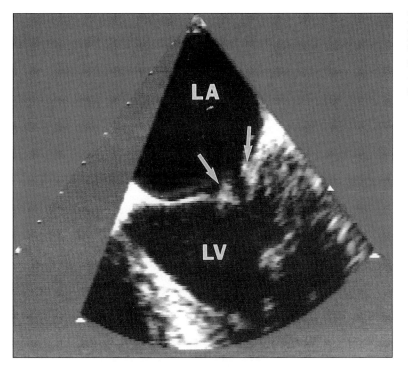

FIGURE 10-8 Transesophageal echocardiogram of patient who presented with fever and bacteremia and transthoracic echocardiogram that was not diagnostic of vegetations. Small, shaggy densities attached to the left atrial surfaces of the mitral valve (*arrows*) showed irregular motion in real-time and were indicative of vegetation. LA—left atrium; LV—left ventricle.

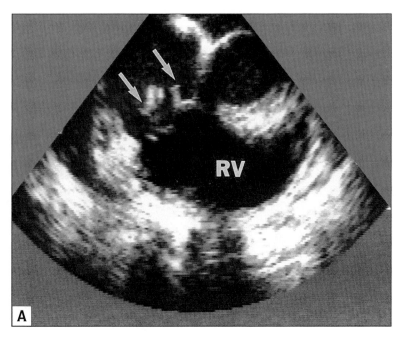

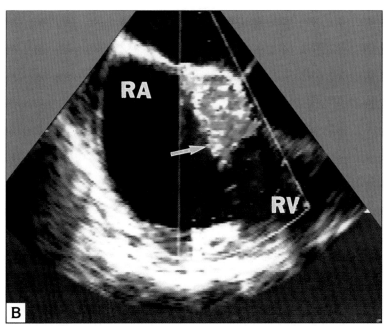

FIGURE 10-9 **A**, Transesophageal two-dimensional echocardiogram of tricuspid valve in an intravenous drug abuser with fever and positive blood cultures. Transthoracic echocardiogram had shown a single vegetation on the tricuspid valve. Two vegetations (*arrows*) were noted by the transesophageal echocardiogram. **B**, Transesophageal view of the tricuspid valve showing jet of tricuspid regurgitation directed toward interatrial septum (*arrow*). RA—right atrium; RV—right ventricle.

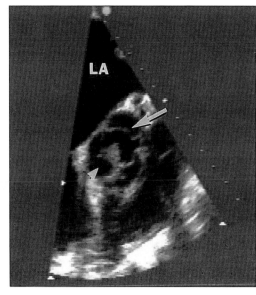

FIGURE 10-10 Close-up transesophageal echocardiographic short-axis view of aortic valve leaflets, showing normal thin anatomy of aortic valve leaflets, including the posterior noncoronary cusp (*arrow*). Between right and left coronary cusps is an echodense mass, indicative of vegetation (*arrowhead*) extending onto body of right coronary leaflet of aortic valve. LA—left atrium.

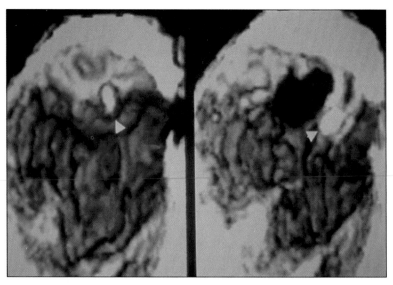

FIGURE 10-11 Systolic (*left panel*) and diastolic (*right panel*) reconstructed three-dimensional echocardiographic views of the mitral valve showing a vegetation (*arrowheads*) on the mitral valve chordae tendineae. Portions of the left ventricular papillary muscles are also visualized. (*From* Nanda *et al.* [8]; with permission.)

FIGURE 10-12 Role of echocardiography in infective endocarditis. Echocardiography often is indicated for its diagnostic utility in suspected or confirmed endocarditis. This figure summarizes the major clinical roles of transthoracic and transesophageal echocardiography in patient settings in which the possibility of infection is entertained and the best way to manage complications must be addressed.

Role of echocardiography in infective endocarditis

TTE
Clinically suspected endocarditis:
To detect a vegetation and confirm the diagnosis
To assess the severity of valve destruction
To assess extension of the infectious process into valvular structures
To assess hemodynamics
Transesophageal echocardiography
Clinically suspected endocarditis and negative TTE
Clinically confirmed endocarditis and suspicion of complications (heart failure, persistent fever, persistent bacteremia)
Evaluation of valvular destruction and extent of infection not readily apparent on TTE
Assessment of preoperative anatomy and postoperative results

TTE—transthoracic echocardiography.

DOPPLER ECHOCARDIOGRAPHY

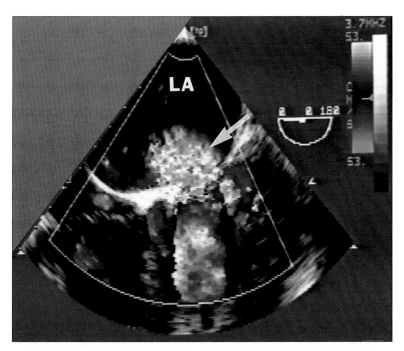

FIGURE 10-13 Transesophageal echocardiographic view of left atrium showing jet of significant mitral regurgitation (*arrow*) in a patient after mitral valve repair who developed postoperative infective endocarditis. Normal flows are demonstrated as blue and red, as visualized in the *color bar* at the right upper corner of the figure. Abnormal flows are high velocity and are depicted as a mosaic of bright colors (*arrow*). LA—left atrium.

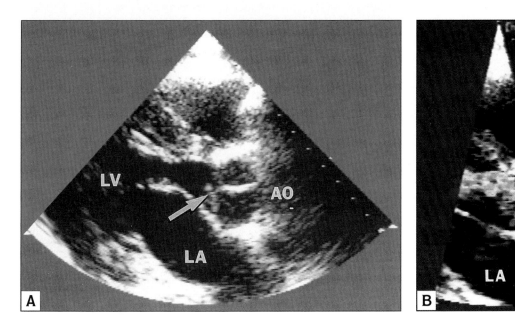

FIGURE 10-14 A, Parasternal long-axis view in a patient with *Staphylococcus aureus* endocarditis showing a completely flail aortic valve leaflet (*arrow*) that failed to coapt properly and prolapsed into the left ventricular outflow tract. **B,** Corresponding view showing color jet of severe aortic insufficiency (*arrow*) originating from this region. AO—aorta; LA—left atrium; LV—left ventricle.

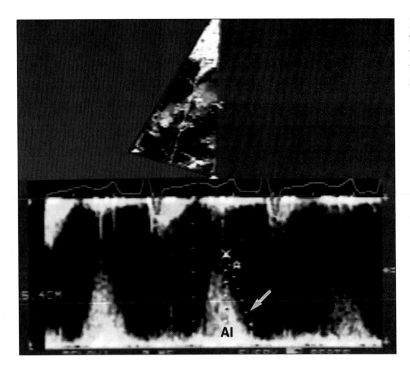

FIGURE 10-15 Continuous-wave Doppler recording from a patient with aortic valve endocarditis showing a fast slope (*arrow*) of the flow velocity profile, indicating rapid equilibration between left ventricular and aortic diastolic pressures consistent with severe aortic insufficiency (AI).

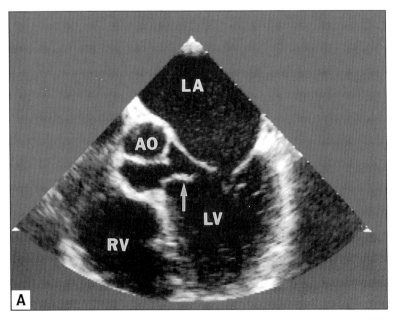

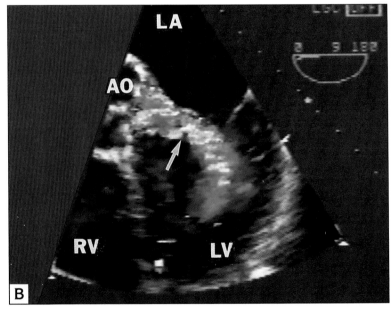

FIGURE 10-16 A, Transesophageal echocardiographic view of a flail aortic valve leaflet (*arrow*) prolapsing into the left ventricular outflow tract. **B,** Corresponding frozen transesophageal echocardio-graphic color-flow Doppler frame (identical projection) showing jet of torrential aortic regurgitation (*arrow*) due to flail aortic valve. AO—aorta; LA—left atrium; LV—left ventricle; RV—right ventricle.

DIAGNOSIS AND COMPLICATIONS

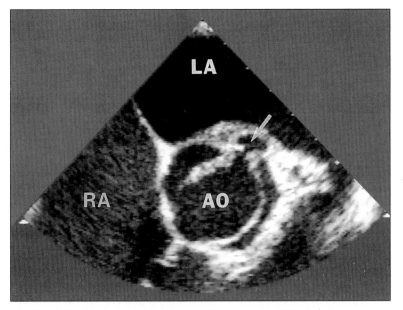

FIGURE 10-17 Transesophageal echocardiographic short-axis view of a patient with congenital bicuspid aortic valve and aortic root abscess, appearing as an echo-free space (*arrow*) adjacent to the aortic valve. AO—aorta; LA—left atrium; RA—right atrium.

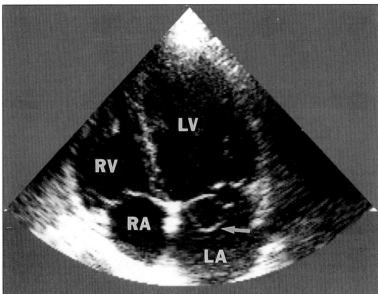

FIGURE 10-18 Transthoracic apical four-chamber recording of an aneurysm (*arrow*) of the mitral valve in a patient with bacterial endocarditis. LA—left atrium; LV—left ventricle; RA—right atrium; RV—right ventricle.

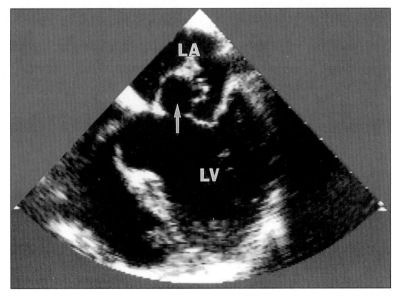

FIGURE 10-19 Transesophageal echocardiogram of a large aneurysm of the anterior mitral valve (*arrow*) in a patient with endocarditis. LA—left atrium; LV—left ventricle.

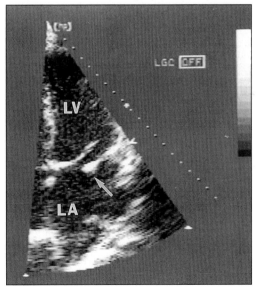

FIGURE 10-20 Apical four-chamber transthoracic view illustrating a healed vegetation on the posterior mitral valve leaflet (*arrow*). Endocarditis has caused the leaflet to become flail (with resultant severe mitral regurgitation). The free leaflet tip points into the left atrial chamber. LA—left atrium; LV—left ventricle.

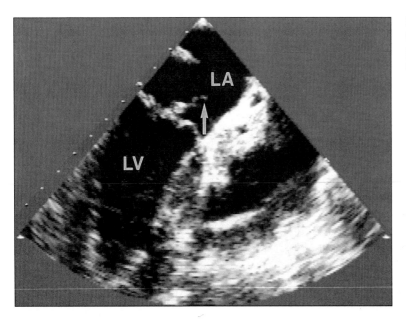

FIGURE 10-21 Transesophageal modified two-chamber view illustrating a small ruptured mitral chordae tendineae (*arrow*) prolapsing into the left atrium (LA) in a patient with mitral valve endocarditis. LV—left ventricle.

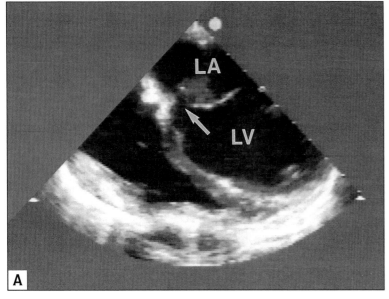

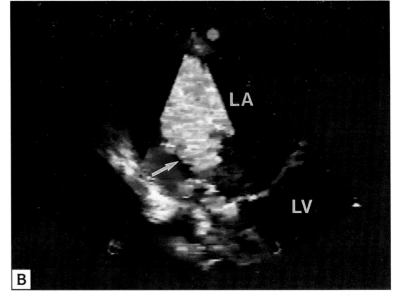

FIGURE 10-22 A, Transesophageal echocardiographic view of a fenestration in the anterior mitral valve leaflet (*arrow*) caused by *Streptococcus viridans* endocarditis. **B,** Frozen close-up color-flow Doppler frame from the same patient revealed that the source of severe mitral regurgitation (*arrow*) was the observed fenestration. LA—left atrium; LV—left ventricle.

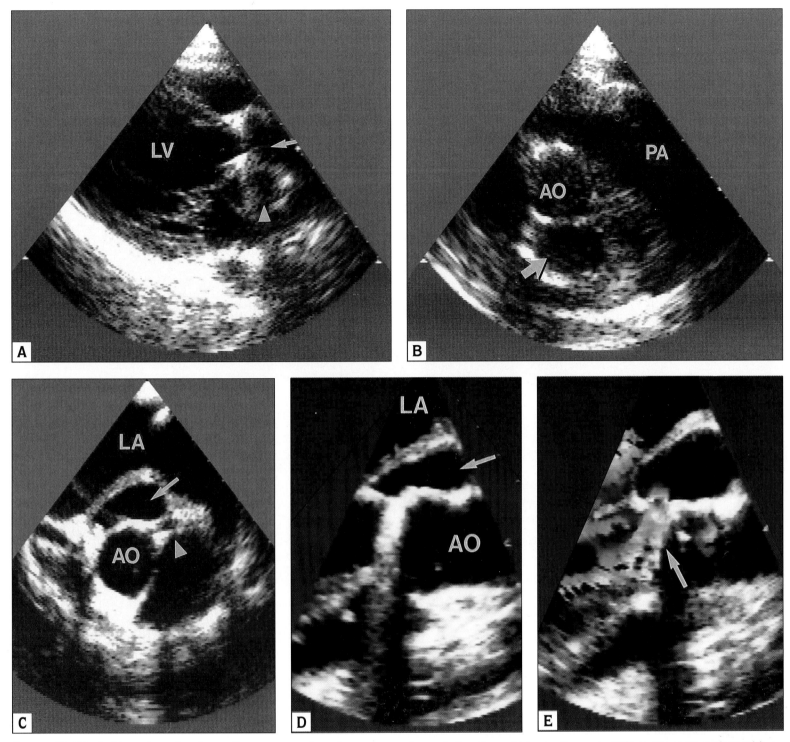

FIGURE 10-23 **A**, Transthoracic echocardiogram, parasternal long-axis view, showing a prosthetic aortic valve (*arrow*) with a large cavity posterior to the prosthesis (*arrowhead*). This cavity is visible even though there is acoustic shadowing artifact from the metallic structure of the prosthesis. **B**, Transthoracic echocardiogram, parasternal short-axis view (perpendicular to previous plane), from the same patient showing large cavity (*arrow*) behind aortic root (AO). **C**, Transesophageal echocardiogram showing large abscess cavity (*arrow*) directly posterior to the aorta (AO) in the same patient with prosthetic aortic valve and a perivalvular abscess. *Arrowhead* indicates left main coronary artery. **D**, Transesophageal echocardiogram, long-axis view, at the level of the aortic valve in the same patient showing abscess cavity (*arrow*) posterior to the aortic valve. **E**, Color-flow Doppler, view angled slightly lateral to *panel 23D*, showing flow exiting abscess cavity (*arrow*) into left ventricular outflow tract. LA—left atrium; LV—left ventricle; PA—pulmonary artery.

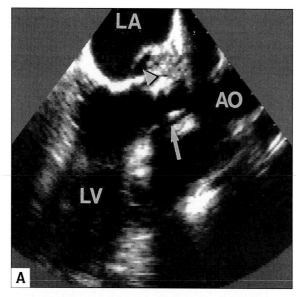

FIGURE 10-24 A, Transesophageal echocardiogram in a patient with a bioprosthetic aortic valve (*arrow*) and abscess cavity (*arrowhead*) located posterior to the valve, between aorta (AO) and left atrium (LA). **B**, Close-up of *panel 24A*. The sewing ring of the prosthesis is evident, as are the leaflets (*arrow*). The abscess cavity is seen directly behind the prosthesis. The cavity is filled with fluid and solid matter (*arrowhead*). **C**, Perpendicular (short-axis) view, similar to *panel 24B*, showing outline of sewing ring of prosthesis (*arrow*) with posteriorly located abscess cavity (*arrowhead*). LV—left ventricle.

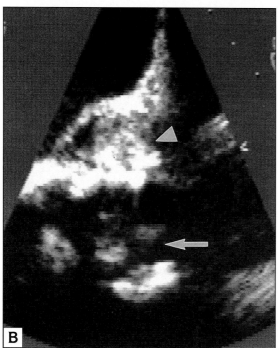

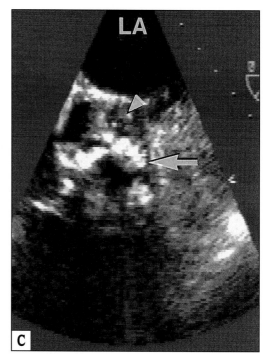

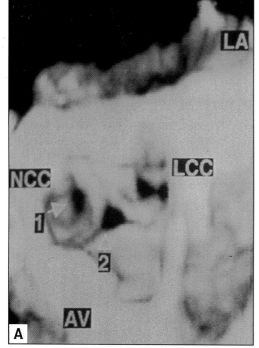

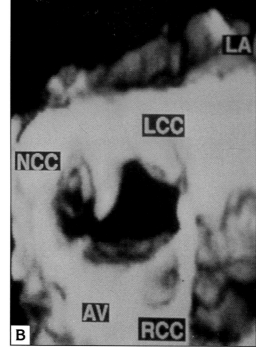

FIGURE 10-25 A and **B**, Three-dimensional reconstructed short-axis view of the aortic valve (AV) in a patient with *Staphylococcus aureus* endocarditis. *Arrow 1* in *panel 25A* shows a perforation in the noncoronary cusp (NCC), destruction of the left coronary cusp (LCC), and an area of noncoaptation (*arrow 2*) of the aortic leaflets in diastole. The systolic frame in *panel 25B* shows a prolapsing vegetation not visualized during diastole due to its position on the aortic side of the valve. LA—left atrium; RCC—right coronary cusp. (*From* Nanda *et al.* [8]; with permission.)

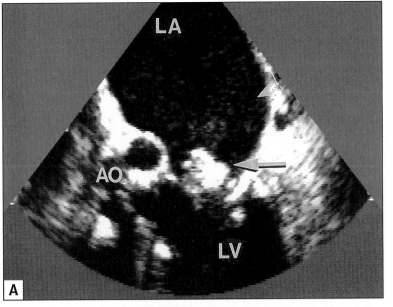

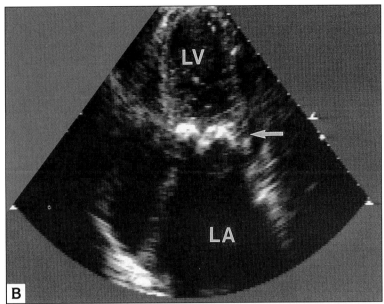

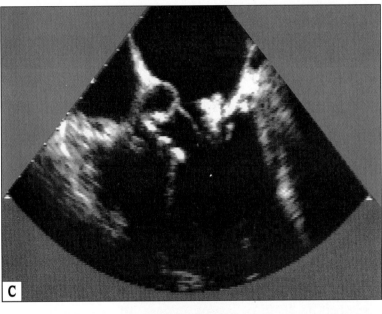

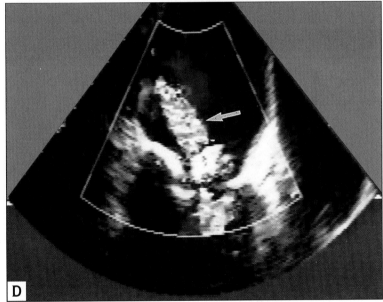

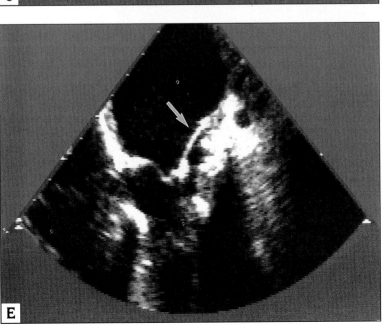

FIGURE 10-26 A, Transesophageal echocardiographic four-chamber view of patient with severe aortic stenosis who presented with fever and bacteremia. A large mobile mass (*arrow*) was seen attached to the posterior mitral valve leaflet. The aortic valve (AO) was stenotic and demonstrated no evidence of endocarditis. Spontaneous echocontrast ("smoke") is seen in the left atrium (LA; *arrowhead*). This phenomenon is a dynamic swirling of smokelike echoes related to low-flow and prethrombotic states. **B,** Transthoracic echocardiography showed a heavily calcified mitral annulus (*arrow*) and was suspicious for additional mitral valve disease, but the vegetation was not clearly evident. A large LA is present. The patient was treated with intravenous antibiotics. **C,** When reimaged at the time of surgery, the appearance of the vegetation was unchanged. **D,** A new jet of mitral regurgitation (*arrow*) was found at the base of the posterior mitral valve leaflet in the vicinity of the vegetation. At surgery, the aortic valve was found to be uninvolved by endocarditis and was replaced with a bioprosthesis. **E,** The mitral valve vegetation was excised, and a fenestration in the posterior leaflet was repaired with a pericardial patch (*arrow*). LV—left ventricle.

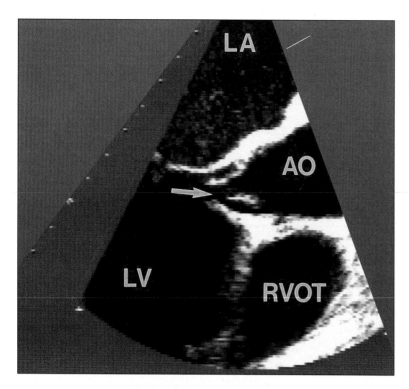

FIGURE 10-27 Transesophageal echocardiogram of a patient in severe cardiogenic shock. View is of aortic valve, which is completely flail (*arrow*) owing to *Staphylococcus aureus* endocarditis. The patient was taken to emergency surgery and did well after aortic valve replacement. AO—aorta; LA—left atrium; LV—left ventricle; RVOT—right ventricular outflow tract.

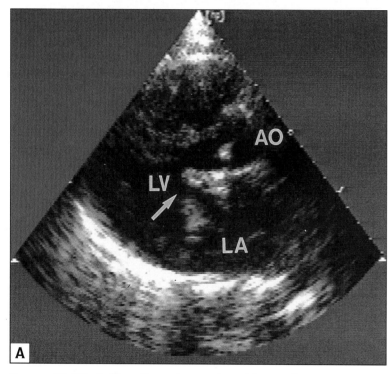

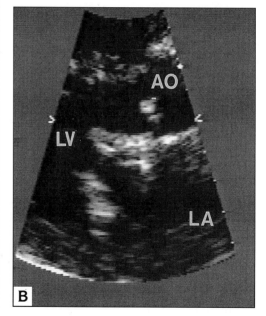

FIGURE 10-28 A, Transthoracic parasternal long-axis view of a patient with a bioprosthetic mitral valve. The struts of the prosthesis are echodense and clearly visible (*arrow*). The aortic valve was mildly thickened, but no overt vegetations were noted. **B,** Close-up of this prosthesis revealed thin leaflets but no gross abnormalities; specifically, no vegetations were seen. (*continued*)

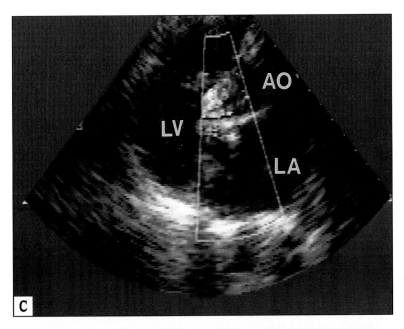

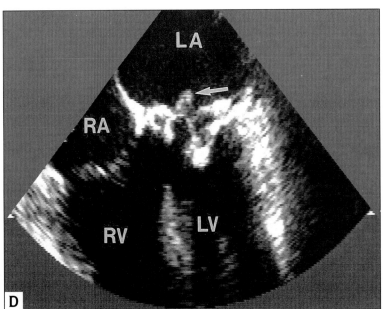

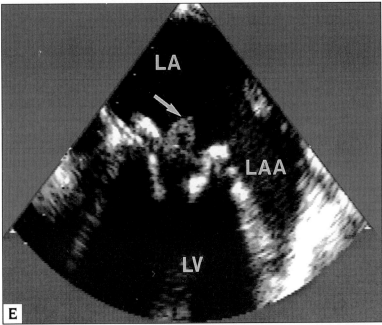

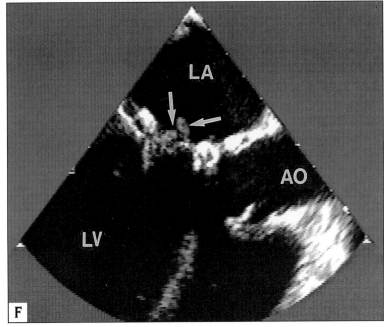

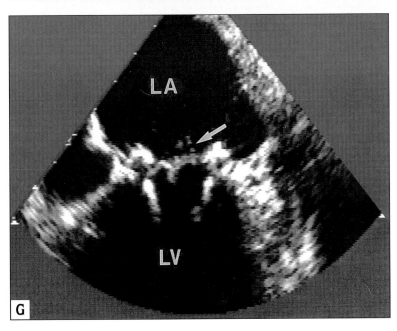

Figure 10-28 (*continued*) **C,** Color-flow Doppler in transthoracic parasternal long-axis view showed a competent mitral valve prosthesis with no evidence of valvular regurgitation. **D,** Transesophageal echocardiogram in same patient shown in *panel 28C* easily revealed a vegetation on the left atrial side of the mitral prosthesis attached to the prosthetic leaflet (*arrow*). **E** and **F,** In the close-up four-chamber (*panel 28E*) and long-axis (*panel 28F*) views, two distinct vegetations were evident (*arrows*). Color-flow Doppler confirmed the absence of mitral regurgitation. The patient subsequently had a stroke despite antibiotic therapy. **G,** A repeat transesophageal echocardiogram after patient's stroke shows remaining strandlike material (*arrow*) on mitral bioprosthetic leaflet, but the large bulk of vegetative matter is no longer present. No valvular destruction was noted, however. AO—aorta; LA—left atrium; LAA—left atrial appendage; LV—left ventricle; RA—right atrium; RV—right ventricle.

Strengths and limitations of echocardiography

	Strengths	Limitations
Transthoracic echocardiography	Noninvasive Readily available Relatively inexpensive Serial studies easy	Relatively insensitive (60%–70%) Not applicable to all patients Limited value for prosthetic valves
Transesophageal echocardiography	High sensitivity (90%–95%) Able to detect smaller vegetations Applicable to all patients Better able to detect abscesses and other complications Improved imaging of prosthetic valves	Invasive Requires sedation Requires physician presence Unable to make histologic diagnosis

FIGURE 10-29 Strengths and limitations of echocardiography. Transthoracic echocardiography is ubiquitous, whereas transesophageal echocardiography is invasive. Listed in the figure are some of the more important features of each technique.

REFERENCES

1. Dillon JC, Feigenbaum H, Konecke LL, et al.: Echocardiographic manifestations of valvular vegetations. *Am Heart J* 1973, 86:698–704.

2. Gilbert BW, Haney RS, Crawford F, et al.: Two-dimensional echocardiographic assessment of vegetative endocarditis. *Circulation* 1977, 55:346–353.

3. Stewart JA, Silimperi D, Harris P, et al.: Echocardiographic documentation of vegetative lesions in infective endocarditis: Clinical implications. *Circulation* 1980, 61:374–380.

4. O'Brien JT, Geiser EA: Infective endocarditis and echocardiography. *Am Heart J* 1984, 106:386–394.

5. Jaffe WM, Morgan DE, Pearlman AS, et al.: Infective endocarditis, 1983–1988: Echocardiographic findings and factors influencing morbidity and mortality. *J Am Coll Cardiol* 1990, 15:1227–1233.

6. Erbel R, Rohmann S, Drexler M, et al.: Improved diagnostic value of echocardiography in patients with infective endocarditis by transesophageal approach: A prospective study. *Eur Heart J* 1988, 9:43–53.

7. Daniel WG, Mügge DA, Martin RP, et al.: Improvement in the diagnosis of abscesses associated with endocarditis by transesophageal echocardiography. *N Engl J Med* 1991, 324:795–800.

8. Nanda NC, Abd-Rahman SM, Khatri G: Incremental value of three-dimensional echocardiography over transesophageal multiplane two-dimensional echocardiography in qualitative and quantitative assessment of cardiac masses and defects. *Echocardiography* 1995, 12:619–628.

SELECTED BIBLIOGRAPHY

Karalis DG, Bansal RC, Hauck AJ, et al.: Transesophageal echocardiographic recognition of subaortic complications in aortic valve endocarditis: Clinical and surgical implications. *Circulation* 1992, 86:353–362.

Khandheria BK, Freeman WK, Sinak LJ: Infective endocarditis: Evaluation by transesophageal echocardiography. In *Transesophageal Echocardiography*. Edited by Freeman WK, Seward JB, Khandheria BK, Tajik AJ. Boston: Little & Brown; 1994:307–338.

Liu F, Ge J, Kupferwasser I, et al.: Has transesophageal echocardiography changed the approach to patients with suspected or known infective endocarditis? *Echocardiography* 1995, 12:637–650.

Mügge A, Daniel WG, Frank G, et al.: Echocardiography in infective endocarditis: Reassessment of prognostic implications of vegetation size determined by the transthoracic and the transesophageal approach. *J Am Coll Cardiol* 1989, 14:631–638.

Sanfilippo AJ, Picard MH, Newell JB, et al.: Echocardiographic assessment of patients with infectious endocarditis: Prediction of risk of complications. *J Am Coll Cardiol* 1991, 18:1191–1199.

Yvorchuk KJ, Chan K-L: Application of transthoracic and transesophageal echocardiography in the diagnosis and management of infective endocarditis. *J Am Soc Echocardiogr* 1994, 14:294–308.

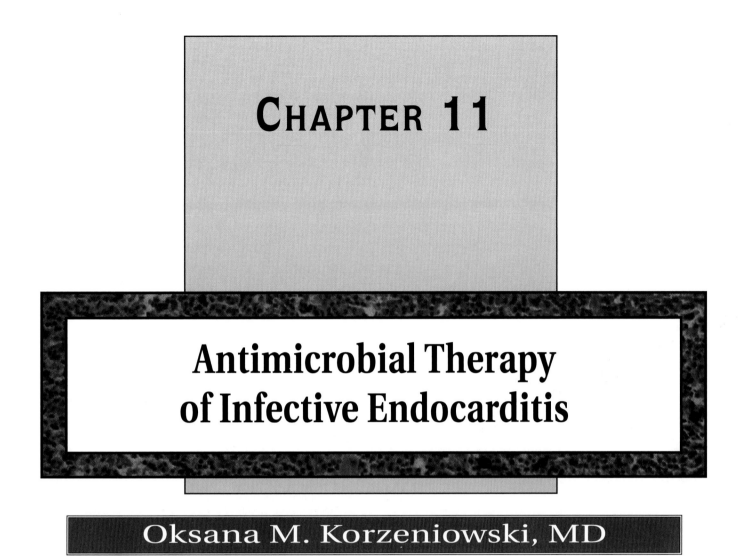

CHAPTER 11

Antimicrobial Therapy of Infective Endocarditis

Oksana M. Korzeniowski, MD

URE OF INFECTIVE ENDOCARDITIS requires sterilization of the vegetations. Inside the vegetation, the
infecting organisms exist at extremely high density
(10^9 to 10^{10}/g of tissue), in a state of reduced metabolic
activity, while protected against host phagocytic cells by a
dense coating of platelets and fibrin. To be effective, antimicrobial therapy must achieve the following goals: 1) therapy
must penetrate within the dense vegetation in concentrations
high enough to be active against the infecting organism, 2)
therapy must be bactericidal to compensate for host defense
deficiencies, and 3) therapy must be administered for a long
enough duration of time to completely eradicate the
microorganisms (in compensation for a slow metabolic rate
of the organisms), or regrowth will occur when the drugs
are withdrawn. Thus, selection of therapy is optimally based
on the identification of the organism, in vitro determination
of its susceptibility to antimicrobial agents, and subsequent
selection of the most active bactericidal agent with the most
favorable pharmacokinetics and least-toxic profile. Tradition-
ally, the most commonly used and most effective agents
have been the cell wall–active antibiotics (penicillins,
cephalosporins, vancomycin) because of their low toxicity,
high achievable serum levels when administered parenterally,
and effective killing of gram-positive organisms, particularly
when combined in synergistic combinations with aminoglycosides. Unfortunately, emergence of strains resistant to β-
lactam agents, vancomycin, and aminoglycosides has complicated the routine therapy of streptococcal and staphylococcal
endocarditis. Isolation of the causative agent and in vitro
determination of the most effective regimen has now
become critical in ensuring optimal therapeutic results.

A definitive diagnosis of infective endocarditis is based
on demonstration of sustained (>1 hour) bacteremia

(three or more positive blood cultures) with organisms
associated with endocarditis in a patient with underlying
susceptible structural heart disease or from demonstration
of bacteria in an embolus or in a vegetation at the time of
surgery or autopsy. Clinical criteria for classification of
suspected endocarditis have been in use since 1981. These
criteria recently have been revised to incorporate the additional diagnostic advantages resulting from advances in
echocardiography.

Substantial morbidity and mortality continues to result
from infective endocarditis despite improvements in diagnostic precision and speed and technologic advances in
medical and surgical therapy. Any measures that prevent
the development of endocarditis are therefore greatly
desired. From animal studies and clinical observation, the
highest risk for infective endocarditis in individuals with
predisposing underlying cardiac conditions is attributed to
exposure to blood-borne bacteria introduced from focal
infectious sites (*eg*, tooth abscesses, cellulitis) or by surgical and dental instrumentation. Although there are no
definitive human trials that have established that antibiotic prophylaxis provides protection against the development of endocarditis during procedures that cause transient bacteremia, analysis of available experimental and
human data on prophylaxis by experts continues to gener-
ate recommendations for prophylactic antibiotic usage.
The classification of risky cardiac lesions, the determination of risky procedures, and the choice of antimicrobial
regimens have evolved over several decades. The most
current published recommendations address the changing
demographics of structural heart disease by analyzing the
risk for infective endocarditis in patients with mitral valve
prolapse.

DIAGNOSIS OF ENDOCARDITIS

A. Proposed new criteria for diagnosis of infective endocarditis

Definite infective endocarditis
  Pathologic criteria
    Microorganisms: demonstrated by culture or histology in a vegetation, *or* in a
      vegetation that has embolized, *or* in an intracardiac abscess, *or*
    Pathologic lesions: vegetation or intracardiac abscess present, confirmed by
      histology showing active endocarditis
  Clinical criteria, using specific definitions listed in *panel 1B*
    Two major criteria, *or*
    One major and three minor criteria, *or*
    Five minor criteria
Possible infective endocarditis
  Findings consistent with infective endocarditis that fall short of "definite," but
    not "rejected"
Rejected
  Firm alternate diagnosis for manifestations of endocarditis, *or*
  Resolution of manifestations of endocarditis, with antibiotic therapy for ≤4 days, *or*
  No pathologic evidence of infective endocarditis at surgery or autopsy, after antibiotic
    therapy for ≤4 days

FIGURE 11-1 A, Modified criteria for clinical classification of suspected endocarditis.
(*continued*)

B. Definitions of terminology used in the proposed new criteria

Major criteria	Minor criteria
Positive blood culture for IE	Predisposition: predisposing heart condition *or* intravenous drug use
Typical microorganism for IE from two separate blood cultures	Fever: ≥38.0°C (100.4°F)
Viridans streptococci,* *Streptococcus bovis,* HACEK† group, *or*	Vascular phenomena: major arterial emboli, septic pulmonary infarcts, mycotic aneurysm, intracranial hemorrhage, conjunctival hemorrhages, Janeway lesions
Community-acquired *Staphylococcus aureus* or enterococci, in the absence of a primary focus, *or*	Immunologic phenomena: glomerulonephritis, Osler nodes, Roth spots, rheumatoid factor
Persistently positive blood culture, defined as recovery of a microorganism consistent with IE from:	Microbiologic evidence: positive blood culture but not meeting major criterion as noted previously‡ or serologic evidence of active infection with organism consistent with IE
1) Blood cultures drawn more than 12 hr apart, *or*	Echocardiogram: consistent with IE but not meeting major criterion as noted previously
2) All of three or a majority of four or more separate blood cultures, with first and last drawn at least 1 hr apart	
Evidence of endocardial involvement	
Positive echocardiogram for IE	
1) Oscillating intracardiac mass, on valve or supporting structures, *or* in the path of regurgitant jets, *or* on implanted material, in the absence of an alternative anatomic explanation, *or*	
2) Abscess, *or*	
3) New partial dehiscence of prosthetic valve, *or*	
New valvular regurgitation (increase or change in preexisting murmur not sufficient)	

*Including nutritional variant strains.

†Includes *Haemophilus aphrophilus/parainfluenzae, Actinobacillus actinomycetemcomitans, Cardiobacterium hominis, Eikenella corrodens, Kingella kingae.*

‡Excluding single positive cultures for coagulase-negative staphylococci and organisms that do not cause endocarditis.

IE—infective endocarditis.

FIGURE 11-1 (*continued*) **B,** Definitions of terminology used in the proposed new criteria. (*From* Durack *et al.* [1]; with permission.)

Antibiotic efficacy in the treatment of infective endocarditis

Host factors	Principles of antimicrobial selection
Vegetation is avascular tissue—antibiotic penetration occurs only through diffusion	High doses to provide high serum levels. Parenteral administration to avoid erratic oral absorption
High intravegetation bacterial densities (10^9–10^{10} organisms/g of tissue)—potential emergence of resistant clones	Appropriate dosing interval to guarantee that microbial multiplication does not occur between doses. Adequate duration of therapy
Organisms in metabolically dormant state are less vulnerable to killing	High doses of antibiotic to compensate for bacterial dormancy. Long duration of therapy
Intravegetation host defenses are compromised—phagocytic cells are absent	Bactericidal regimens; synergistic combinations

FIGURE 11-2 Antibiotic efficacy in the treatment of infective endocarditis. Host factors: Optimal antimicrobial therapy is based on selection of the least-toxic antibiotic with the highest killing capacity at serum levels achievable with parenteral therapy. The objectives for effective treatment of endocarditis are eradication of the organism from all sites of infection and control of intra- and extracardiac complications. Failure to sterilize the vegetation or the extracardiac sites of seeding will result in bacterial regrowth, relapse of the bacteremia, and reappearance of symptoms. Principles of antimicrobial selection: Ideal therapy utilizes antimicrobial agents that can overcome the unfavorable therapeutic milieu of the vegetation. Best results are achieved with bactericidal agents given in high enough doses parenterally to ensure adequate concentration in the vegetation and administered for a long enough period to sterilize 10^{10} organisms per gram of tissue.

In vitro determinants of antimicrobial efficacy

	Susceptibility testing	Clinical significance
MIC	Lowest concentration of antibiotic that inhibits growth of organisms in vitro	Should be performed for all isolates to determine susceptibility to antimicrobial agents
MBC	Lowest concentration of antibiotic that results in a 99.9% kill of a standard inoculum within 24 hr	Not clinically significant in treatment of streptococci and staphylococci with penicillins, cephalosporins, or vancomycin—MIC and MBC are frequently the same Important for selection of appropriate therapy of gram-negative organisms
Tolerance	Slower rate of kill of organisms with MBC greatly (10–32-fold or more) divergent from MIC	No clinical significance for streptococci or staphylococci
Synergy	Enhanced killing efficacy of a combination of antimicrobial agents against an organism only inhibited by the individual components of the regimen	Synergistic bactericidal effect is required for enterococci and relatively penicillin-resistant streptococci

MBC—minimal bactericidal concentration; MIC—minimal inhibitory concentration.

FIGURE 11-3 In vitro determinants of antimicrobial efficacy. Laboratory assays for susceptibility to antimicrobial agents guide selection of the most appropriate therapy for individual isolates in infective endocarditis. In vitro demonstration of tolerance has not correlated with adverse outcomes.

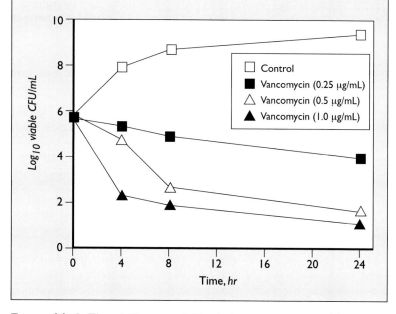

FIGURE 11-4 Time-kill assay of *Staphylococcus aureus* with vancomycin at increasing concentrations. Higher concentrations of vancomycin result in faster and more complete killing of the organism and can guide selection of route of administration. CFU—colony-forming units. (*From* Knapp and Moody [2]; with permission.)

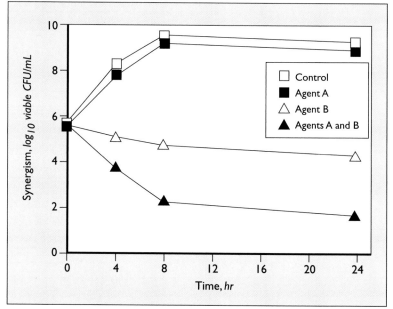

FIGURE 11-5 Time-kill assay showing synergism between antimicrobial agents. CFU—colony-forming units. (*From* Knapp and Moody [2]; with permission.)

Therapy for native valve endocarditis caused by penicillin-susceptible viridans streptococci and *Streptococcus bovis*

Regimen	Antibiotic	Dosage and route (for patients with normal renal function)	Duration, *wk*
A	Aqueous penicillin G	12–18 MU/24 hr IV, continuously or in 6 divided doses	4
B	Ceftriaxone sodium	2 g once daily IV or IM	4
C	Aqueous penicillin G +	12–18 MU/24 hr IV, continuously or in 6 divided doses	2
	Gentamicin sulfate	1 mg/kg IM or IV every 8 hr	2
D	Vancomycin hydrochloride	30 mg/kg/24 hr IV in 2 divided doses; NOT to exceed 2 g/24 hr unless serum levels are monitored	4

IM—intramuscularly; IV—intravenously.

FIGURE 11-6 Therapy for native valve endocarditis caused by penicillin-susceptible (minimum inhibitory concentration ≤0.1 µg/mL) viridans streptococci and *Streptococcus bovis*. Penicillin-susceptible viridans streptococci and *S. bovis* are most easily treatable with β-lactam agents alone. Cure rates of 97% to 98% are achieved with all the recommended regimens. The choice of regimen is based on comorbid conditions, duration of illness, and associated complications. Regimen A is preferred for elderly patients or those with renal or eighth nerve impairment. Regimen B is adaptable for outpatient therapy. Regimen C is appropriate for patients with uncomplicated infective endocarditis (*ie*, no extracardiac foci of infection, intracardiac abscesses, prosthetic valves, or nutritionally variant isolates). Gentamicin is preferable to streptomycin because of its wide clinical use, intravenous administration, easily measurable serum levels, and the more common appearance of high-level resistance to streptomycin among clinical isolates. Dosage reduction is needed in patients with renal failure. Monitoring of serum concentration is desirable (peak level 3 µg/mL, trough <1 µg/mL). Regimen D is recommended for patients with immediate-type hypersensitivity to β-lactam antibiotics. Dosage reduction is needed in patients with renal failure. Desirable peak serum level should be 30 to 45 µg/mL 1 hour after completion of infusion. (*Adapted from* Wilson *et al.* [3].)

Therapy for native valve endocarditis due to strains of viridans streptococci and *Streptococcus bovis* relatively resistant to penicillin G

Regimen	Antibiotic	Dosage and route (for patients with normal renal function)	Duration, *wk*
E	Aqueous penicillin G +	18–24 MU/24 hr IV, continuously or in 6 divided doses	4
	Gentamicin sulfate	1 mg/kg IM or IV every 8 hr	2
F	Vancomycin hydrochloride	30 mg/kg/24 hr IV in 2 equally divided doses; NOT to exceed 2 g/24 hr unless serum levels are monitored	4

IM—intramuscularly; IV—intravenously.

FIGURE 11-7 Therapy for native valve endocarditis due to strains of viridans streptococci and *Streptococcus bovis* relatively resistant to penicillin G (minimum inhibitory concentration >0.1 µg/mL and <0.5 µg/mL). Streptococci with intermediate sensitivity to penicillin are killed slowly by penicillin alone. The addition of gentamicin enhances eradication of organisms from tissue. Regimen E is recommended for all patients with viridans streptococcal or *S. bovis* infections involving prosthetic valves or other prosthetic material. Penicillin administration should be prolonged to 6 weeks. First-generation cephalosporin may be substituted for penicillin. Regimen F is recommended for patients with immediate-type hypersensitivity to penicillin. The addition of gentamicin is not necessary. (*Adapted from* Wilson *et al.* [3].)

Therapy for infective endocarditis caused by *Streptococcus pneumoniae*

Penicillin susceptible (MIC <0.1 µg/mL)
  Aqueous penicillin G 18 MU/24 hr IV, continuously or in
  6 divided doses
Penicillin resistant (intermediate [MIC = 0.1–1.0 µg/mL] or
  high [MIC ≥2.0 µg/mL])
  Ceftriaxone sodium 2 g once daily IV if susceptible
  Vancomycin hydrochloride 30 mg/kg/24 hr IV in 2 equally
  divided doses

IV—intravenously; MIC—minimum inhibitory concentration.

FIGURE 11-8 Therapy for infective endocarditis caused by *Streptococcus pneumoniae*. Pneumococcal infection is an uncommon cause of infective endocarditis (<1% of native valve infective endocarditis). Because of a fulminant course and the emergence of resistance to penicillin, vancomycin (with or without ceftriaxone) has replaced penicillin as empiric treatment. (*Adapted from* Wilson *et al.* [3].)

Therapy for infective endocarditis caused by *Streptococcus pyogenes* (group A) and group B, C, or G streptococci

Streptococcus pyogenes
  Susceptible to penicillin
  Aqueous penicillin G or first-generation cephalosporins intravenously for 4–6 wk
Group B, C, or G streptococci
  Relatively resistant to penicillin
  Aqueous penicillin G or first-generation cephalosporin for
  4–6 wk plus gentamicin for first 2 wk

FIGURE 11-9 Therapy for infective endocarditis caused by *Streptococcus pyogens* (group A) or group B, C, or G streptococci. Nonviridans streptococci are uncommon and most often encountered in patients with underlying malignancy or diabetes. (*Adapted from* Wilson *et al.* [3].)

General considerations in selection of therapy for enterococcal endocarditis

Antimicrobial resistance of enterococci is increasing:
  Gentamicin (10%–25% *Enterococcus faecalis*, 45%–50%
  E. faecium)
  Intrinsic resistance to penicillin (MIC >16 µg/mL),
  β-Lactamase production
  Vancomycin resistance (*E. faecium* >>> *E. faecalis*)
  Moderate (MIC ≥16 µg/mL) *or*
  High level (MIC ≥256 µg/mL)
Synergistic interaction of a cell wall–active agent (penicillin
  or vancomycin) with an agent that inhibits protein synthesis
  (aminoglycoside) is needed to kill the enterococcus (standard
  therapy in nonresistant strains)
Cephalosporins are inactive
High-level aminoglycoside–resistant organisms (MIC to
  streptomycin 2000 µg/mL; MIC to gentamicin 500–2000
  µg/mL) are not killed synergistically in vitro or in vivo
All isolates must be tested for antimicrobial susceptibility

MIC—minimum inhibitory concentration.

FIGURE 11-10 General considerations in selection of therapy for enterococcal endocarditis. Therapy of enterococcal endocarditis is complicated by the emergence of resistance to previously active antibiotics.

Standard therapy for endocarditis due to enterococci and nutritionally variant viridans streptococci

Antibiotic	Dosage and route	Duration, wk
Aqueous penicillin G	18–30 MU/24 hr IV, continuously or in 6 divided doses	4–6
or		
Ampicillin sodium	12 g/24 hr IV, continuously or in 6 divided doses	4–6
or		
Vancomycin hydrochloride	30 mg/kg/24 hr IV in 2 divided doses; NOT to exceed 2 g/24 hr	4–6
+		
Gentamicin sulfate	1 mg/kg IM or IV every 8 hr	4–6

IM—intramuscularly; IV—intravenously.

FIGURE 11-11 Standard therapy for endocarditis due to enterococci and nutritionally variant viridans streptococci. Enterococci are intrinsically inhibited but not killed by penicillin or vancomycin. Addition of an aminoglycoside is needed to promote a synergistic bactericidal effect. Because nutritionally variant viridans streptococci are difficult to grow and test for penicillin susceptibility in vitro, recommendations for therapy include the addition of aminoglycosides for 4 weeks as for the treatment of enterococci. Standard regimens are only applicable to endocarditis caused by penicillin and aminoglycoside-susceptible strains. A 4-week regimen is recommended for patients with symptoms lasting <3 months; a 6-week regimen is recommended for patients with a prosthetic valve and/or symptoms lasting >3 months. Vancomycin is indicated for patients allergic to β-lactam antibiotics. Vancomycin may enhance the nephrotoxic potential of gentamicin. Serum levels of vancomycin and aminoglycosides should be followed. Peak recommended serum level for gentamicin is 3 to 5 µg/mL. Peak serum level for streptomycin 1 hour after 7.5 mg/kg intramuscular injection every 12 hours should be approximately 20 µg/mL. (*Adapted from* Wilson *et al.* [3].)

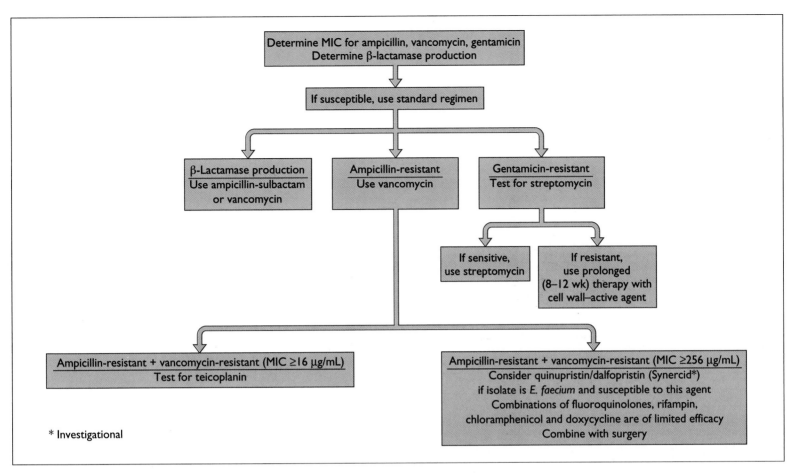

FIGURE 11-12 Strategy for selection of an antimicrobial regimen when high-level resistance of enterococcus to components of the standard regimen is encountered. MIC—minimum inhibitory concentration.

Therapy of staphylococcal endocarditis in the absence of prosthetic material

Antibiotic	Dose and route	Duration
Methicillin susceptible		
Nafcillin or oxacillin with	2 g IV every 4 hr	4–6 wk
optional gentamicin	1 mg/kg IM or IV every 8 hr	3–5 days
Cefazolin (or other first-generation cephalosporin in equivalent doses)	2 g IV every 8 hr	4–6 wk
with optional gentamicin	1 mg/kg IM or IV every 8 hr	3–5 days
Vancomycin	30 mg/kg/24 hr IV in 2 divided doses; NOT to exceed 2 g unless serum levels monitored	4–6 wk
Methicillin resistant		
Vancomycin	30 mg/kg/24 hr IV in 2 divided doses; NOT to exceed 2 g unless serum levels monitored	4–6 wk

IM—intramuscularly; IV—intravenously.

FIGURE 11-13 Therapy of staphylococcal endocarditis in the absence of prosthetic material. Clinical cures and mortality differ in patients with right- vs left-sided *Staphylococcus aureus* endocarditis. Uncomplicated right-sided endocarditis in intravenous drug abusers responds to less aggressive therapy and may be treated effectively with 2 weeks of nafcillin plus gentamicin. Substitution of vancomycin for nafcillin is ineffective. In standard therapy, the optional addition of gentamicin is associated with more rapid clearance of bacteremia but no improvement in cure rates. Vancomycin is recommended only for patients with immediate hypersensitivity to β-lactam antibiotics or those infected with methicillin-resistant strains. Clearance of bacteremia is delayed when compared with penicillins. Treatment options for patients intolerant of vancomycin are suboptimal. (*Adapted from* Wilson et al. [3].)

Therapy of staphylococcal endocarditis in the presence of a prosthetic valve or other prosthetic material

Antibiotic	Dosage and route	Duration, *wk*
Methicillin resistant		
Vancomycin	30 mg/kg/24 hr IV in 2 divided doses; NOT to exceed 2 g unless serum levels monitored	≥6
+		
Rifampin	300 mg orally every 8 hr	≥6
+		
Gentamicin	1 mg/kg IM or IV every 8 hr	2
Methicillin susceptible		
Nafcillin or oxacillin	2 g IV every 4 hr	≥6
+		
Rifampin	300 mg orally every 8 hr	≥6
+		
Gentamicin	1 mg/kg IM or IV every 8 hr	2

IM—intramuscularly; IV—intravenously.

FIGURE 11-14 Therapy of staphylococcus endocarditis in the presence of a prosthetic valve or other prosthetic material. The majority of prosthetic valve endocarditis is caused by *Staphylococcus aureus* and coagulase-negative staphylococci. Most coagulase-negative strains are methicillin resistant. Curative therapy frequently involves surgical replacement of prosthetic material. Right-sided catheter/pacemaker–associated infections may respond to antimicrobial therapy alone. Rifampin resistance develops rapidly if used as monotherapy. If an isolate is aminoglycoside resistant, aminoglycoside treatment should be omitted; if susceptible, a fluoroquinolone may be used instead of the aminoglycoside. First-generation cephalosporins or vancomycin can be used in patients allergic to β-lactam antibiotics and infected with methicillin-susceptible strains of staphylococci. (*Adapted from* Wilson *et al.* [3].)

Therapy for endocarditis due to HACEK* microorganisms

Antibiotic	Dosage and route	Duration, *wk*
Ceftriaxone sodium	2 g IV or IM daily	4
Ampicillin sodium *with*	12 g/24 hr IV, continuously or in 6 divided doses	4
Gentamicin	1 mg/kg IM or IV every 8 hr	4

*Includes *Haemophilus aphrophilus/parainfluenzae, Actinobacillus actinomycetemcomitans, Cardiobacterium hominis, Eikenella corrodens, Kingella kingae.*

IM—intramuscularly; IV—intravenously.

FIGURE 11-15 Therapy for endocarditis due to HACEK (*Haemophilus aphrophilus/parainfluenzae, Actinobacillus actinomycetemcomitans, Cardiobacterium hominis, Eikenella corrodens, Kingella kingae*) microorganisms. Gram-negative bacilli of the HACEK group grow slowly in standard blood culture media and may require prolonged incubation (≥2 weeks). Blood cultures may be intermittently positive. Emergence of HACEK resistance to ampicillin has been identified. Because susceptibility testing is difficult, all strains should be considered resistant. All strains are susceptible to third-generation cephalosporins. Duration of therapy for prosthetic valve endocarditis should be 6 weeks. Alternative regimens based on in vitro data include trimethoprim-sulfamethoxazole, fluoroquinolones, and aztreonam. (*Adapted from* Wilson *et al.* [3].)

Treatment of unusual organisms

Enterobacteriaceae
  In vitro susceptibility testing
  Most likely third-generation cephalosporin, imipenem,
    ciprofloxacin + gentamicin (4–6 wk)
Pseudomonas aeruginosa
  In vitro susceptibility testing
  Most likely third- or fourth-generation cephalosporin,
    piperacillin, ciprofloxacin, imipenem + gentamicin (6 wk)
Fungi
  Amphotericin B acutely 6–8 wk
  Consider long-term suppression with an active imidazole
    (fluconazole for *Candida* spp; itraconazole for *Aspergillus* spp)

FIGURE 11-16 Treatment of unusual organisms. Therapy of Enterobacteriaceae, fungi, and *Pseudomonas* species must be based on individual susceptibility testing of isolates. Regimens should utilize the most bactericidal agents.

Therapy for culture-negative endocarditis

Native valve
  Ampicillin + gentamicin as per standard regimen for
    enterococci
Prosthetic valve
  Ampicillin + gentamicin + vancomycin

FIGURE 11-17 Therapy for culture-negative endocarditis. Culture-negative infective endocarditis on a native valve most commonly results from preculture use of antibiotics. Empiric antimicrobial regimen should be directed at the most resistant strain of likely bacteria, *ie*, enterococcus. Empiric therapy for prosthetic valve endocarditis takes into account the high likelihood of a staphylococcal species as the etiologic agent.

Outpatient therapy for endocarditis

Patient selection:
Documented response to initial therapy
Afebrile
Hemodynamically stable
Not experiencing any threatening complication
Compliant
Capable of managing the technical aspects of therapy

FIGURE 11-18 Outpatient therapy of endocarditis. New technologic developments (*eg*, multilumen central lines and infusion pumps) and availability of antibiotics with prolonged half-lives have made management of infective endocarditis outside the hospital an increasingly common practice. Patients to be treated in an outpatient setting must be carefully selected and followed closely so that any adverse events can be immediately addressed.

PROPHYLAXIS OF INFECTIVE ENDOCARDITIS

Relative risk for endocarditis by underlying cardiac lesions

Endocarditis prophylaxis recommended	Endocarditis prophylaxis not recommended
High-risk category Prosthetic cardiac valves, including bioprosthetic and homograft valves Previous bacterial endocarditis Complex cyanotic congenital heart disease (*eg*, single ventricle states, transposition of the great arteries, tetralogy of Fallot) Surgically constructed systemic-pulmonary shunts or conduits **Moderate-risk category** Most other congenital cardiac malformations (other than those in the high- and low-risk categories) Acquired valvular dysfunction (*eg*, rheumatic heart disease) Hypertrophic cardiomyopathy Mitral valve prolapse with valvar regurgitation and/or thickened leaflets*	**Low- or negligible-risk category** Isolated secundum atrial septal defect Surgical repair of atrial septal defect, ventricular septal defect, or patent ductus arteriosus (without residua beyond 6 mo) Previous coronary artery bypass graft surgery Mitral valve prolapse without valvar regurgitation* Physiologic, functional, or innocent heart murmurs* Previous Kawasaki disease without valvar dysfunction Previous rheumatic fever without valvar dysfunction Cardiac pacemakers and implanted defibrillators

*See Fig. 11-20 for discussion.

FIGURE 11-19 Relative risk for endocarditis by underlying cardiac lesions. Structural cardiac lesions have variable predispositions for the development of endocarditis and for the severity of the evolving disease. In general, areas of turbulent blood flow with large pressure variations are at greatest risk (*see* Chapter 3, "Pathology: Anatomy and Predisposing Cardiac Lesions"). Prophylaxis is recommended only for individuals who have cardiac lesions identified in the high- or moderate-risk categories. (*Adapted from* Dajani *et al.* [4]; with permission.)

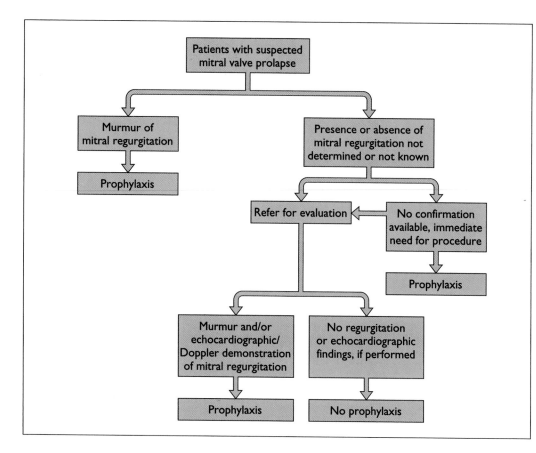

Figure 11-20 Clinical approach to determination of the need for prophylaxis in patients with suspected mitral valve prolapse. The most controversial area of prophylaxis is the stratification of risk among patients with different clinical and echocardiographic manifestations of mitral valve prolapse. An increased likelihood of endocarditis is associated with the sheer forces and flow abnormalities due to the jet of mitral insufficiency (if present) and not because of abnormal valve motion. Controversy arises over whether all patients with mitral valve prolapse or only those with demonstrable regurgitation should undergo prophylaxis and whether clinical or ultrasound criteria of regurgitation have a better predictive value for the risk of endocarditis. Current recommendations from the experts are outlined in the figure. (*Adapted from* Dajani *et al.* [4]; with permission.)

A. Relative risks of invasive procedures for endocarditis: Endocarditis prophylaxis recommended*

Oral tract
  Dental extractions
  Periodontal procedures including surgery, scaling and
    root planing, probing, recall maintenance
  Dental implant placement and reimplantation of avulsed teeth
  Endodontic (root canal) instrumentation or surgery only
    beyond the apex
  Subgingival placement of antibiotic fibers/strips
  Initial placement of orthodontic bands but not brackets
  Intraligamentary local anesthetic injections
  Prophylactic cleaning of teeth or implants where bleeding
    is anticipated
Respiratory tract
  Surgical operations that involve respiratory mucosa
  Bronchoscopy with a rigid bronchoscope
Gastrointestinal tract
  Sclerotherapy for esophageal varices
  Esophageal stricture dilation
  Endoscopic retrograde cholangiography with biliary
    obstruction
  Biliary tract surgery
  Surgical operations that involve intestinal mucosa
Genitourinary tract
  Prostatic surgery
  Cystoscopy
  Urethral dilation

*Prophylaxis is recommended for patients with high- and moderate-risk cardiac conditions.

Figure 11-21 A and **B,** Relative risks of invasive procedures for infective endocarditis. Prophylaxis is recommended for surgical and dental procedures that are known to induce bacteremias by organisms commonly associated with endocarditis. These bacteremias include the oral streptococci, enterococci, and staphylococci. If a series of procedures requiring prophylaxis is planned, an interval between procedures and between prophylaxis of 9 to 14 days is recommended to reduce the potential emergence of organisms resistant to the antimicrobial regimen. (*Adapted from* Dajani *et al.* [4]; with permission.) (*continued*)

B. Relative risks of invasive procedures for endocarditis: Endocarditis prophylaxis not recommended

Oral tract
Restorative dentistry* (operative and prosthodontic) with or without retraction cord†
Local anesthetic injections (nonintraligamentary)
Intracanal endodontic treatment; postplacement and buildup
Placement of rubber dams
Postoperative suture removal
Placement of removable prosthodontic/orthodontic appliances
Taking of oral impressions
Fluoride treatments
Taking of oral radiographs
Orthodontic appliance adjustment
Shedding of primary teeth
Respiratory tract
Endotracheal intubation
Bronchoscopy with a flexible bronchoscope, with or without biopsy‡
Tympanostomy tube insertion

Gastrointestinal tract
Transesophageal echocardiography‡
Endoscopy with or without gastrointestinal biopsy‡
Genitourinary tract
Vaginal hysterectomy‡
Vaginal delivery‡
Cesarean section
In uninfected tissue:
Urethral catheterization
Uterine dilatation and curettage
Therapeutic abortion
Sterilization procedures
Insertion or removal of intrauterine devices
Other
Cardiac catheterization, including balloon angioplasty
Implantation of cardiac pacemakers, implanted defibrillators, and coronary stents
Incision or biopsy of surgically scrubbed skin
Circumcision

*Includes restoration of decayed teeth (filling cavities) and replacement of missing teeth.
†Clinical judgment may indicate antibiotic use in selected circumstances that may create significant bleeding.
‡Prophylaxis is optional for high-risk patients.

FIGURE 11-21 (*continued*)

A. Prophylactic regimens for dental, oral, respiratory tract, and esophageal procedures

Situation	Agent	Regimen*
Standard general prophylaxis	Amoxicillin	Adults: 2.0 g Children: 50 mg/kg PO 1 hr before procedure†
Unable to take oral medications	Ampicillin	Adults: 2.0 g IM/IV Children: 50 mg/kg IM/IV Within 30 min before procedure†
Penicillin-allergic	Clindamycin or	Adults: 600 mg Children: 20 mg/kg PO 1 hr before procedure†
	Cephalexin‡ or cefadroxil‡ or	Adults: 2.0 g Children: 50 mg/kg PO 1 hr before procedure†
	Azithromycin or clarithromycin	Adults: 500 mg Children: 15 mg/kg PO 1 hr before procedure†
Penicillin-allergic Unable to take oral medications	Clindamycin or Cefazolin‡	Adults: 600 mg Children: 25 mg/kg IV within 30 min before procedure† Adults: 1.0 g Children: 25 mg/kg IM/IV within 30 min before procedure†

*Total children's dose should not exceed adult dose.
†For patients in the high-risk category for endocarditis, half the dose may be repeated 6 hr after the initial dose (except for azithromycin—second dose is not necessary).
‡Cephalosporins should not be used in individuals with immediate-type hypersensitivity reaction (urticaria, angioedema, or anaphylaxis) to penicillins.
IM—intramuscularly; IV—intravenously; PO—orally.

FIGURE 11-22 A and **B**, Prophylactic regimens for dental, oral, respiratory tract, and esophageal procedures (*panel 22A*) and genitourinary and gastrointestinal (excluding esophageal) procedures (*panel 22B*). Prophylaxis is most effective when serum antibiotic levels during and after the procedure are adequate to inhibit the bacteremia expected from that procedure. The antibiotics should be directed against the flora most likely to be introduced into the bloodstream and most capable of causing endocarditis. The most common flora for dental procedures are viridans streptococci and HACEK (*Haemophilus aphrophilus/parainfluenzae, Actinobacillus actinomycetemcomitans, Cardiobacterium hominis, Eikenella corrodens, Kingella kingae*) organisms, whereas the genitourinary procedure risks for endocarditis result from enterococcal bacteremia. Antibiotics should be initiated shortly before the procedure is started and continued only during the perioperative period to minimize emergence of resistance. (*Adapted from* Dajani *et al.* [4]; with permission.) (*continued*)

B. Prophylactic regimens for genitourinary and gastrointestinal (excluding esophageal) procedures

Situation	Agents(s)*	Regimen[†]	
High-risk patients	Ampicillin + gentamicin	Adults:	Ampicillin 2.0 g IV/IM Gentamicin 1.5 mg/kg (not to exceed 120 mg) within 30 min of starting the procedure 6 hr later, ampicillin 1 g IM/IV or amoxicillin 1 g PO
		Children:	Ampicillin 50 mg/kg IM/IV (not to exceed 2.0 g) Gentamicin 1.5 mg/kg within 30 min of starting the procedure 6 hr later, ampicillin 25 mg/kg IM/IV or amoxicillin 25 mg/kg PO
High-risk patients allergic to ampicillin/amoxicillin	Vancomycin + gentamicin	Adults:	Vancomycin 1.0 g IV over 1–2 hr Gentamicin 1.5 mg/kg IV/IM (not to exceed 120 mg) Complete injection/infusion within 30 min of starting the procedure
		Children:	Vancomycin 20 mg/kg IV over 1–2 hr Gentamicin 1.5 mg/kg IV/IM Complete injection/infusion within 30 min of starting the procedure
Moderate-risk patients	Amoxicillin *or* ampicillin	Adults:	Amoxicillin 2.0 g PO 1 hr before procedure *or* Ampicillin 2.0 g IV/IM within 30 min of starting the procedure
		Children:	Amoxicillin 50 mg/kg PO 1 hr before procedure *or* Ampicillin 50 mg/kg IV/IM within 30 min of starting the procedure
Moderate-risk patients allergic to ampicillin/amoxicillin	Vancomycin	Adults:	Vancomycin 1.0 g IV over 1–2 hr Complete infusion within 30 min of starting the procedure
		Children:	Vancomycin 20 mg/kg IV over 1–2 hr Complete infusion within 30 min of starting the procedure

* No second dose of vancomycin or gentamicin is recommended.

[†]Total children's dose should not exceed adult dose.

IM—intramuscularly; IV—intravenously; PO—orally.

FIGURE 11-22 (*continued*)

REFERENCES

1. Durack DT, Lukes AS, Bright DK, and the Duke Endocarditis Service: New criteria for diagnosis of infective endocarditis: Utilization of specific echocardiographic findings. *Am J Med* 1994, 96:200–209.

2. Knapp C, Moody J: Antimicrobial susceptibility testing. In *Clinical Microbiology Procedures Handbook*, vol 1. Edited by Isenberg H. Washington, DC: American Society for Microbiology; 1992:5.16.1–5.16.33.

3. Wilson W, Karchmer AW, Dajani AS, *et al.*: Antibiotic treatment of adults with infective endocarditis due to streptococci, enterococci, staphylocci, and HACEK microorganisms. *JAMA* 1995, 274:1706–1713.

4. Dajani AS, Taubert KA, Wilson W, Bolger AF, and the Committee on Rheumatic Fever, Endocarditis, and Kawasaki Disease, Council on Cardiovascular Disease in the Young: *Prevention of Bacterial Endocarditis: Recommendations by the American Heart Association*. Dallas, TX: American Heart Association; in press.

SELECTED BIBLIOGRAPHY

Dajani AS, Bawdon RE, Berry MC: Oral amoxicillin as prophylaxis for endocarditis: What is the optimal dose? *Clin Infect Dis* 1994, 18:157–160.

Hoen B, Beguinot I, Rabaud C, *et al.*: The Duke criteria for diagnosing infective endocarditis are specific: Analysis of 100 patients with acute fever or fever of unknown origin. *Clin Infect Dis* 1996, 23:298–302.

Karchmer AW: Infective endocarditis. In *Heart Disease: A Textbook of Cardiovascular Medicine*, 5th ed. Edited by Braunwald, E. Philadelphia: WB Saunders; 1997:1077–1104.

Mathew J, Addai T, Anand A, *et al.*: Clinical features, site of involvement, bacteriologic findings, and outcomes of infective endocarditis in intravenous drug users. *Arch Intern Med* 1995, 155:1641–1648.

Muehrcke DD: Fungal prosthetic valve endocarditis. *Semin Thorac Cardiovasc Surg* 1995, 7:20–24.

Van der Meer JT, Van Wijk W, Thompson J, *et al.*: Efficacy of antibiotic prophylaxis for prevention of native-valve endocarditis. *Lancet* 1992, 339:135–139.

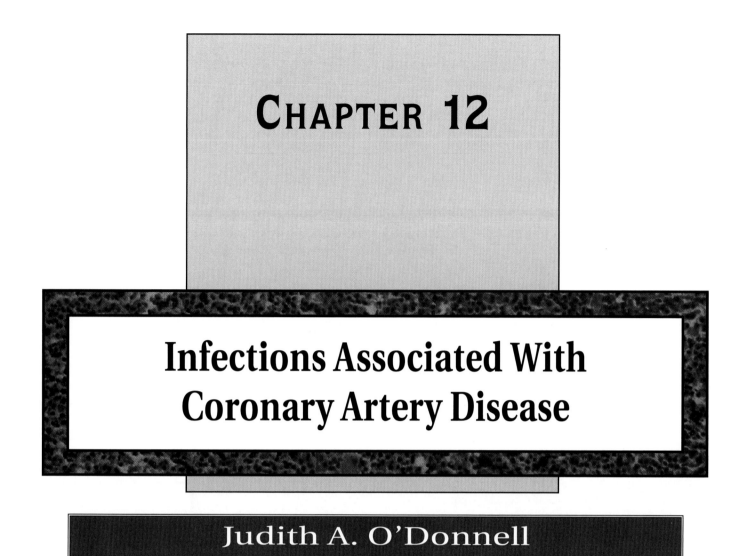

CHAPTER 12

Infections Associated With Coronary Artery Disease

Judith A. O'Donnell

ATHEROSCLEROTIC CORONARY ARTERY DISEASE (CAD) continues to be the leading cause of death in the United States and in other industrialized nations. Billions of healthcare dollars are spent yearly on diagnostic tests, surgical procedures, invasive techniques, and pharmacologic treatments of CAD. The classic risk factors for CAD, such as hypertension, hypercholesterolemia, and smoking, are now well recognized and have been made the target for interventions designed to lower the risk of CAD and to decrease the subsequent risk of recurrence in those individuals with known CAD. However, since the 1980s, a number of intriguing studies have been published suggesting an association between a few specific infectious diseases and CAD. Could an infectious pathogen, or pathogens, be in some way responsible for the formation of atherosclerotic plaques and the eventual development of CAD and myocardial infarction? Although it may seem an unlikely scenario, who could have predicted that the large majority of peptic ulcer disease was caused by a gram-negative bacterium named *Helicobacter pylori*?

This chapter presents a compilation of all of the currently available data regarding the link between infectious diseases and CAD. It also provides insight into current pathogenetic theories. There is much work yet to be done before a definitive causal relationship between CAD and pathogens such as *Chlamydia pneumoniae* and cytomegalovirus can be established. However, if such a relationship is proved, the diagnosis, management, and prevention of atherosclerotic CAD will be radically changed.

Infectious pathogens associated with atherosclerotic coronary artery disease		
Pathogen	Seroepidemiologic association	Presence identified within atherosclerotic plaque tissue
Chlamydia pneumoniae	Yes	Yes
Cytomegalovirus	Yes	Yes
Helicobacter pylori	Yes	No
Herpes simplex virus	No	Rare

FIGURE 12-1 The association between atherosclerotic coronary artery disease and infectious diseases. Within the past 10 years there have been studies linking the bacterium *Chlamydia pneumoniae* and the herpes virus cytomegalovirus to atherosclerotic coronary artery disease (CAD) [1–5]. Although Koch's postulates have yet to be fulfilled, it appears that both of these pathogens are associated in some way with atherosclerotic plaques. In separate studies each pathogen has been shown to have serologic and/or direct tissue evidence of infection. Additionally, one study in the United Kingdom that examined antibody evidence of infection in patients with CAD found an association between *Helicobacter pylori* infection and increased risk of CAD [6]. This potential association requires further investigation. Herpes simplex virus has also been investigated as a possible risk factor. Seroepidemiologic studies do not suggest an association, but herpes simplex viral RNA has been identified in a few coronary artery tissue samples [7].

CHLAMYDIA PNEUMONIAE INFECTION

Serologic evidence of *Chlamydia pneumoniae* infection in individuals with atherosclerotic CAD
Individuals with known atherosclerotic CAD are much more likely to have serologic evidence of *C. pneumoniae* infection
C. pneumoniae infection appears to be an independent risk factor for CAD
The association is strong and statistically significant only in those individuals with CAD and a past or current history of smoking
CAD—coronary artery disease.

FIGURE 12-2 Serologic evidence of *Chlamydia pneumoniae* infection in individuals with atherosclerotic coronary artery disease (CAD). Chronic *C. pneumoniae* infection may be a significant independent risk factor for the development of atherosclerotic CAD. Serologic case-control studies of patients in Helsinki, Finland; Seattle, Washington; and Great Britain have shown that patients with atherosclerotic CAD are more likely than controls to have serologic evidence of *C. pneumoniae* infection [1,2,6,8,9]. IgG, IgA, and/or IgM titers, along with measurement of circulating lipopolysaccharide-containing immune complexes, were variably performed in these studies. All studies controlled for the presence of CAD risk factors such as age, hypertension, smoking, and cholesterol levels. *C. pneumoniae* infection was found in all studies to be a statistically significant risk factor for CAD, and the risk was independent of the classic CAD risk factors. Interestingly, this strong association was only seen in individuals who had a current or past history of smoking. One study in Brooklyn, New York, failed to find an association between *C. pneumoniae* infection and CAD [10].

Evidence of the presence of *Chlamydia pneumoniae* in atherosclerotic plaque tissue

C. pneumoniae has been identified in atherosclerotic plaques removed during atherectomies and at autopsy

The presence of *Chlamydia* spp or *C. pneumoniae* in such tissues has been confirmed with a variety of tests, including
  Direct immunofluorescence
  Immunohistochemical staining
  Polymerase chain reaction
  Transmission electron microscopy

C. pneumoniae has only rarely been cultured from atherosclerotic plaque tissue

FIGURE 12-3 Detection of *Chlamydia pneumoniae* in atherosclerotic plaque tissue. A variety of diagnostic techniques have been used to confirm the presence of either *Chlamydia* species or *C. pneumoniae* specifically in atherosclerotic plaque tissue [3–5]. Tissue has been obtained from both living patients undergoing atherectomy and cadavers undergoing autopsy. Culture of the organism from such tissues has been attempted many times, but only rarely has it been successful [11]. It should be noted that a solitary study of atherectomy patients in Brooklyn, New York, failed to identify the presence of *C. pneumoniae* in all but one patient's coronary artery tissue sample [10].

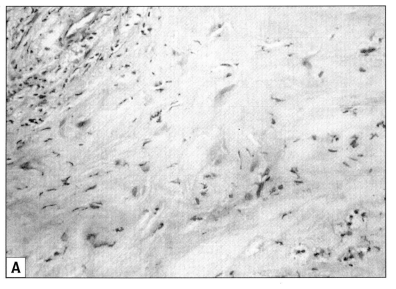

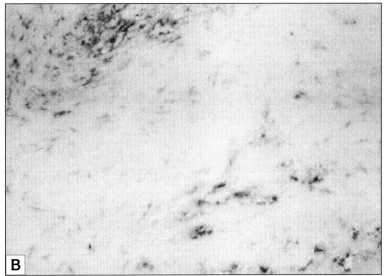

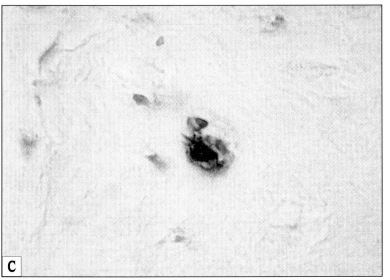

FIGURE 12-4 Immunocytochemical stain of *Chlamydia pneumoniae* in atherectomy tissue. **A**, Section of atherectomy tissue under low power stained with hematoxylin-eosin, depicting small vessels and a surrounding inflammatory infiltrate. **B**, A parallel tissue section stained for the presence of mononuclear cells and macrophages (dark stain) within the lesion. **C**, A macrophage within the mononuclear inflammatory infiltrate that has stained positive (dark stain) for the presence of *Chlamydia pneumoniae*. (Panels 4A and 4B, original magnification, ×200; panel 4C, ×1000.) (*From* Campbell *et al.* [4]; with permission.)

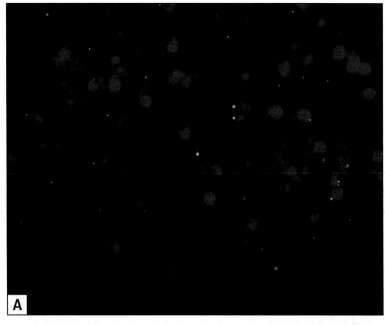

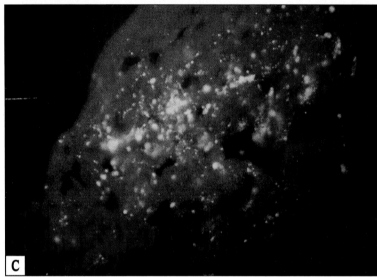

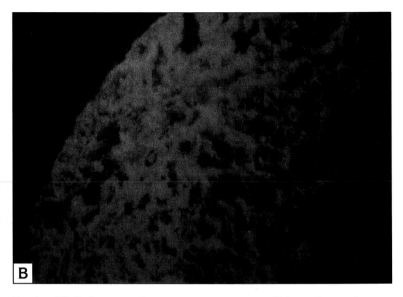

FIGURE 12-5 Immunofluorescent testing for *Chlamydia* species in atherectomy tissue. **A,** The positive control specimen shows the *Chlamydia* species staining apple-green in color. **B,** A section of atherosclerotic plaque staining negatively for the presence of *Chlamydia* species. **C,** A section of atherosclerotic plaque with a strongly positive pattern. (*From* Muhlestein *et al.* [5]; with permission.)

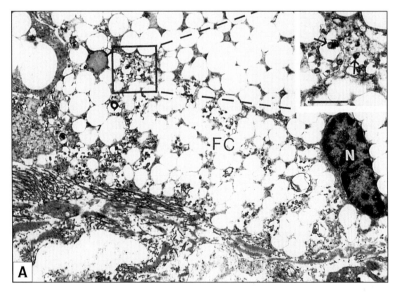

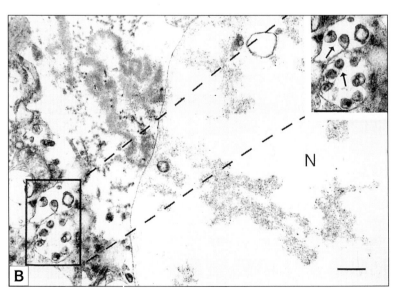

FIGURE 12-6 Transmission electron micrographs of *Chlamydia pneumoniae* in atherectomy tissue. **A,** A foam cell (FC) within an atheromatous lesion. The nucleus (N) of the cell is also seen. The *boxed area* represents typical *C. pneumoniae* inclusions. The *inset* represents an enlargement of the boxed area and depicts the pear-shaped elementary bodies (*arrows*) of *C. pneumoniae*. *Bar*=1 μm. **B,** Endosomes within a foam cell of an atheromatous lesion with the pear-shaped elementary bodies of *C. pneumoniae* binding to the endosomal membranes. *Bar*=0.5 μm. (*From* Kuo *et al.* [3]; with permission.)

A. The facts about *Chlamydia pneumoniae* and the proposed mechanisms by which it may lead to atheroma formation

Characteristics of *C. pneumoniae* that may contribute to its role in atherosclerosis

Chlamydiae are known to be capable of inducing chronic infection

C. pneumoniae has been shown in vitro to be capable of infecting and multiplying within human macrophages

Chlamydial lipopolysaccharide can bind to low-density lipoprotein cholesterol in vitro

Chlamydiae and their lipopolysaccharides are active inducers of tumor necrosis factor and other inflammatory cytokines

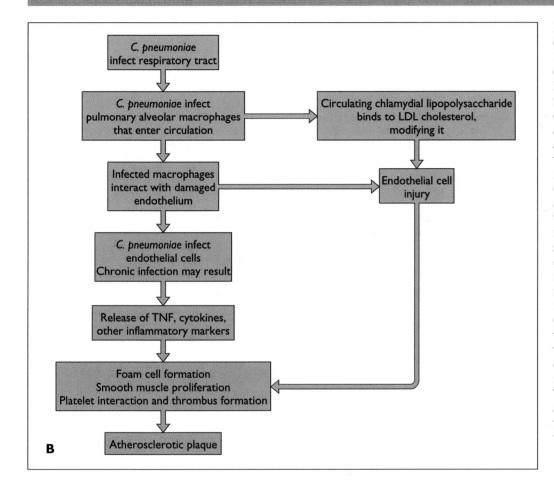

FIGURE 12-7 A and **B,** Proposed pathogenetic mechanisms through which *Chlamydia pneumoniae* could induce atherosclerotic coronary artery disease. Chlamydiae are known for causing chronic infections, with resultant chronic inflammation. The development of atherosclerosis is known to be an ongoing inflammatory and fibroproliferative process. Chlamydiae have been shown to multiply within a variety of human cells, including macrophages, smooth muscle cells, and endothelial cells. These cell types are among those involved in atheroma formation according to the currently held response-to-injury hypothesis of atherosclerosis. This theory also proposes that circulating low-density lipoprotein (LDL) molecules may be modified and that the modified complex may be capable of inducing or promoting endothelial injury. Chlamydiae may bind to LDL, allowing it to be modified to cause such injury and to begin the cascade of events. Finally, chlamydiae are known inducers of tumor necrosis factor (TNF) and other cytokines. These compounds are also believed to play a role in the sequence of events that eventually can lead to atherosclerotic plaque formation [12,13].

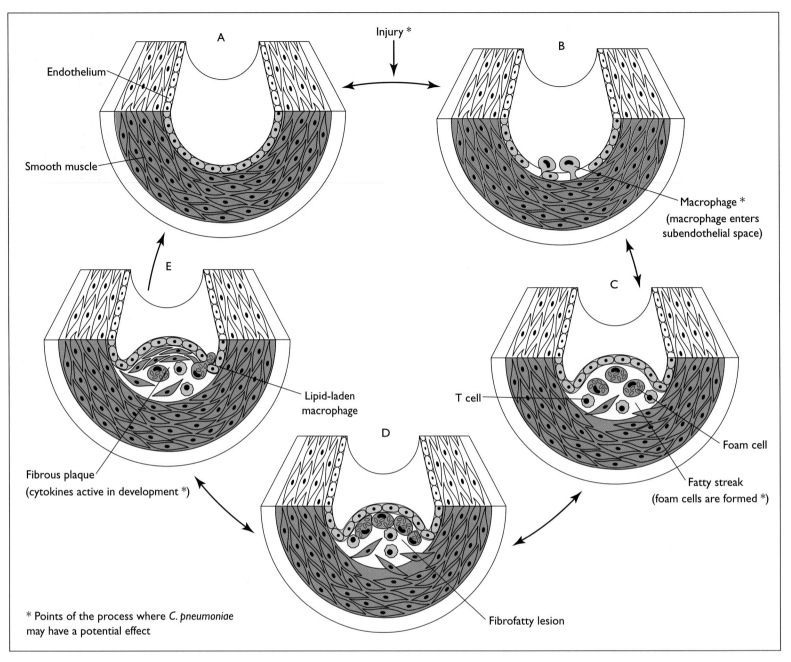

FIGURE 12-8 Schematic illustrating the response-to-injury hypothesis of atherosclerosis and the various points in the process where *Chlamydia pneumoniae* may pay a role. Normal cross-section through a vessel wall is shown (*A*). With injury to the endothelium from a variety of sources, including chlamydial infection, comes increased adherence of monocytes, macrophages, and T lymphocytes (*B*). These cells can migrate through the endothelium and situate themselves within the subendothelial layer. Chlamydiae within the macrophages may gain access to the vessel wall in this way. Macrophages accumulate lipids and become large foam cells. Chlamydiae may contribute to foam cell formation (*C*). Foam cells, T cells, and smooth muscle cells eventually form the fatty streak. Chlamydiae may infect and replicate within all of these cells, potentially propagating the process. The fatty streak becomes a fibrofatty lesion (*D*). Fibrous plaque formation is complete (*E*). Cytokines are active here. Chlamydiae can activate cytokines. Some of the lipid-laden macrophages may return to the bloodstream, and when this occurs at sites of vessel branching, platelet mural thrombi may form. Each of the stages of lesion formation is potentially reversible. If the cause of injury is removed, or if the inflammatory or fibroproliferative process is reversed, lesions may regress at any stage. (*Adapted from* Ross [13].)

Future direction for research regarding the association between *Chlamydia pneumoniae* and atherosclerotic CAD
A causal relation between *C. pneumoniae* and atherosclerotic plaque formation must still be proved or disproved
If the causal relationship is verified, *C. pneumoniae* treatment or vaccine development may be used to impact on the incidence of CAD
CAD—coronary artery disease.

FIGURE 12-9 Future direction for research regarding the association between *Chlamydia pneumoniae* and atherosclerotic coronary artery disease (CAD). More research into the association between *C. pneumoniae* and atherosclerotic CAD is needed. Although serologic evidence of infection and direct evidence of *C. pneumoniae* within atherosclerotic lesions have been verified, it remains to be proved that chronic infection with this organism leads to atherosclerosis. If *C. pneumoniae* infection was definitively shown to be a cause of CAD, the public health implications could be far-reaching. CAD, like peptic ulcer disease, may in some—or many—cases be amenable to treatment with antimicrobials or be potentially preventable with an as-yet-to-be-developed vaccine.

CYTOMEGALOVIRUS INFECTION

Association between CMV infection and atherosclerosis
Evidence of CMV has been documented in tissues taken from individuals with atherosclerosis
CMV infection in cardiac transplant recipients is associated with an increased likelihood of cardiac allograft vasculopathy
CMV infection increases the risk of restenosis after atherectomy in normal hosts with coronary artery disease
CMV—cytomegalovirus.

FIGURE 12-10 The association between cytomegalovirus (CMV) infection and atherosclerosis. CMV infection has been detected through a variety of diagnostic techniques in tissues of patients with atherosclerotic coronary artery disease and in the arterial walls of some normal individuals. Cardiac transplant recipients can develop a unique form of coronary artery atherosclerosis, called *cardiac allograft vasculopathy*, in their transplanted organs. This form of atherosclerosis is the major cause of late death in transplant recipients. No definitive cause for this process has been established, however, CMV infection appears to be associated with an increased risk of cardiac allograft vasculopathy. Prior CMV infection in nontransplant patients undergoing coronary atherectomy has been shown to be a strong independent risk factor for restenosis within 6 months of the procedure. CMV DNA has also been identified in atheromas from patients with restenosis [14–20].

CMV infection and the development of atherosclerosis
An animal model of herpesvirus-induced atherosclerosis exists among chickens with Marek disease
CMV antigens and DNA sequences have been identified in arterial smooth muscle cells from patients with and without atherosclerotic coronary artery disease
Presence of CMV antibodies has been associated with increased risk of atherosclerosis
Virus has never been cultured from the lesions
CMV—cytomegalovirus.

FIGURE 12-11 Evidence of the association between cytomegalovirus (CMV) infection and atherosclerosis. An animal model in chickens exists in which Marek disease virus, a herpesvirus, causes atherosclerosis. Although it remains to be proved that infection with CMV induces atheroma formation and eventually coronary artery disease in humans, there are a number of interesting findings suggesting an association. CMV antigens and DNA sequences have been identified through different laboratory methods in human arterial smooth muscle cells. One seroepidemiologic study suggests that higher levels of CMV IgG antibody titers may be associated with an increased risk of severe atherosclerosis. Although viral DNA and gene sequences have been found in human arterial smooth muscle and endothelial cells, attempts at culturing the virus from atheromas have failed [20,21].

CMV infection and cardiac allograft vasculopathy

CMV infection is associated with earlier onset of graft coronary artery disease and cardiac allograft vasculopathy

The role of CMV infection in producing these lesions or in contributing to the development of these lesions has yet to be elucidated

Characteristics of CMV infection that may contribute to development of lesions include
  Interaction with endothelial cells
  Alteration of lipid metabolism by smooth muscle cells
  Promotion of T cell–mediated immune response against infected endothelial cells

CMV—cytomegalovirus.

FIGURE 12-12 CMV infection and cardiac allograft vasculopathy (CAV). Cytomegalovirus (CMV) infection plays a role in the development of posttransplant CAV, but the exact mechanism of CAV is unknown. CMV infection is associated with an increased likelihood and earlier onset of CAV. It is postulated that CMV may promote this unique form of atherosclerosis by infecting or reactivating latent infection within endothelial cells, expressing viral receptors on the cell surface, and causing cell damage. CMV infection of human smooth muscle cells in vitro has been shown to cause the cells to accumulate lipids. This process may occur in vivo as well, contributing to CAV development. Additionally, CMV infection causes a cellular immune response that may release cytokines and further promote atherogenesis and CAV [14–17,22].

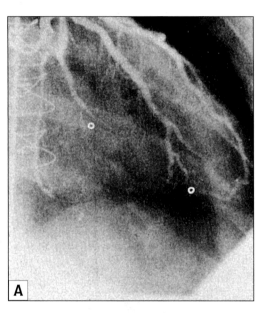

A

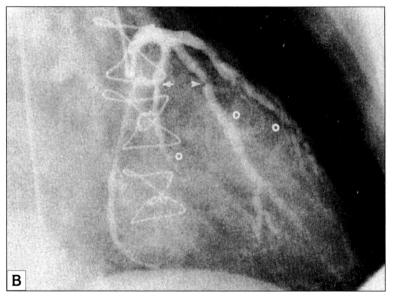

B

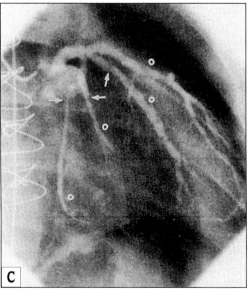

C

FIGURE 12-13 Sequential coronary artery angiograms in a cardiac allograft recipient who developed cytomegalovirus infection and cardiac allograft vasculopathy. **A–C**, Left coronary artery angiograms are shown at 1 year (*panel 13A*), 2 years (*panel 13B*), and 4 years (*panel 13C*) after cardiac transplantation. Already after the first postoperative year, diffuse disease (*o*) was seen in distal parts of the left anterior descending artery (LAD) and in the left obtuse marginal branches (LOM I and II) (score 6). A dramatic acceleration of cardiac allograft vasculopathy occurred during the subsequent year; severe discrete stenosis (*arrows*) developed in the LOM I and II. The angiogram showed marked concentric narrowing with irregular vessel boundaries and loss of fine branches in the proximal, middle, and distal parts of the LAD and LOM I and II (score 14). Four years after transplantation, the acceleration of cardiac allograft vasculopathy had leveled off and a new mild stenosis was seen in the left circumflex coronary artery (LCX). LAD, LOM I and II, and the middle and distal parts of LCX were diffusely affected (score 16). (*From* Koskinen *et al.* [15]; with permission.)

CMV infection and restenosis

CMV DNA sequences have been identified in restenosed
atherectomy tissue

Patients who develop restenosis after atherectomy are more
likely to have had past infection with CMV

CMV may promote restenosis through one of its early gene
protein products by
   Allowing proliferation of smooth muscle cells to be enhanced
   Inhibiting cell apoptosis

CMV—cytomegalovirus.

**Future direction for research regarding the association
between cytomegalovirus and atherosclerosis**

Cytomegalovirus must be proved conclusively or disproved
to be the causative agent of atherosclerosis, coronary artery
vasculopathy, and restenosis
Further study into the mechanisms by which it induces
atherosclerosis must be performed
If a causal relationship is verified, prevention of infection
will be of paramount importance because treatment options
are very limited

FIGURE 12-14 Role of cytomegalovirus (CMV) infection in
restenosis of coronary arteries. Recent studies have shown that
CMV DNA is present within the atherectomy tissue removed from
restenosed lesions. In addition, early CMV gene products also have
been identified within the smooth muscle cells from these lesions.
One specific early CMV gene product, the protein IE84, binds to
and inhibits a particular human protein, p53 tumor-suppressor
gene product. Through this interaction, it is postulated that CMV
may allow the unchecked proliferation of arterial smooth muscle
cells and apoptosis, both of which lead to restenosis [18,19].

FIGURE 12-15 Future direction for research regarding the
association between cytomegalovirus (CMV) and atherosclerosis.
Although the current evidence is interesting, it still must be
shown that CMV induces atherosclerosis. If a causal relationship
is identified, the next steps will be to elucidate how CMV induces
atheromas and how this mechanism can be blocked or the
infection prevented.

REFERENCES

1. Saikku P, Leinonen M, Tenkanen L, *et al.*: Chronic *Chlamydia pneumoniae* infection as a risk factor for coronary heart disease in the Helsinki heart study. *Ann Intern Med* 1992, 116:273–278.

2. Thom DH, Grayston JT, Siscovick DS, *et al.*: Association of prior infection with *Chlamydia pneumoniae* and angiographically demonstrated coronary artery disease. *JAMA* 1992, 268:68–72.

3. Kuo C, Shor A, Campbell LA, *et al.*: Demonstration of *Chlamydia pneumoniae* in atherosclerotic lesions of coronary arteries. *J Infect Dis* 1993, 167:841–849.

4. Campbell LA, O'Brien ER, Cappuccio AL, *et al.*: Detection of *Chlamydia pneumoniae* TWAR in human coronary atherectomy tissues. *J Infect Dis* 1995, 172:585–588.

5. Muhlestein JB, Hammond EH, Carlquist JF, *et al.*: Increased incidence of *Chlamydia* species within coronary arteries of patients with symptomatic atherosclerotic versus other forms of cardiovascular disease. *J Am Coll Cardiol* 1996, 27:1555–1561.

6. Patel P, Mendall MA, Carrington DP, *et al.*: Association of *Helicobacter pylori* and *Chlamydia pneumoniae* infections with coronary heart disease and cardiovascular risk factors. *BMJ* 1995, 311:711–714.

7. Visser MR, Vercellotti GM: Herpes simplex virus and atherosclerosis. *Eur Heart J* 1993, 14(suppl K):39–42.

8. Linnamaki E, Leinonen M, Mattila K, *et al.*: *Chlamydia pneumoniae*–specific circulating immune complexes in patients with chronic coronary heart disease. *Circulation* 1993, 87:1130–1134.

9. Mendall MA, Carrington D, Strachan D, *et al.*: *Chlamydia pneumoniae*: Risk factors for seropositivity and association with coronary disease. *J Infect* 1995, 30:121–128.

10. Weiss SM, Roblin PM, Gaydos CA, *et al.*: Failure to detect *Chlamydia pneumoniae* in coronary atheromas of patients undergoing atherectomy. *J Infect Dis* 1996, 173:957–962.

11. Ramirez JA, and the *Chlamydia pneumoniae*/Atherosclerosis Study Group: Isolation of *Chlamydia pneumoniae* from the coronary artery of a patient with coronary atherosclerosis. *Ann Intern Med* 1996, 125:979–982.

12. Gaydos CA, Summersgill JT, Sahney NN, *et al.*: Replication of *Chlamydia pneumoniae* in vitro in human macrophages, endothelial cells, and aortic artery muscle cells. *Infect Immun* 1996, 64:1614–1620.

13. Ross R: The pathogenesis of atherosclerosis: A perspective for the 1990s. *Nature* 1993, 362:801–809.

14. Everett JP, Hershberger RE, Norman DJ, *et al.*: Prolonged cytomegalovirus infection with viremia is associated with development of cardiac allograft vasculopathy. *J Heart Lung Transplant* 1992, 11:S133–S137.

15. Koskinen PK, Nieminen MS, Krogerus LA, *et al.*: Cytomegalovirus infection accelerates cardiac allograft vasculopathy: Correlation between angiographic and endomyocardial biopsy findings in heart transplant patients. *Transpl Int* 1993, 6:341–347.

16. Koskinen PK, Nieminen MS, Krogerus LA, *et al.*: Cytomegalovirus infection and accelerated cardiac allograft vasculopathy in human cardiac allografts. *J Heart Lung Transplant* 1993, 12:724–729.

17. Gao SZ, Hunt SA, Schroeder JS, *et al.*: Early development of accelerated graft coronary artery disease: Risk factors and course. *J Am Coll Cardiol* 1996, 28:673–679.

18. Zhou YF, Leon MB, Waclawiw MA, *et al.*: Association between prior cytomegalovirus infection and the risk of restenosis after coronary atherectomy. *N Engl J Med* 1996, 335:624–630.

19. Speir E, Modali R, Huang ES, *et al.*: Potential role of human cytomegalovirus and p53 interaction in coronary restenosis. *Science* 1994, 265:391–394.

20. Melnick JL, Adam E, Debakey ME: Cytomegalovirus and atherosclerosis. *Eur Heart J* 1993, 14:Suppl K:30–38.

21. Melnick JL, Adam E, Debakey ME: Possible role of cytomegalovirus in atherogenesis. *JAMA* 1990, 263:2204–2207.

22. Ventura HO, Mehra MR, Smart FW, Stapleton DD: Cardiac allograft vasculopathy: Current concepts. *Am Heart J* 1995, 129:791–799.

SELECTED BIBLIOGRAPHY

Campbell LA, O'Brien ER, Cappuccio AL, *et al.*: Detection of *Chlamydia pneumoniae* TWAR in human coronary atherectomy tissues. *J Infect Dis* 1995, 172:585–588.

Muhlestein JB, Hammond EH, Carlquist JF, *et al.*: Increased incidence of *Chlamydia* species within coronary arteries of patients with symptomatic atherosclerotic versus other forms of cardiovascular disease. *J Am Coll Cardiol* 1996, 27:1555–1561.

Ross R: The pathogenesis of atherosclerosis: A perspective for the 1990s. *Nature* 1993, 362:801–809.

Speir E, Modali R, Huang ES, *et al.*: Potential role of human cytomegalovirus and p53 interaction in coronary restenosis. *Science* 1994, 265:391–394.

Zhou YF, Leon MB, Waclawiw MA, *et al.*: Association between prior cytomegalovirus infection and the risk of restenosis after coronary atherectomy. *N Engl J Med* 1996, 335:624–630.

INDEX